211 234 69 72 74 14 120 123

THE NEW HEALING HERBS

Critical Praise
for the Original *Healing Herbs*

". . . a welcome and candid assessment of medicinal herbs and their uses. One of the best-researched and most readable herb guides. [Michael] Castleman, a health writer of broad experience, has produced an objective, insightful, and easy-to-read blend of herbal history, lore, research, applications, safety data, and gardening information."

—*HerbalGram*

". . . breaks new ground in the literature on self-care with herbs. Outlines when [herbal] self-care is appropriate and when it is not. Castleman does a good job of putting the possible dangers of herbs in perspective. Strikes a refreshingly healthy balance between traditional herbalism and modern science."

—*Natural Health*

". . . a must-read. Answers every question you ever had about herbs and their medicinal value. Explores herbal folklore, science, uses, caveats, and side effects, with historical anecdotes and gardening tips."

—*Modern Maturity*

". . . demonstrates Castleman's love of herbs and willingness to do homework far beyond the call of duty. Describes the boundaries of appropriate self-care. Balances tradition with modern scientific research. Written with flair, humor, and insight."

—*Herb Quarterly*

". . . valuable information not available elsewhere. Intelligent discussion of the toxicology and contraindications of each herb, [which] is rare."

—*Medical Herbalism*

". . . the most authoritative and user-friendly herbal guide currently available. If one were to have only one book on [medicinal] herbs, this should be it."

—*Utne Reader*

THE NEW HEALING HERBS

THE **CLASSIC GUIDE**
TO NATURE'S BEST MEDICINES

FEATURING THE TOP 100 TIME-TESTED HERBS

Michael Castleman

RODALE

Notice
This book is intended as a reference volume only, not as a medical manual. The information given here is designed to help you make informed decisions about your health. It is not intended as a substitute for any treatment that may have been prescribed by your doctor. You should consult your physician or a physician with expertise in herbs before treating yourself with herbs or combining them with any medications. Women who are pregnant or who are considering becoming pregnant should not use herbs or other medications without seeking the approval of their doctors. If you suspect that you have a medical problem, we urge you to seek competent medical help.

The Healing Herbs by Michael Castleman was first published in 1991 by Rodale Inc.

Printed in the United States of America
Rodale Inc. makes every effort to use acid-free ♺ , recycled paper ∞

Cover and book design by Christina Gaugler
Cover photograph by Rodale Images
Illustrations by Wayne Michaud

Library of Congress Cataloging-in-Publication Data

Castleman, Michael.
    The new healing herbs : the classic guide to nature's best medicines featuring the top 100 time-tested herbs / Michael Castleman.
       p.   cm.
    Rev. ed. of: The healing herbs. c1991.
    Includes bibliographical references and index.
    ISBN 1–57954–304–9   paperback
    1. Herbs—Therapeutic use.
    [DNLM: 1. Plants, Medicinal—Popular Works.   2. Medicine, Herbal—Popular Works.   QV766 C353n 2001]
    I. Castleman, Michael. Healing herbs.   II. Title.
    RM666.H33 C39   2001
    615'.321—dc21   00–011434

Distributed to the book trade by St. Martin's Press

2 4 6 8 10 9 7 5 3   paperback

Visit us on the Web at www.rodalebooks.com, or call us toll-free at (800) 848-4735.

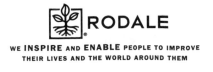

RODALE

WE **INSPIRE** AND **ENABLE** PEOPLE TO IMPROVE
THEIR LIVES AND THE WORLD AROUND THEM

Acknowledgments

At home: Anne Simons, M.D., and Jeffrey and Maya Castleman.

At Rodale Inc.: Anne Alexander, Susan Massey, Tami Booth, Ed Claflin, Susan Berg, Jane Sherman, Christina Gaugler (revised edition); Alice Feinstein, Debora Yost, William Gottlieb, and Sharon Faelten (first edition).

At John Brockman and Associates: Katinka Matson and John Brockman.

And: Harriet Beinfield, L.Ac., herbalist and author; Paul Bergner, editor of *Medical Herbalism*; Mark Blumenthal, executive director of the American Botanical Council and editor of *Herbal-Gram*; Wade Boyle, N.D., historian and author; Alan Brauer, M.D.; Maureen Buehrle, executive director of the International Herb Growers and Marketers Association; Susan Clotfelter, editor of *Herbs for Health*; Lyle E. Craker, Ph.D., editor of *Herb, Spice, and Medicinal Plant Digest*; Ara der Marderosian, Ph.D., pharmacognosist and author; James A. Duke, Ph.D., ethnobotanist and author; Eclectic Medical Publications; Peter Finkle, research director of Yerba Prima; Steven Foster, herbalist and author; Alan Gaby, M.D.; H. Winter Griffith, M.D., author; Sheldon Saul Hendler, M.D., Ph.D., author; Christopher Hobbs, L.Ac., herbalist and author; *Lawrence Review of Natural Products*; Kathi Keville, herbalist and author; Efrem Korngold, L.Ac., O.M.D., herbalist and author; Lawrence Liberti, M.S., pharmacognosist and author; Albert Y. Leung, Ph.D., pharmacognosist and author; Lloyd Library; Robert McCaleb, president of the Herb Research Foundation; Daniel Mowrey, Ph.D., herbalist and author; Michael Murray, N.D., naturopath; Paula Oliver, herb grower and author; Joseph Pizzorno, N.D., naturopath; Jeanne Rose, herbalist and author; Lynda Sadler, research director of Traditional Medicinals; Emma Segal, editor; Linda Sparrowe, editorial director of *The Herb Quarterly*; Varro E. Tyler, Ph.D., pharmacognosist and author; Susun Weed, herbalist and author; Michael Weiner, Ph.D., herbalist and author; Rudolph Fritz Weiss, M.D., herbal physician and author; Melvyn Werbach, M.D.; Linda White, M.D., herbalist and author; and all the good people at *Herb Companion*, *Herbs for Health*, and *Herb Quarterly* magazines.

Contents

Chapter 6

Introduction to the Revised Edition
EVERYTHING OLD IS NEW AGAIN

Ten years ago, when I wrote the original edition of *The Healing Herbs*, I knew that herbal medicine was growing in popularity. But I had no idea that the book would become an international bestseller, with more than 1 million copies in print in English, Spanish, French, Italian, and Finnish. Nor did anyone involved in herbal healing in the late 1980s anticipate the explosion of interest that would embrace the discipline by the dawn of the 21st century.

Herbal medicine is now a $3-billion-a-year industry, about five times larger than when the original *Healing Herbs* was published in 1991. In 1998 and 1999, according to a national survey commissioned by *Prevention* magazine, some 49 percent of American adults—more than 100 million people—tried herbal remedies. And 24 percent—some 25 million people—considered themselves regular herb users.

Perhaps even more significant, many of today's herb users are mainstream M.D.'s. A decade ago, the medical profession was at best skeptical of herbal medicine. Today, many physicians don't hesitate to recommend echinacea to treat the common cold, garlic to control cholesterol, cranberry to prevent urinary tract infections, or St. John's wort to lift depression.

Doctors have become more open to herbal medicine in part because family members, friends, and patients have reported success with herbs. In addition, they've been influenced by the changing opinions of mainstream medical journals.

A decade ago, the major journals published only those reports detailing the hazardous side effects of herbs, ignoring information about the benefits of medicinal plants. Today, they're publishing a steady stream of studies in support of herbal healing. (You'll read more about the latest herb research throughout this revised edition.)

• A report in the *British Medical Journal* was largely responsible for popularizing St. John's wort as an antidepressant.
• A major review in the *Journal of Family Practice* concluded that echinacea is an effective cold treatment.
• Studies published in *Lancet* have demonstrated the effectiveness of feverfew in migraine prevention.
• A study reported in the *New England Journal of Medicine*, which was once openly hostile to herbs, showed that cranberry juice helps protect against urinary tract infections.
• Recent reports in the *Journal of the American Medical Association*, another traditional herb basher, support ginkgo for Alzheimer's disease and saw palmetto for benign prostate enlargement.

In other words, herbal medicine has gone mainstream. It's still not as widely accepted in the

United States as in some other countries, notably Germany. Nor is it as mainstream as it was in 19th-century America, before the pharmaceutical industry took disease treatment and prevention out of the herb garden and into the laboratory. But herbal medicine is no longer the fringe practice that it was a decade ago.

Herbal products have also come a long way in the last 10 years. Many more products are on the market. They're more widely available, sold not just in health food stores but also in many pharmacies and even some supermarkets. And they've become more reliable with the advent of standardized extracts.

Standardized extracts are made from plants that have been bred to contain certain concentrations of pharmacologically active compounds. These plants are grown, harvested, stored, and prepared under controlled conditions to produce reliable dose uniformity. Standardized extracts are not quite as dose-controlled as laboratory-synthesized pharmaceuticals, but they're close. And they're considerably more dose-controlled than bulk herbs.

The past decade has produced a few reports of safety problems with herbs. Most notable were the estimated 30 deaths attributed to Chinese ephedra (ma huang) after thrill seekers began taking megadoses of the herb—hundreds of times more than a responsible herbalist would recommend—in pursuit of amphetamine-like intoxication.

With this one exception, the news about herb safety has been quite good. Even though more Americans are using more medicinal herbs than at any time in U.S. history, few serious incidents have been reported, especially when compared with the side effects and even deaths caused by pharmaceuticals.

Nonetheless, safety concerns seem destined to remain the most pressing issue in herbal medicine. This is largely because the FDA has so far refused to reopen its review of over-the-counter drugs, a process that would allow manufacturers to seek government approval for their herb products.

The good news is that for the first time in the agency's history, considerable numbers of FDA staff support the use of healing herbs. I'm cautiously optimistic that over the next decade, the agency will adopt labeling regulations for medicinal herbs that are more appropriate to the needs of consumers.

In the meantime, you have this volume for your reference. Completely revised, updated, and expanded, it should enable you to use medicinal herbs confidently, effectively, and above all, safely.

Introduction to the First Edition
ANCIENT REMEDIES AND MODERN MEDICINE

The World Health Organization estimates that healing herbs are the primary medicines for two-thirds of the world's population, some 4 billion people. Herb critics concede herbal healing's leading role in third-world health care but say it's obsolete in today's high-technology, laboratory-based American medicine.

That's hardly the case. Even in the United States, 25 percent of all prescriptions still contain active ingredients derived from plants, and the average physician writes eight herb-based prescriptions every day. Even the most vociferous herb critics use healing herbs all the time—usually without realizing it.

Coffee, Coke, and Clorets

When was the last time you used a healing herb? Perhaps you started your day with a cup of coffee or tea. Not only is coffee America's favorite morning stimulant, but scientists have also shown that it's an effective bronchial decongestant. Try a cup or two the next time you have a cold or flu or as part of an asthma management program in consultation with your physician. Or use coffee to increase your stamina, assist in weight loss, or minimize jet lag. Tea is less stimulating than coffee, but it's also an effective decongestant. In addition, tea is a good source of fluoride, so it helps prevent tooth decay. Animal studies suggest that it also may help reduce cholesterol.

Do you enjoy soft drinks? Most of today's carbonated beverages were originally herbal medicines. Thousands of years ago, the ancient Chinese drank ginger tea for indigestion, a use validated by modern science. During Elizabethan times, the British developed their own ginger-based stomach soother, ginger beer, which evolved into today's ginger ale.

Coca-Cola began as an attempt to develop an herbal headache remedy. Coke was invented in the 1880s by an Atlanta pharmacist who stocked the tropical kola nut because 19th-century physicians prescribed it to treat respiratory ailments. An article in the *Journal of the American Medical Association* suggested giving cola drinks to children with asthma because they prefer them to standard asthma medication.

The last time you dined out, did your plate come with a sprig of parsley? Parsley garnishes are another echo of herbal healing. People used to munch this herb to freshen their breath after meals. Parsley is rich in the breath-sweetening plant pigment chlorophyll, the "Clor" in Clorets breath mints and one of the active ingredients in Certs.

And speaking of restaurants, perhaps your check arrived with an after-dinner mint. These candies harken back to ancient times, when people sipped mint tea after feasts to settle their stomachs, another traditional medicinal use confirmed by modern science.

Aspirin, Sudafed, and Listerine

America's medicine cabinets are filled with drugs. Did you know that the very word *drug* links us to herbal healing? *Drug* comes from the early German *droge*, meaning to dry, as in drying herbs, which is the first step in processing herbs into medicines. But the link goes beyond word origins. Many drugs in home medicine cabinets have herbal roots.

Aspirin was originally created from two healing herbs, white willow bark and meadowsweet. In fact, meadowsweet's old genus name, *Spirea*, gave us the "-spirin" in "aspirin."

For the congestion of colds, flu, or hay fever, millions of Americans reach for Sudafed. Its active ingredient, pseudoephedrine, was developed from the world's oldest healing herb, Chinese ephedra (ma huang), which Chinese physicians have prescribed for 5,000 years to treat chest congestion.

Thousands of years ago, people noticed that several aromatic herbs helped treat tooth pain. We now know that tooth decay and gum disease are caused by oral bacteria, and science has shown that the herbs traditionally used to treat dental ailments kill these germs. One antibacterial herb is peppermint, which is why peppermint oil (menthol) is an ingredient in many toothpastes. Another is thyme, whose active chemical (thymol) is an ingredient in Listerine.

Constipation is one of America's most common health complaints, and most laxatives are herbal products. Metamucil is almost entirely psyllium seed. Cascara sagrada is the active ingredient in Stimulax, Comfolax, and Cas Evac. And Movicol owes its laxative action to buckthorn.

If there are children in your home, chances are there's a cherry-flavored cough syrup in your medicine cabinet. The cherry flavor is no accident. Native Americans treated coughs with wild cherry bark, and we're still using it today.

The Blind Spot in Medical Training

British and European physicians often prescribe herbal medicines along with—or instead of—pharmaceuticals. Some American physicians support herbal healing, but most remain skeptical. Some are downright hostile. Why?

The answer has to do with a major blind spot in American medical training. Medical schools ignore the history of healing, so most physicians have no idea that until this century, most medicines were herbal. And pharmacology professors rarely mention that 25 percent of all U.S. prescription medications are still derived from plants.

From time to time, a leading medical journal reports an herb's effectiveness. For example, a report in the *Journal of the National Cancer Institute* suggested that garlic prevents stomach cancer. But most herb studies are published in obscure journals (many in German)—publications that the typical physician never sees. As a result, most American doctors are unfamiliar with the vast scientific literature demonstrating herbs' safety and effectiveness for an enormous number of ills.

The sad fact is, the typical American physician's only real exposure to herbal healing involves the small but steady stream of medical journal articles reporting harm from the irresponsible use of healing herbs. The number of people harmed by herbs is only a tiny fraction of the number harmed by pharmaceuticals and accepted medical procedures. Nonetheless, the majority of what physicians know about herbs is decidedly negative, so it's no wonder that they feel skeptical of herbal healing.

Fortunately, this situation is changing as herb studies make their way into more prestigious journals. Headache specialists now recommend feverfew to prevent migraines because several well-publicized studies have shown its effectiveness. Many physicians now suggest ginger to prevent motion sickness and the nausea associated with cancer chemotherapy because a study in the respected British medical journal *Lancet* showed it prevents nausea better than a standard treatment, diphenhydramine (Dramamine). Many cardiologists now recommend a diet high in garlic based on studies showing that it is remarkably effective in reducing cholesterol and other risk factors for heart disease. Surgeons routinely spur the healing of surgical incisions with preparations containing a chemical extracted from comfrey (allantoin). And some gastroenterologists now recommend a slightly modified form of licorice for ulcers based on studies that show it to be about as effective as the standard treatment cimetidine (Tagamet).

Healing herbs even play a role in cancer chemotherapy. Two substances extracted from the Madagascar periwinkle, vincristine and vinblastine, are now used to treat childhood leukemia and Hodgkin's disease.

How to Use This Book

Some people become so enamored of herbal healing that they reject mainstream medicine entirely. This is a serious mistake. Herbal healing can make an important contribution to human well-being, but it also has its limits. Responsible herbalists consult physicians and use pharmaceuticals appropriately. In general, if an ailment does not respond to herbal self-treatment within 2 weeks, consult a physician.

For some conditions, all you need is an herbal remedy: aloe for minor burns, dill for infant colic, or clove oil for fast, temporary toothache relief.

For others, you can mix and match several approaches. Consider upset stomach. You might change what you eat: fewer hard-to-digest fats and more easily digestible fresh fruits and vegetables. You might change how you eat: more slowly, in a relaxed setting, chewing more thoroughly. You might take a pharmaceutical antacid. Or you might try one of the many herbs that help soothe the stomach, such as fennel, caraway, peppermint, or ginger.

Of course, many conditions require professional care, including high blood pressure, diabetes, heart disease, and congestive heart failure. But healing herbs can still play an important role in your overall treatment plan as complements to standard therapies in consultation with your physician.

Before you start using healing herbs:

• Read chapter 1 to gain an appreciation of herbal history. According to legend, the world's first herbalist, China's mythological emperor Shen Nung (c. 3400 B.C.), died when he took too much of a poisonous herb. Those who ignore herbal history sometimes live to regret it. They also miss the richness and beauty of humanity's deep relationship with these incredible plants.

• Read chapter 2 to gain a basic understanding of herbal safety issues. All the herbs discussed in this book can be used safely if they are used responsibly. However, when used improperly, some may cause harm.

• Before you ingest any healing herb, read chapters 3 and 4 to make sure you understand how to obtain and prepare it. For example, an infusion is not a tea.

• Before you attempt to treat any health problem herbally, read the appropriate herb profile in chapter 5. These profiles provide basic information that the well-informed herbalist should know. Pay special attention to the sections headlined "Rx Recommendations," "The Safety Factor," and "Wise-Use Guidelines."

• To find an herb for a specific health concern, refer to the charts in chapter 6.

• The reference section on page 442 lists additional books on the subject of herbal medicine that may be of interest to you. If you'd like to know the scientific sources of the information on each herb, they are also available.

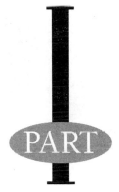

PART I

There is nothing in the most advanced contemporary medicine whose embryo cannot be found in the medicine of the past.

—Maximilien E. P. Littre
French lexicographer

CHAPTER 1

From Magic to Medicine

5,000 YEARS OF HERBAL HEALING

In 1991, on a glacier in the Italian Alps that had melted back to an unusual extent, hikers stumbled on a dead body. It turned out to be the naturally mummified body of a prehistoric man who had frozen to death some 5,300 years before and whose remains were preserved in the ice.

Dubbed the Iceman, he's been studied by Italian anthropologists ever since. He wore straw-lined leather shoes, leather clothing, a thick coat made from woven grass, and a bearskin cap. He carried a wooden bow, a leather quiver filled with stone-tipped arrows, a flint-bladed knife, a wood-handled ax with a copper blade, and a food pouch that still contained dried deer meat and a prune.

The Iceman's pouch also contained two mysterious corklike lumps about the size of walnuts that were pierced through and strung together on a leather thong, indicating that they were of value. The lumps turned out to be bracket fungus (*Piptoporus betulinus*), one of many mushrooms that grow in shelflike plates on tree trunks. This species of fungus contains agaric acid, a potent laxative, and an oily resin that is toxic to some bacteria and intestinal parasites.

The scientists studying the Iceman had no idea why he would have carried bracket fungus until, in 1998, a painstaking autopsy of his digestive tract turned up the eggs of an intestinal parasite (*Trichuris trichiura*) in his rectum.

It now appears that the Iceman knew he carried the parasite, which causes abdominal pain, and was using bits of bracket fungus to treat his condition. Given its laxative and antiparasitic action, the fungus probably provided some benefit.

This discovery ranks as the world's oldest documented example of the practice of medicine, and it suggests that prehistoric humanity was more medically sophisticated than previously believed. After all, the Iceman or someone else had diagnosed his malady correctly and had recommended a reasonably appropriate treatment—an herbal treatment—around 3300 B.C.

Animal Attractions

Just what is a healing herb? The word *herb* comes from the Latin for "grass." Technically, herbs are plants that wither each autumn, plants other than shrubs or trees. But many woody perennials are used in herbal healing, such as slippery elm, tea tree, and white willow. To an herbalist, the phrase "healing herbs" applies to *every* plant with medicinal value.

Prehistoric sites in Iraq show that the Neanderthals used yarrow, marshmallow, and other herbs some 60,000 years ago. What attracted them to these plants?

Animals played a key role. Prehistoric humans were keen observers of the world around them. No doubt our ancestors noticed that when animals appeared ill, they sometimes ate plants that they ordinarily ignored. Humans sampled these plants, in many cases noticing curious effects—wakefulness, sleepiness, laxative action, increased urination, and so on. The herbs that caused these effects were incorporated into prehistoric shamanism, and later into medicine.

Animal-inspired herbalism has continued into modern times. The controversial herbal cancer therapy marketed by Harry Hoxsey was reportedly inspired by a cancer-stricken horse who ate unusual herbs (more on this later).

Aromatic Magic

Early humans were also attracted to healing herbs' aromas. They rubbed strong-smelling herbs on their bodies to repel insects and to hide their human scent from animals that they feared or hunted. They also adorned themselves with sweet-smelling herbs to please their mates.

Fragrant herbs evolved into the first perfumes and embalming mixtures. Demand for them spurred ancient trade. During the Middle Ages, when Europeans believed that bathing was unhealthy and farm animals often shared human living quarters, homemakers spread aromatic "strewing herbs" to freshen the air. Herbalists still prepare scent baskets (potpourris) today, and the perfume industry still creates most of its fragrances from herbal essences.

But foul odors, not fragrant ones, were key to the development of herbal healing. Early humans used plants such as rosemary, thyme, dill, and virtually all of today's culinary spices to mask the stench of rotting meats. Today, we use culinary herbs and spices only as flavor enhancers, but to prehistoric humanity, flavor enhancement was incidental to food preservation.

Prehistoric humanity had no refrigeration, and meats spoiled quickly. Spoilage destroyed precious reserves, and early humans learned the hard way that eating rotten meats caused illness and sometimes death. No doubt some prehistoric homemaker happened to lay some rotting meat on a bed of wild mint, sage, basil, or some other aromatic herb, hoping the herb's fragrance would mask the meat's malodorousness. It did, and as a bonus, the meat didn't spoil as quickly.

Our ancestors began wrapping meats in aromatic herbs to preserve them, which led to other astonishing discoveries. Those who ate preservative herbs along with meats suffered less illness. As an added benefit, the meats tasted better.

Surely, our ancestors must have decided, aromatic herbs were magic. As time passed and magic was incorporated into religion, ancient civilizations came to view aromatic herbs as gifts from the gods. This is why many herbs figure prominently in ancient myths and religions.

Thanks to modern science, we know that the oils that give aromatic herbs their fragrance and flavor contain antimicrobial compounds that kill many food-spoiling, disease-causing microorganisms. In fact, rosemary and sage have food-preservative action comparable to that of the commercial preservatives BHA and BHT.

Trial and Error

Our ancestors also discovered many healing herbs simply by trial and error. They learned through experience that some plants healed, while others harmed. They had little control over their world or their bodies. Their average life expectancy was barely 30 years. Because their lives were so full of threatening, often fatal, surprises, *anything* that made life more predictable acquired an aura of magic and healing.

It's no coincidence that shamans from prehistoric times down to the present day have relied heavily on herbs, such as ipecac, buckthorn, and wormwood, that cause vomiting, purging, and hallucinations. Any predictable effect was better than none, and the ability to induce vomiting, purging, or visions made shaman/herbalists appear to possess magic powers.

The allure of predictable action remained central to medicine for thousands of years. Herbs that induced vomiting (emetics) or had powerful laxative action were used routinely in medicine until well into the 19th century.

Major effects made big impressions, but early humans also recognized herbs' more subtle benefits. We'll never know what possessed some ancient Chinese peasant to brew a tea from the small, ungainly stalks of ma huang (Chinese ephedra), but several thousand years ago, someone did. In the process, that person stumbled upon one of the world's oldest medicines, a decongestant whose laboratory analog, pseudoephedrine, is still an ingredient in cold formulas today.

Similarly, we'll never know how many roots ancient Asians dug up before they discovered ginger. Or why Native Americans had a hunch that black cohosh might be useful in gynecology. All over the world, however, ancient peoples dug, dried, chewed, pounded, rubbed, and brewed the plants around them. In this way, they discovered the vast majority of healing herbs still in use today.

Isolated Cultures, Similar Herbs

Herbal trial and error becomes even more remarkable when we consider that cultures separated by thousands of miles arrived at similar uses for many healing herbs. What's more, they apparently did so independently of one another.

There are four major herbal traditions: Chinese, Ayurvedic (in India), European (including Egyptian), and Native American. The spice trade clearly introduced Asian herbs such as garlic, ginger, and cinnamon into Europe thousands of years ago. And a few ancient herbalists—notably the 1st-century Greek Dioscorides—traveled extensively, spreading knowledge around the ancient world.

Nonetheless, early Chinese, Indian, and European herbalists were largely isolated from one another. In modern times, it's difficult to comprehend just how isolated they were. Until the 1st century A.D., it took *2 years* for spice traders to make the round trip from Greece to India's black-pepper-producing region.

Even in this age of instant global communication, different healing systems still operate relatively independently of one another. During the 1970s and early 1980s, ginkgo became an important medicine in France and Germany for aging-related ailments, with sales topping $500 million a year. Most U.S. medical school libraries stocked the German and French journals showing ginkgo's remarkable effectiveness, yet American physicians virtually ignored ginkgo well into the 1990s. So how connected could the ancient herbalists have been?

Even granting a nearly impossible level of herbal cross-fertilization between Asia and Europe, the land bridge between Asia and North America became the Bering Sea about 10,000 years ago. Until the 15th century, Old World cultures were almost entirely isolated from the Americas, but nonetheless, Old and New World herbalists used many herbs similarly.

• Angelica and licorice: Asians, Europeans, and Native Americans relied on these herbs as treatments for respiratory ailments.
• Hop and the mints: All of the ancient herbal traditions used these herbs as stomach soothers.
• Blackberry and raspberry: Around the world, these herbs played a role in treating diarrhea.
• Uva-ursi: Asians, Europeans, and Native Americans all discovered this herb's diuretic properties.
• White willow: All of the herbal healing disciplines used this herb to treat pain and inflammation.

During the 19th century, chemists homed in on this "herbal convergence" to point them to the plants whose extracts became the first pharmaceuticals. According to a report in the journal *Science*, about 75 percent of the pharmaceuticals derived from plants came to drug companies' attention because of their use in traditional herbal medicine.

Homage to the "Wise Women"

Most medical histories chronicle great achievements by great men: Hippocrates, the father of medicine; Galen, Rome's leading physician; William Harvey's explanation of blood circulation; Edward Jenner's inoculations against smallpox; Louis Pasteur's Germ Theory; Alexander Fleming's discovery of penicillin.

The contributions of these men unquestionably changed the world. But from ancient times down to the present day, a relatively small number of male physicians made the great discoveries and ministered to the rich and royal. An enormous number of women herbalists took care of everyone else.

Women healers have gone by many names: midwives, wise women, green women, witches, old wives, and nurses. Most physicians have never taken women's folk healing very seriously, and scientists often dismiss folk wisdom as "old wives' tales."

The reality is, though, that medically untrained women still provide most of the world's primary care. Even in the United States, most people view physicians as the health care choice of last resort. The medical profession promotes the idea that family doctors are our primary providers, but studies show that before people call health professionals, about *90 percent* consult a friend or family member. These informal heath advisers are overwhelmingly women.

Ancient physicians officially recognized women's leading role in obstetrics and gynecology more than 2,000 years ago in the Hippocratic Oath, which many graduating medical students still recite today: "I will prescribe no . . . pessary [contraceptive device] to produce abortion." Anti-abortion activists have seized on this statement as a condemnation of abortion. In fact, it withdrew male doctors from gynecology and gave the field—including abortion—to the midwives.

Whatever your personal opinion of abortion, there's no doubt that women have always sought to control their fertility. After all, until about 150 years ago, childbirth was a leading cause of death among women.

Midwives completely dominated obstetrics and gynecology until about a century ago. It's no coincidence that many herbs were traditionally used to calm the womb, trigger menstruation, induce abortion, promote or dry up mothers' milk, and treat infant colic and infectious diarrhea (still a leading cause of infant death in third-world nations). These were the daily concerns that women patients presented to their women healers.

Sometimes medically unschooled women herbalists introduced university-trained physicians to powerful medicines, such as the heart drug digitalis from foxglove. By and large, though, physicians looked down on folk healers as ignorant practitioners of inferior medicine.

Nonetheless, women herbalists have played a key—and largely undocumented—role in medical history. Just as herbs are the forgotten sources of many medicines, the "wise women" represent the forgotten healers whose thousands

of years of collective experience taught us how to use herbs safely and effectively.

The wise women were particularly adept at contraception. Around 700 B.C., an oracle sent Greek colonists to the coast of what is now Libya to found a colony, Cyrene. It was located in a dry, desolate, inhospitable place, but the colonists soon discovered a plant that made them wealthy—silphion (in Latin, *silphium*), a species of fennel.

Silphium was a remarkably effective contraceptive. When women ate it, they did not conceive. The herb quickly became the contraceptive of choice around the Mediterranean. Cyrenian coins depicted the plant, often held by a woman. Poets wrote of its powers. And overharvesting eventually wiped it out.

Shen Nung and
The Classic of Herbs

The origins of Chinese herbalism are lost in the mists of time. Legend has it that around 3400 B.C. (the time of the Iceman), "the divine farmer," mythical emperor-sage Shen Nung, invented agriculture and discovered that many plants have medicinal value. He tested herbs on himself and recorded their effects, then died after consuming too much of one that turned out to be poisonous.

Chinese herbalists credit Shen Nung as the author of China's first great herbal, the *Pen Tsao Ching* (*The Classic of Herbs*), which listed 237 herbal prescriptions using dozens of herbs, including ephedra, rhubarb, and opium poppy. Most authorities agree, however, that the *Pen Tsao Ching* was not written down until the Han dynasty, around A.D. 100. It chronicles not the discoveries of one mythical emperor but rather the collected insights of generations of Chinese herbalists.

Chinese herbalists discovered many medicinal plants, notably ginseng, tea, sesame, garlic, and cinnamon. Starting around A.D. 500, it became customary for Chinese emperors to commission updates of Shen Nung's herb guide, or herbal. Over the centuries, these became increasingly elaborate—and contradictory. By 1590, when Li Shih-Chen published his landmark 52-volume *Pen Tsao Kang Mu* (*The Catalogue of Medicinal Herbs*), he included 1,094 medicinal plants and an astounding 11,000 herbal formulas.

Chinese herbalists still study Li's work, but they have simplified his art. Today, Chinese medicine employs about 300 herbs, 150 of which are considered indispensable. These include Chinese angelica (dang gui), burdock, chrysanthemum, cinnamon, dandelion, garlic, gentian, ginger, ginseng, hawthorn, licorice, lotus, mint, rhubarb, scullcap, senna, and tea.

Starting in the mid-19th century, European colonialists introduced Western medicine into China, dismissing traditional Chinese herbalism and acupuncture as nonsense. The Chinese felt the same way about the "foreign devils'" medicine, and the two systems seemed irreconcilable.

Shortly after the establishment of the People's Republic in 1949, however, the Chinese government decided that China's huge, medically underserved population could benefit from the integration of Western and Chinese medicine. Today, in many places in China, Western-trained physicians practice alongside traditional herbalists and acupuncturists. Chinese and Western physicians examine the same patients, confer with each other, and often coordinate their recommendations.

A turning point in American acceptance of Chinese medicine occurred in 1972, when President Richard Nixon first visited China. Network news broadcast astonishing footage of a woman having abdominal surgery while fully conscious, her only anesthesia being a few acupuncture needles in her earlobes and feet.

While accompanying President Nixon to China, *New York Times* columnist James Reston developed appendicitis and had surgery. Afterward, he decided to try acupuncture for post-surgical pain control, and he was pleased with the results. His testimonial account in the nation's most influential newspaper helped open the United States to acupuncture and Chinese herbalism.

Jivaka and the Vedas

According to legend, around the time of the Hebrew exodus from Egypt (1200 B.C.), a poor Indian boy named Jivaka went to study medicine under the great Punarvasu Atreya, founder of India's first medical school at the University of Taxila in the Punjab. Having no money, the lad offered to become Atreya's servant in exchange for training.

After 7 years, Jivaka asked his teacher when his studies would be completed. Instead of answering, Atreya challenged him to scour the countryside and collect all the plants that he considered medically useless. Jivaka searched for many days. When he finally returned, he was sullen and empty-handed. He told his mentor that he was unable to find a single plant without healing power. Atreya replied, "Go! You now have the knowledge to be a physician."

Centered in the Indus Valley near the present India-Pakistan border, ancient Indian civilization was quite advanced. Excavations at Harappa and Mohenjo Daro dating to about 2500 B.C. have revealed municipal water and sewerage systems more advanced than the ones the Romans developed 2,000 years later.

Ancient Indians called their medicine Ayurveda, from two Sanskrit words: *ayur,* "life," and *veda,* "knowledge." Ayurvedic medicine developed from the Vedas, India's four books of classic wisdom.

The oldest, the 4,500-year-old *Rig Veda,* is a collection of 1,028 Hindu hymns, recited orally starting around 2500 B.C. and written down 1,000 years later. The *Rig Veda* contains astonishingly detailed descriptions of eye surgery, limb amputation, and formulas for medicines using 67 medicinal herbs, including ginger, cinnamon, and senna. The 3,200-year-old *Atharva Veda* also discusses many healing herbs.

Around 700 B.C. (4 centuries before Hippocrates), Charaka, a professor at the University of Taxila, wrote Ayurvedic medicine's first medical encyclopedia. Called the *Charaka Samhita,* it listed 500 herbal formulas. A century later, another famous Ayurvedic, Susruta, wrote the *Susruta Samhita,* which also emphasized herbal healing.

In 250 B.C., India's King Asoka converted to Buddhism and launched a 1,000-year golden age of Ayurvedic medicine. Asoka sent Buddhist monk-physicians around the country to heal the sick and convert them to Buddhism. As the centuries passed, pilgrims came from as far away as China and Persia to receive Ayurvedic treatment.

One herb that Ayurvedic healers introduced was *Rauwolfia serpentina.* It's the source of resperine, which was used until recently in Western medicine to manage high blood pressure.

After A.D. 600, Ayurvedic healing influenced Arab medicine, which combined Greco-Roman, Middle Eastern, and Asian therapies. Arab physicians in turn introduced some Ayurvedic practices into Europe.

During the 19th century, the British introduced Western medicine into India, but a majority of Indians and Pakistanis still rely on Ayurvedic medicine or homeopathy, both of which emphasize medicinal herbs instead of drugs.

10,000 Healing Herbs

The land between the Tigris and Euphrates rivers in present-day Iraq was at one time home to the Sumerians, Assyrians, Babylonians, and Persians. The earliest Sumerians had no physicians. Sick people congregated in public squares, and passersby gave them advice.

As Sumerian culture developed, so did its medicine. In late Sumerian mythology, the gods give Sumeria's original healer, Thrita, a golden knife, 10,000 healing herbs, and the medical wisdom to use them. One of the world's oldest surviving prescriptions is a Sumerian clay tablet from around 2100 B.C. that mentions several herbs, including myrrh, cypress, and opium poppy.

By 1000 B.C., the Assyrians had three kinds of healers: herb doctors (internists), knife doctors (surgeons), and word doctors (psychiatrists). Herb doctors were the most numerous and prominent, in part because Assyria was strategically placed along the ancient Spice Route (also known as the Silk Route) from Asia to Egypt. Archeologists have unearthed the remains of an Assyrian pharmacy that stocked 230 herbs, including almond, anise, caraway, coriander, juniper, saffron, sesame, turmeric, and willow.

The Assyrians, and later the Babylonians and Persians, played a major role in the ancient spice trade, one of the world's oldest forms of commerce. Spices had many advantages over other trade goods. Great demand made herbs as precious as jewels, which meant high profits. When properly dried and stored, spices could travel great distances without spoiling. They didn't have to be fed like cattle and slaves. In addition, they took up little space, which meant they could be transported easily.

No wonder that in the biblical story, when Joseph's jealous brothers sold him into slavery, he was purchased by "a caravan . . . coming from Gilead [Jordan], their camels bearing gum, balm, and myrrh on their way to carry it down to Egypt" (Genesis 37:25).

Imhotep and the "Stinking Ones" of the Nile

In 1874, in the Valley of the Tombs near Luxor, the German Egyptologist Georg Ebers discovered the world's oldest surviving medical text, a 65-foot papyrus dating from shortly after the time of Joseph, around 1500 B.C. The *Ebers Papyrus* listed 876 herbal formulas from more than 500 plants, including aloe, caraway, castor, chamomile, cinnamon, coriander, cardamom, fennel, fenugreek, garlic, gentian, ginger, juniper, mint, myrrh, opium poppy, onion, sesame, saffron, sage, and thyme. This represents about one-third of the herbs in today's Western herbal pharmacopoeia.

Some Ebers formulas strike the modern reader as bizarre, such as a shampoo made from a dog's paw, decayed palm leaves, and a donkey hoof, all boiled in oil and then rubbed on the head. Others sound surprisingly contemporary, such as the recommendation to bandage moldy bread over wounds to prevent infection. Modern antibiotics were originally derived from molds.

In Egyptian mythology, medicine was created by Thoth, the god of knowledge. Thoth also invented writing and the arts and sciences. The most notable Egyptian physician was Imhotep, who was also the architect to Pharaoh Zoser (3000 B.C.).

Imhotep is credited with designing one of the first pyramids, but as time passed, he was remembered mostly as a healer. Imhotep became deified, and around 700 B.C., Egypt's medical school at Memphis was dedicated to him, as was a nearby school for midwives.

The Egyptians imported enormous quantities of herbs for perfumes, embalming mixtures, and medicines. They also considered plants important spoils of war. In 1475 B.C., when Pharaoh Thutmose III conquered what is now Syria, he demanded as tribute specimens of all Syrian plants not found in Egypt.

The Egyptians loved aromatic herbs. The ancient kingdom's access to both the Mediterranean and Arabian seas allowed them to import aromatics from as far away as Spain to the west and the Spice Islands (Indonesia) to the east.

The Egyptians' affection for fragrant herbs paled next to their obsession with two herbs that many ancients considered foul-smelling: garlic and onion. The Egyptians believed that garlic and onion strengthened the body and prevented disease (a view supported by modern science). They ate so much that the Greek historian Herodotus called them "the stinking ones." Six cloves of garlic were found in the tomb of King Tut.

The Egyptians also gave their slaves daily

rations of garlic and onions to keep them strong and healthy. In 450 B.C., Herodotus wrote of an inscription inside the Cheops Pyramid at Gisa (built in 2900 B.C.) that said "1,600 talents of silver" (about $4 million) had been spent on garlic and onions for its builders.

According to legend, a garlic shortage once forced the Egyptians to cut their slaves' rations. The slaves were so incensed that they refused to work. If this story is true, it was the world's earliest recorded strike.

Egyptian farmers could not satisfy the demand for garlic and onions, so the Egyptians turned to the Philistines, who lived in nearby Canaan (Israel). The Philistine city of Askelon became a major garlic and onion trading center, not only for the Egyptians but also for the Greeks and Romans. The Romans favored the Philistines' small green onions, calling them *ascalonia* after Askelon. The word evolved into *escallon*, and finally into our *scallion*.

By about 500 B.C., Egyptian herbalists were considered the finest in the Mediterranean, and rulers from Rome to Babylon recruited them as court physicians. Aspiring physicians—Galen among them—went to Egypt to study with the medical masters of the Nile.

From Aesculapius to Hippocrates

The early Greeks viewed illness as a divine curse and prayed to Apollo, god of medicine, for recovery. In Greek mythology, Apollo had a son, Aesculapius, a physician-god like Imhotep, who treated the sick with help from his daughters, Hygeia and Panacea. Hygeia, the source of our word *hygiene*, represented healthy living, while Panacea, whose name means cure-all, treated disease.

When ill, early Greeks visited temples dedicated to Aesculapius, where physician-priests treated them with baths, exercise, massage, fasting, prayer, herbs, and counseling. Treatment culminated in animal sacrifices to entice Aesculapius's spirit into patients' dreams to tell them how to get well. The program was similar to the regimens at many of today's health spas, except for the sacrifices—and the snakes.

Snakes were sacred to Aesculapius, and they slithered freely around his temple grounds. One omen of imminent recovery was to have a snake lick a patient's wounds. Snakes' tongues thus became symbols of healing, and they remained ingredients in medicinal potions well into the Middle Ages.

An echo of the snake-as-healer belief survives today. Aesculapius was often pictured carrying a staff with a snake wrapped around it, and the snake-staff combination became the caduceus, the symbol of medicine.

The Aesculapian priesthood was a family affair, with sons following their fathers into the healing temples. On the island of Kos, off the coast of Turkey, one Aesculapian family produced Hippocrates (460–377 B.C.), the father of medicine. Hippocrates rebelled against Aesculapius, however, by secularizing Greek medicine. He believed that diseases came not from the gods but from natural causes: the environment, climate, and diet.

Homer wrote in the *Iliad* that Greek medicine came from Egypt. Kos is located only a short voyage from the land of Imhotep. But Hippocrates clearly elaborated on Egyptian practices. From his seat under a plane tree (of the sycamore family), he was the first physician to examine patients closely and the first to use case studies in medical training, a method that's still in practice today.

Hippocrates never wrote a word, but his students compiled the 72-volume *Corpus Hippocraticum*. It mentions 350 medicinal plants, including mint, rosemary, thyme, anise, clove, cinnamon, and burdock.

Hippocrates taught that health depended on a balance among the body's four fluids, or "humors": blood, phlegm, yellow bile, and black bile. Hippocrates' Humoral Theory of illness remained a cornerstone of European medicine until the mid-19th century, when Pasteur's Germ Theory supplanted it.

The humors had four qualities: hot, cold, dry, and wet. Hippocrates prescribed warming herbs such as ginger for diseases that he believed were caused by cold, and cooling herbs such as mint for ailments brought on by heat. All of the classic herbals assigned Hippocratic qualities to healing herbs—warming, cooling, and so on—and listed the "foul humors" that they supposedly relieved.

Aesculapian priests and later Greek physicians grew and gathered many herbs. They also bought medicinal plants from herbalists known as root gatherers or rhizomists. (In botany, a rhizome is an underground stem.) The rhizomists were peasant herbalists who sold medicinal plants in market towns.

Hippocrates had no women students, but many midwives were also rhizomists. Homer mentions one named Agamede, who was famous for her knowledge of healing herbs.

Shortly before Hippocrates' death, Theophrastus (372–285 B.C.), the father of botany, was born. He wrote *Historia Plantarum* (*An Inquiry into Plants*) and *De Causis Plantarum* (*The Growth of Plants*), which remained standard references for more than 1,000 years. Many of the 550 plants that Theophrastus discussed were used in healing.

Theophrastus owned a prominent herb shop in Athens. He was also a friend of Aristotle. When the noted philosopher died, he bequeathed Theophrastus his garden.

Roman Herbalists: Dioscorides, Pliny, and Galen

The first true medical botanist was Pedanius Dioscorides (A.D. 40–90). Born in Turkey, he was Greek, but he served as a physician with the Roman legions of Emperor Nero.

Dioscorides traveled from Germany to the Middle East with the army. In A.D. 78, he published *De Materia Medica* (*On Medicines*), Europe's first real herbal. It discussed 600 plants, including aloe, anise, chamomile, cinnamon, dill, marjoram, poppy, rhubarb, and thyme.

As an army physician, Dioscorides concentrated on soldiers' medicine, particularly wounds. But *De Materia Medica* also included a great deal of herbal folk wisdom, so it's clear that he sought out herbalists during his travels.

De Materia Medica remained a standard medical reference for 1,500 years. Virtually every herbal published through the 17th century referred to it. After the invention of printing in the 1450s, *De Materia Medica* was one of the first books published. The oldest copy in the United States, from 1547, is in the Lloyd Library collection in Cincinnati (more on the Lloyd brothers later).

It's fitting that Rome's legions produced a great herbalist, because part of their mission was to protect Rome's Spice Routes from barbarian incursions and provincial revolts. By the

1st century A.D., the herb and spice trade was a cornerstone of Roman commerce. Roman demand for medicinal, culinary, and perfume herbs was almost insatiable.

Shortly before the publication of *De Materia Medica*, Greek merchants discovered the secret of the Indian Ocean's shifting monsoon winds, which blew toward India part of the year and toward Egypt the rest. Capitalizing on this new insight, spice merchants were able to reduce by half—from 2 years to 1—the round trip from Rome to India's black-pepper-producing Malabar region. As a result, the price of black pepper came down to the modern equivalent of about $100 per ounce. Many other herbs were equally costly.

While Dioscorides traveled the Empire, back in Rome, Caius Plinius Secundus, or Pliny the Elder (A.D. 23–79), was busy compiling ancient scientific knowledge into his 37-volume *Historia Naturalis* (*Natural History*). Volumes 12 through 19 dealt with botany, and 20 through 27 specifically addressed healing herbs.

Pliny made some wild assertions. For colds, he advised "kissing the hairy muzzle of a mouse." Nevertheless, many of his herbal recommendations guided physicians for centuries.

In August of A.D. 79, Pliny traveled to Pompeii upon learning that Mount Vesuvius was rumbling. When the volcano exploded on August 24, Pliny was perched on a nearby hill, taking notes. He died of asphyxiation.

Fifty years after Pliny, Claudius Galenus, better known as Galen (A.D. 131–200), became Rome's leading physician. Born into a wealthy family in Pergamum (now Bergama), Turkey, Galen studied medicine in Greece and Alexandria, then worked for several years as a physician to Pergamum's gladiators. At age 30, he moved to Rome, and eventually he became the physician to Emperor Marcus Aurelius.

Galen was notoriously arrogant, boastful, and dogmatic. He rebelled against the Hippocratic idea of examining patients and practiced a highly theoretical form of medicine that dominated physician training in Europe for more than 1,000 years.

At a time when midwife-herbalists used single herbs or formulas with only a few ingredients, Galen insisted on "polypharmacy"—complex concoctions of herbs, animal parts, and minerals called galenicals. Galen's wealthy patients liked galenicals because they were expensive and therefore exclusive. As the centuries passed, Europe's nobility came to favor costly galenicals, while the peasantry stuck with single herbs or simple formulas, which became known as simples.

Roman rhizomists—or *herbarii*, in Latin—congregated around Capitoline Hill. They were a motley crew. Physicians accused them of mislabeling and adulterating their herbs. Pliny and Galen boycotted them and urged physicians to grow and gather their own medicinal plants. The *herbarii* grew so troublesome that several emperors attempted to control them with a licensing system. These attempts failed, however.

Roman Assassins: From Mithridates to *Theriaca*

Roman herbalists were as likely to be killers as healers. The Imperial court seethed with murderous intrigue. Among the available assassination methods—knifing, "accidents," and poisoning—the herbal approach was most popular.

Political notables were typically surrounded

by bodyguards, making knifings and accidents difficult to arrange. Physical assault also involved considerable risk of capture. By comparison, poisoning could be carried out from a safe distance. Death occurred some time after the deed, allowing for escape or alibi. And in an age before autopsy, when apparently healthy people often sickened and died suddenly, wily poisoners might remain above suspicion.

As a result, rulers throughout the Roman empire became obsessed with the identification of herbal poisons and the development of antidotes known as *theriaca* (in English, "theriacs"). The word comes from the Greek *theriakon*, meaning remedies for venomous bites.

The ancient world's most poison-paranoid ruler was Mithridates Eupator (120–66 B.C.), king of Pontus, on the Black Sea. Mithridates governed by terror and was convinced (probably rightly) that he was destined to be poisoned. As a result, he delved into botany, believing that familiarity with both poisonous and medicinal plants was his best defense. His botanical expertise is commemorated in the genus name of boneset, *Eupatorium*.

In addition to formulating dozens of theriacs, Mithridates supposedly ordered his court physician, Krateus, to concoct the ultimate herbal poison. The ancient king took increasing doses to develop a tolerance and make himself immune.

Then, in 66 B.C., the Romans attacked. Facing capture and execution, Mithridates tried to poison himself, but he'd become so tolerant that no poison could kill him. Finally, he ordered a slave to stab him to death. To this day, the word *mithridatism* means an acquired tolerance to poisons.

Mithridates made a big impression in Rome, where the nobility offered to pay enormous sums for any antidotes attributed to the King of Pontus. Needless to say, Rome's unscrupulous *herbarii* were only too happy to peddle bogus mixtures as "Mithridates' Theriac."

A century after the unpoisonable king's death, Emperor Nero became nearly insane with fear of poisoning, in part because he'd gained the throne by poisoning his stepbrother. Nero ordered his physician, Andromachus of Crete, to improve on Mithridates' Theriac. Andromachus mixed 78 herbal, animal, and mineral ingredients—including opium, a lizard, and snake flesh (in homage to Aesculapius)—to create Andromachus's Theriac. The antidote became popular throughout Rome.

Slave midwife-herbalists were highly valued as poisoners. They could often be placed as concubines in the bedrooms of their intended victims, beyond the reach of bodyguards and "tasters," who sampled rulers' food and drink before they ate, just in case. The slave herbalist Locusta became famous for her skill as a poisoner. After one important murder, she received her freedom and a gift of land.

Not to be outdone by Andromachus, Galen wrote a book containing more than 100 theriac recipes. He also developed his own, Galene, a polypharmaceutical brew of 70 ingredients, including dozens of herbs, honey, wine, minerals, and animal parts. It took 40 days to prepare.

When Rome fell, the barbarians seized not only Rome's lands and wealth but also its vast stores of herbs and spices. During one attack, the barbarians demanded horses, money—and 3,000 pounds of black pepper.

Theriaca eventually evolved into the Elizabethan English word *treacle*. The Elizabethan peasantry used garlic as an all-purpose medicine and antidote, and it became known as the poor man's treacle.

Avicenna and the Invention of Pharmacy

As Rome collapsed, Arab civilization filled the intellectual vacuum. From A.D. 600 to 800, Islamic armies forged an empire stretching from Spain across Northern Africa to India. Unlike the barbarians who seized Roman Europe, the Arabs venerated Greco-Roman culture and learning. Along with the spoils of conquest, they sent tens of thousands of Greco-Roman books to Baghdad, where they were translated into Arabic and studied.

Ibn-Sina, or Avicenna (A.D. 980–1037), was the leading Arab physician. While still quite young, he cured an Arab prince of a serious illness. Afterward, his services were in great demand. A follower of Galen, he wrote the *Canon of Medicine*, the West's medical bible for 600 years. Book Two discussed the healing herbs, including nutmeg, senna, sandalwood, rhubarb, myrrh, cinnamon, clove, and rosewater.

The Arabs revered Galen but were not ruled by polypharmacy. They simplified Galen's medicines and developed pharmacy as a field distinct from medicine. The first modern pharmacies appeared in Baghdad in the 9th century.

Arab pharmacists replaced galenicals with syrups, ointments, and tinctures (alcohol extracts). They were the first to distill pure alcohol, whose name is derived from the Arabic *al-kohl*, or "quintessence." Arab medicine also gave us the terms *alkalai*, from *al-qali*, or "ashes," and *sugar*, from *sukkar*, meaning "grain or pebble."

From A.D. 800 until it was recaptured by the Christians in the 1400s, Spain rivaled Baghdad as a center of Arab herbalism. One influential herbalist was Abul-Kasim Khalef ibn Abbas—in Spanish, Abulcasis (A.D. 936–1013). He lived in Cordoba and wrote *Liber Servitoris* (*The Book of Simples*), an important source for later European herbals.

The other prominent herbalist was Ibn al-Baitar (A.D. 1197–1248), a botanist from Malaga who collected 1,500 plants from Spain to Syria. He also wrote the most complete Arab herbal, the *Corpus of Simples*. It introduced 200 new healing herbs (and poisons), including tamarind, aconite, and nux vomica (strychnine).

Monasteries and Liqueurs

After the fall of Rome, European medicine was dominated by the Catholic Church, which adopted the pre-Hippocratic Greek belief that illness was a punishment from God and was treatable only by prayer and penance. But Catholic monks preserved Greco-Roman herbalism by copying the ancient texts.

Among the monastic orders, the Benedictines were the most avid herbalists. They were the first Europeans to adopt the Arab practice of making tinctures. They flavored wine with digestion-promoting herbs and created the forerunners of today's liqueurs, one of which is still known as Benedictine.

Charlemagne (A.D. 742–814) was so impressed by the Benedictines' herb gardens that he ordered all of the monasteries in his vast realm to plant "physic gardens" to ensure an adequate supply of healing herbs. Charlemagne described herbs as "friends of the physician and cook."

Around A.D. 820, the Benedictines designed

their ideal monastery, known as the Plan of St. Gall. In one corner was a medical area that included an infirmary, bath, doctor's room, and bloodletting room. It also featured a 1,000-square-foot physic garden that contained two dozen herbs, among them cumin, fennel, fenugreek, mint, pennyroyal, rose, rosemary, rue, sage, savory, and watercress.

In another corner was a kitchen garden that also contained many herbs. Among them was dill, which was commonly mixed with salt water to preserve vegetables, particularly cucumbers. We enjoy them today as dill pickles.

The most notable Benedictine herbalist was Hildegard of Bingen (1098–1179), abbess of the Rupertsburg convent in the German Rhineland. Hildegard was a Renaissance woman centuries before the Renaissance—a nun, administrator, composer, writer, and herbalist. She wrote religious music that is still performed today.

Hildegard claimed that visions of God commanded her to treat the sick and compile herbal formulas. Her book, *Hildegard's Medicine*, combined mystical Catholicism and early German folk medicine, along with the author's own extensive herbal experience. Hildegard's favorite herbs included aloe, apple, basil, bay, blackberry, caraway, celery, clove, dill, fennel, garlic, hyssop, licorice, marjoram, myrrh, nettle, nutmeg, onion, oregano, parsley, raspberry, rosemary, rue, thyme, and watercress.

Hildegard's herbal is unique. She wrote an original medical work based on her own experience at a time when the few literate Europeans—mostly monks—were content to copy the Greeks, Romans, and Avicenna. What's more, she was the only medieval woman who left any account of the "wise women" healing practices.

Some of Hildegard's advice sounds silly. For poor vision, she advocated rubbing the eyes with a topaz soaked in wine. Many of her recommendations were quite sensible, however. She advocated eating a balanced diet and brushing the teeth with aloe and myrrh, both of which have antibacterial, decay-preventive properties.

While Hildegard relied on simples, galenicals continued to be valued, largely by the nobility, who had access to galenically inclined physicians and the wealth to afford all the ingredients that Galen's polypharmaceuticals required. The men who mixed medieval galenicals were the first alchemists.

Around the time that the Benedictines invented liqueur, Germanic Angles and Saxons were settling England. They brought European herbalism with them, and they learned how the native Celts and their priests, the Druids, used healing herbs.

Around A.D. 950, a nobleman named Bald persuaded England's King Alfred to commission the first British herbal. The book combined Anglo-Saxon and Celtic herbalism with Greco-Roman and Arab practices sent by the Patriarch of Jerusalem. It was called the *Leech Book of Bald*. (*Leech* comes from *laece*, the Anglo-Saxon word for "doctor.") It discussed 500 plants, including vervain and mistletoe, both sacred to the Druids. A surviving copy is on display at the British Museum in London.

With the Renaissance, European medicine took a secular turn. After the invention of printing, monks stopped copying the ancient herbals, but they continued to tend their gardens. In 1868, an Austrian monk, Gregor Mendel, published *Plant Hybridization*, an account of his experiments with peas. It launched the modern science of genetics.

Wise Women: From Healers to Witches

Hildegard of Bingen was lucky to have lived in the 12th century. Had she practiced herbalism from 1300 to 1650, she probably would have been burned as a witch.

It's not clear what led to Europe's 350 years of witch-hunts. Feminists link the practice to the rise of secular medicine as a male-dominated profession. Others blame the hysteria on bubonic plague (the Black Death), which swept Europe in waves and killed half of its population.

A more recent theory holds that European rulers and the Catholic Church became alarmed by a decline in population, which they blamed on the contraceptive herbalism of the wise women. The leading medieval contraceptive herbs were all abortifacients, or "morning-after" plants, in modern parlance. The most popular were pennyroyal, artemesia, and rue. Modern research shows that all three stimulate uterine contractions and abortion.

Whatever the cause of the witch-hunts, after 1300 the image of the folk herbalist changed from helpful wise woman to evil witch. Witch-hunts started in Germany and eventually reached all of Europe. Accusations of "sexual intercourse with the Devil" were typically accompanied by testimony that the alleged witch practiced herbal medicine and made healing mixtures, cosmetics, love potions, aphrodisiacs, abortifacients, and poisons.

Accusations of poisoning were particularly damning. It's quite possible that some women herbalists continued the Roman tradition of herbal assassination, but this was the era before the discovery of the dose-response relationship: the idea that the greater the dose, the greater the effect. Many so-called witches' plants, poisonous in large amounts, caused no harm in therapeutic or cosmetic amounts. Nonetheless, the witch-hunters considered them poisons.

One plant associated with witchcraft was called devil's herb. Large amounts are lethal when taken internally. The juice causes the pupils to dilate when placed in the eyes, and medieval women used devil's herb cosmetically. Eventually, the plant was renamed belladonna, or "beautiful woman."

Then there was witch's bells. Large amounts are poisonous, but small amounts stimulate the heart. After the witch-hunt era, the plant's name was changed to foxglove, source of the heart drug digitalis.

Conviction of witchcraft meant death. At the height of the witch-hunts, as many as 600 women a year—about two a day—were executed in parts of Germany. At Toulouse, France, 400 were put to death in a single day.

North America did not escape the hysteria. The Salem witch trials in Massachusetts (1692) resulted in 20 women being executed. Records suggest that they, too, were wise women herbalists.

After the witch-hunts, the saintly Hildegard was forgotten, replaced by the witches of Shakespeare's *Macbeth*, who threw mandrake, belladonna, and other evil herbs into their bubbling cauldron. Witches were also vilified in the stories that have become today's fairy tales. In "Snow White," for example, the evil queen-witch concocts an herbal poison, coats an apple with it, and slips it to Snow White, who falls into a coma, thus following a tradition of herbal assassination dating back to the Romans.

The witch-hunts failed to eradicate women's herbalism, but they succeeded in driving it underground. More than a century after the last witch-hunts, the "old woman" who helped popularize foxglove said that it was a "secret family recipe." Her forebears had good reason to keep their use of witch's bells a secret.

A World Hungry for Spices

The fall of Rome devastated the spice trade. Arab merchants continued to import Asian herbs into Europe, but the commerce declined and prices soared. During the Middle Ages, a pound of ginger could buy a fat sheep. Black pepper was counted out corn by corn and used to pay rents, taxes, and dowries. One pound of pepper could buy a serf his freedom.

Then came the Crusades. From 1095 until 1291, European armies attempted to wrest the Holy Land from Islamic control. Their efforts failed militarily, but while in the Middle East, the Crusaders tasted Asian spices and returned home craving more.

The 1296 publication of Marco Polo's travelogue heightened European fascination with the Orient and its herbs. Polo's father and uncle were merchants who set out from Venice to China in 1271, taking the 17-year-old Marco with them. The young Italian became a favorite of Kublai Kahn, and when he returned in 1295, his famous memoir was filled with mouthwatering accounts of Asia's wonderful spices.

The ancient Spice Routes slowly reopened. Around 1300, British spice dealers obtained a royal charter to become the Guild of Pepperers. They bought black pepper and other herbs from brokers in Venice, who traded with Arab importers. By 1400, Venice alone imported 2,500 tons of ginger and black pepper a year. European demand seemed insatiable.

Then something terrible happened. During the 1400s, the Mongols, who supported trade with Europe, lost Western Asia to the Ottoman Turks, who closed the trade routes. In Venice and Genoa, cities enriched by the spice trade, Italian merchants grew desperate for new avenues to the East. If the world was round, as some claimed, it might be possible to sail west across the Atlantic and reach the Indies.

It was no coincidence that Christopher Columbus hailed from Genoa. He never reached the East Indies, but he returned from the New World with allspice and red pepper, which the Caribbean Indians called *kian*, or "cayenne."

In 1498, when the Portuguese explorer Vasco da Gama succeeded in sailing around Africa to India, his first words in Calcutta were, "We come in search of Christians and spices."

The Portuguese and Dutch took an early lead in world exploration. They monopolized the sea route around Africa to India and the Spice Islands (Indonesia), as well as the trade in cinnamon, cloves, tea, and black pepper.

The Spanish concentrated on the New World and its gold. Sometimes they found the precious metal, sometimes other valuables.

In 1519, Hernando Cortez watched as Mexico's Aztec ruler, Montezuma, toasted his arrival by sipping from a golden goblet. Cortez coveted the goblet—but the herbal beverage that it contained, *chocolatl* or "chocolate," eventually became more important than the Aztec's gold.

In addition to chocolate, Spanish conquistadors returned home with corn, tobacco, potatoes, carrots, strawberries, lima beans, tomatoes, sarsaparilla, passionflower, and the most important new healing herb of all, cinchona (Jesuit or Peruvian bark). Cinchona was the first effective treatment for malaria (also known as ague, intermittent fever, and swamp fever), which had plagued the Mediterranean area and Europe since ancient times. Centuries later, cinchona became the source of the antimalarial drug quinine.

The Spanish may also have returned from the New World with something else: syphilis. A doctor in Seville claimed that he had treated Columbus's crew in 1493. It's possible that they became infected in Haiti. Or perhaps increased trade spread a disease that had existed for ages in isolated pockets around the Mediterranean.

In any event, an epidemic of unusually virulent syphilis swept through Europe in 1494, killing thousands. Europeans considered the disease an import from the New World and looked across the Atlantic for a cure. They focused on sarsaparilla, which was widely used until well into the 19th century. The herb turned out to be ineffective against the disease.

Another syphilis treatment was mercury. It played a key role in the schism that developed in the early 19th century between pro-mercury "regular" physicians and anti-mercury herbal "Eclectics."

Spain kept chocolate, cinchona, and other New World plants secret for years. Eventually, they were revealed in a book by Spanish physician-botanist Nicolas Monardes. The book became a huge bestseller. It was published in English in 1577, with the title *Joyful Newes out of the Newe Founde Worlde*.

Twenty years after *Joyful Newes*, the British still played a minor role in world exploration. That changed in 1599, when the Dutch suddenly tripled the price of black pepper. The British were outraged. Eighty London merchants pooled their capital and established the British East India Company, which began importing pepper and other herbs directly from India.

The British eventually took control of the subcontinent and Ceylon (Sri Lanka). The East India Company also imported Chinese tea, which quickly became as British as the Union Jack.

The East India Company's tea was very popular in England's North American colonies. In 1773, when Parliament tried to tax it, New England tea lovers dumped several tons into Boston Harbor in protest. The Boston Tea Party helped ignite the American Revolution.

Paracelsus and the Doctrine of Signatures

Around 1500, Italian mathematician Giambattista della Porta of Naples conceived the first new medical philosophy since Galen. Called the Doctrine of Signatures, it claimed that a plant's physical appearance revealed its healing value. As British herbalist William Coles explained in his *Art of Simpling* (1656), God had not only "stamped upon plants . . . a distinct forme but also given them particular signatures whereby a Man may read the use of them."

According to Coles, "Wall-nuts [walnuts] have the perfect signature of the Head. The outer husk represents the Pericranium or outward skin of the skull, whereon the hair groweth, and therefore those husks are exceedingly good for wounds in the head. The inner woody shell hath the Signature of the Skull . . . and the Kernel hath the very figure of the Brain. If the Kernel be bruised, moistened with wine, and laid upon the Head, it comforts the head and brain mightily." Some herbals still suggest walnuts for headache.

The most vocal champion of the Doctrine of Signatures was Phillippus Aureolus Theophrastus Bombastus von Hohenheim (1493–1541), the son of a Swiss alchemist/physician. A brilliant, arrogant student of medicine, he lived up to his name, Bombastus. But he changed it to Paracelsus ("greater than Celsus"), convinced that he was more brilliant than the Roman physician Celsus (53 B.C.–A.D. 7), then considered on a par with Galen.

Paracelsus taught at the University of Basel in Switzerland in the 1520s. At a time when medical students studied only Hippocrates, Galen, Celsus, and Avicenna, Paracelsus publicly burned their books to symbolize his rejection of Galenic dogma. He also replaced the ancient Humoral Theory of illness with the Doctrine of Signatures.

Strange as it sounds today, the doctrine was based on experience with healing herbs, although it overgeneralized that experience badly. For instance, the leaves of garlic and onion are hollow, allowing air to pass through them. In addition, they both had been used for centuries as decongestants. Based on these characteristics, the doctrine declared that any plant with hollow leaves or stems was a respiratory remedy.

The Doctrine of Signatures quickly became the new medical dogma. Bile has a yellowish tinge, and jaundice, a liver problem, turns the skin yellow. Under the doctrine, any yellow flower or root was considered a liver medicine. Similarly, any plant with long, snaking roots was used to treat snakebite. Plants with heart-shaped leaves were considered heart remedies. Juicy plants were used as diuretics and lactation promoters.

In addition to promoting the insurgent medical philosophy, Paracelsus further offended the professional medical community by writing in the vernacular instead of in Latin, thus opening medicine to those unschooled in the language of the universities. He correctly predicted the discovery of "active principles" in plants and pioneered the chemical extraction of plant oils.

Paracelsus also discovered the dose-response relationship. "It depends only on the dose," he wrote, "whether a poison is a poison or not." This insight came too late to save thousands of alleged witches executed in part for possession of "poisons," but it allowed Paracelsus to introduce many potentially toxic minerals into medicine in very small doses. He used arsenic, sulphur, lead, antimony, and particularly mercury, not just for syphilis but also for many other diseases. In time, physicians came to view mercury as a panacea.

The Age of the Herbals

With the invention of printing in the 1450s, herbals proliferated, and England's university-trained physicians began to fear the loss of their medical monopoly. Emboldened by the witch-hunts, they lobbied their influential patients in the British Court to outlaw the practice of medicine by the "rogues, horse-gelders, rat catchers, idiots, and witches" and restrict it to them.

In a 1511 decree, Henry VIII reserved the practice of medicine for university-trained physicians and barber-surgeons who had completed apprenticeships. Anyone else had to pass a test administered in Latin by the Bishop of London and a committee of prominent doctors.

Of course, folk herbalists could not read Latin. Many didn't read English. Some stopped practicing. Many became "green men and women," latter-day rhizomists who supplied herbs to the physicians and the early pharmacists, or apothecaries, often while continuing to practice herbal healing stealthily and illegally.

In time, England's herbalists rebelled against the suppression of folk medicine by publishing two anonymous herbals. *Bancke's Herball* (1525), a compilation of English herb lore, was the first herbal printed in English. *The Grete Herball* (1526) was a translation of French and German books.

Henry VIII's edict eventually led to a major shortage of doctors. In 1543, he rescinded it with the Herbalists' Charter: "From henceforth, it shall be lawful for every . . . King's subject, having knowledge and experience of . . . Herbs and Roots . . . to practice, use, and minister to any Sore, Wound, Swelling, or Disease any Herbs, Ointments, Baths, Pulsters (poultices) and Emplaisters (plasters), according to their Cunning, Experience, and Knowledge . . . without Suit, Vexation, Trouble, Penalty, or Loss of their Goods."

The Herbalists' Charter came just 1 year after German botanist Leonhard Fuchs (1501–1566) published *De Historia Stirpium* (*On Plants*), the first original book of medical botany since Dioscorides' treatise almost 1,500 years earlier. Illustrated with detailed woodcuts, it discussed 500 healing herbs, including 100 from the New World.

In 1546, the University of Padua in Italy planted the first academic botanical garden, which helped launch the modern science of botany. In time, most major universities and many physicians and apothecaries planted their own physic gardens.

William Turner, the father of British botany, published his *New Herball* in 1551. Turner supported both Paracelsus's Doctrine of Signatures, still an insurgent philosophy at the time, and his dose-response concept. He advised against taking large amounts of healing herbs.

In 1554, the Belgian physician-botanist Rembert Dodoens (1517–1585) published a Dutch herbal, which was revised and re-released in Latin in 1583. A London publisher commissioned Dr. Robert Priest to translate the herbal into English, but Dr. Priest died before completing the project, and his translation disappeared.

Enter John Gerard (1545–1612), who had apprenticed as a barber-surgeon but loved horticulture. He established a noted physic garden in Fetter Lane, London, that contained more than 1,000 species, including England's first potatoes. In 1586, Gerard was appointed curator of the College of Physicians' Physic Garden, and soon after, he became herbalist to King James I.

In 1597, Gerard published his *Herball or Generall Historie of Plantes*, in which he displayed the College of Physicians' characteristic contempt for "overbold apothecaries, and foolish women." Gerard apparently had nothing against plagiarism, however. He obliquely acknowledged Dr. Priest, leading to accusations that he'd obtained Priest's lost translation of Dodoens's herbal and published it as his own.

Although Gerard denied any wrongdoing, and his herbal contained a good deal of original information on herb gardening, most authorities believe that he stole Priest's work.

John Parkinson (1567–1650) was another pioneering British herbalist. In 1640, he published *Theatrum Botanicum* (*The Theater of Plants*), subtitled *The Universall and Complete Herball*. It was no understatement. The 1,800-page book discussed 3,800 plants, which Parkinson organized into 17 "Classes or Tribes," including "Venomous, Sleepy, and Hurtfull Plants, and Their Counter Poysons"; "Hot and Sharpe Biting Plantes"; and "Strange and Outlandish Plants."

Parkinson's classification system appears quaint today, but during the 17th century, it was taken quite seriously. Many scientists proposed similar systems, but none stuck until 1737. That's when Swedish naturalist Carl Linne, also known as Carolus Linnaeus (1707–1778), developed his Latin binomial genus-and-species system based on reproductive characteristics. After Darwin, scientists adopted evolutionary criteria, but to this day, plants and animals are still named using Linnaeus's binomial formula.

As university medicine slowly became more scientific, leading physicians stopped growing their own herbs. They turned instead to the increasing number of apothecaries, who used mortars and pestles to powder healing herbs. The mortar and pestle remain symbols of pharmacy today.

In 1673, London's apothecaries established Britain's finest medicinal herb garden, the 3.8-acre Chelsea Physic Garden. Today, it contains 5,000 species of herbs from around the world. Located 2 miles west of Picadilly Circus, it is open to the public.

Nicholas Culpeper: England's Herbal Robin Hood

Nicholas Culpeper was by far England's most influential herbalist. His *Complete Herbal and English Physician*, first published in 1652, has been in print ever since. It has appeared in more than 100 editions, a record surpassed by only the Bible and Shakespeare. A century after Culpeper's death, literary lion Dr. Samuel Johnson wrote, "Culpeper . . . undoubtedly merits the gratitude of posterity."

Culpeper was—and still is—loathed as well as loved. His herbalist contemporary, William Coles, denounced him as "a man very ignorant in simples." More than 250 years later, in *The Old English Herbals* (1922), Elinour Rohde wrote, "The infamous Nicholas Culpeper was a false prophet of herbalism . . . [author of] an absurd book." And today, scientists scoff at Culpeper's devotion to astrology.

Egotistical and brash, Culpeper came of age during the English Civil War (1642–1648), which pitted King Charles I and the monarchist aristocracy against Oliver Cromwell and the Puritan Parliament. The Puritans won, abolished the monarchy, and executed Charles.

Culpeper came from an aristocratic family, but he was a Puritan and fought for Cromwell. He took a musket ball in the chest, which left him in poor health for the rest of his life and influenced his decision to study medicine.

As an aristocrat, Culpeper attended Cambridge, where he fell in love and planned to elope. But his fiancée was killed when lightning struck her carriage on her way to their secret rendezvous. Beside himself with grief, Culpeper left Cambridge and became an apothecary's apprentice, a major social step downward for anyone who had attended the university.

Culpeper was an anomaly. Trained at Cambridge, he could read Greek and Latin as well as the physicians. He resented the snobbery of former classmates who became doctors and looked down on apothecaries. Furthermore, as a Puritan, he was outraged that the monarchist College of Physicians ignored the medical needs of the largely Puritan lower classes. Culpeper's solution was to become England's medical Robin Hood.

In 1649, Culpeper translated the College of Physicians' Latin manual, the *Pharmacopoiea Londinensis*, into English, calling it *The London Dispensatory and Physical Directory*. It gave apothecaries and others illiterate in Latin their first look at the 1,600 simples and 1,100 other formulas that constituted the state of the art in 17th-century British medicine.

Culpeper's audacity earned him the physicians' undying hatred. Apothecaries, midwives, and the common people, however, lionized him for giving them access to professional medical information.

Culpeper's apothecary shop in Spitalfields, near London, became wildly popular. He often treated the poor for free. The College of Physicians attacked him relentlessly, and in response, he became increasingly combative.

Culpeper wrote a series of essays, "The Epistles," in which he accused the physicians of greed for their high fees and stupidity for their outdated devotion to Galen and Avicenna: "[We have] a company of proud, domineering doctors whose wits were born 500 years before themselves. . . . College, College, thou art Diseased, and I will tell thee the Cause. The Cause is Mammon [greed]. The Cure: Fear God. Love the Saints. Be Studious. Hate Covetousness. Regard the Poor."

To make herbal medicine even more accessible, Culpeper published his herbal in 1652. It was revolutionary because it gave equal weight to the official herbalism of the ancient masters and the homegrown folk wisdom of England's country people.

Today, critics dismiss Culpeper because of his devotion to astrology. In his herbal, Mars owned garlic, lavender was under Mercury, and the sun claimed rosemary under the celestial Ram. But astrology was considered a legitimate science in Culpeper's day. All the universities taught it, and the College of Physicians routinely factored it into diagnosis and treatment decisions. In fact, one reason that the college hated Culpeper was that he accused them of making astrological errors.

Culpeper's real problem was that he rarely met an herb that he didn't consider a panacea. He touted dozens of herbs "to heal all inward and outward hurts." He called about a third of the herbs in his herbal sure cures for "the bites and stings of venomous creatures." He also promoted scores of herbs to "bring down women's courses" (promote menstruation), many more than midwives of that era considered abortifacient.

Perhaps Culpeper can be forgiven his exaggerations. In the 1650s, very little was known about the body, and statements that seem to be gross misrepresentations today may not have been all that far-fetched.

Physicians call most medical problems "self-limiting"—that is, if you wait long enough, they go away by themselves. Take almost any herb for "inward or outward hurts," and most clear up, with or without all the herbs Culpeper recommended. The same goes for attacks by "venomous creatures." Few bites and stings are fatal. Most eventually resolve on their own.

Unfortunately, Culpeper's promotion of every herb for every ill has haunted herbalism ever since. Some recent herbals still tout Culpeper's exaggerations as truth, providing easy—and legitimate—targets for attacks by herb skeptics.

Nicholas Culpeper was a seminal figure in botanical medicine, but his herbal should be viewed as history, not as a guide to herbal healing for the 21st century.

Dr. Withering's Wise Woman

In 1767, 26-year-old William Withering had barely begun practicing medicine in Stafford, England, when he was called to treat 17-year-old Helena Cookes. She was bedridden with a lingering illness that kept her from her favorite pastime, painting watercolors of wildflowers.

Like every other medical student, Withering had studied botany. He hated it. Still, he was quite taken with the young Miss Cookes. He gathered wildflowers for his patient to paint while in bed, and he married her 5 years later. Along the way, he developed a passion for medical botany.

"In the year 1775," he later wrote, "my opinion was asked concerning a recipe for the cure of dropsy [congestive heart failure]. I was told it had been a family secret of an old woman in Shropshire, who sometimes made cures after regular practitioners had failed." The old woman's recipe contained 20 herbs, but Withering quickly decided that the heart stimulator was foxglove. Withering began using foxglove himself and gained a reputation for treating the heart problem.

In 1776, Dr. Erasmus Darwin (Charles's grandfather) asked Withering to treat a woman with dropsy. Withering gave her foxglove, and she improved. Darwin submitted a report to a British medical journal claiming that he himself had cured the woman using foxglove. He did not mention Withering.

Furious, Withering published his *Account of the Foxglove and Its Medical Uses*, which summarized his results in 163 cases. The drug derived from foxglove, digitalis, has only recently been surpassed by other medications as a treatment for congestive heart failure.

Sickly Colonists, Robust Indians

Europeans considered Indians "ignorant savages"—except when it came to health and healing. Explorers and colonists were all too familiar with the plagues, pestilence, and suffering back in Europe. They marveled at the Indians' good health, physical stamina, and fine teeth. Not surprisingly, many became eager students of Indian herbal medicine.

Each tribe had its own medical mythology, but this Cherokee tale is typical. Long ago, humanity grew too numerous. Hunters killed so much game that the animals feared for their survival. The bears, deer, birds, and other creatures decided to unleash diseases to reduce hunting. But the plants decided that the animals had acted unfairly. The trees, shrubs, grasses, and flowers showed humanity how they could cure the diseases that the animals had unleashed.

One of the first Europeans to appreciate Indian medicine was Jacques Cartier, the French explorer who discovered Canada's St. Lawrence River. In 1536, he sailed to the site of present-day Quebec, where he and his crew dug in for the winter. Within a few months, 25 of his 100 men had died of the "sailors' disease" (scurvy), and most of the rest were gravely ill.

Scurvy was a terrible scourge during the Age of Exploration. On his famous voyage around Africa, Vasco da Gama lost 100 of his 160 crew members to it. During the 16th and 17th centuries, ships were sometimes sighted adrift on the high seas, their entire crews dead from scurvy.

Fortunately for Cartier, an Indian gave the sickly explorers a tea brewed from yellow cedar bark and leaves. Everyone recovered. Later, the tea was shown to contain vitamin C, which prevents and cures scurvy.

In Boston, Puritan minister-physician Cotton Mather (1663–1728) wrote that Indian healers produced "many cures that are truly stupendous." And when John Wesley (1703–1791), founder of Methodism, visited America in the 1730s, he wrote that the Indians had "exceedingly few" diseases and that their medicines were "quick and generally infallible."

Later, even ardent Indian haters in the U.S. Army marveled at the effectiveness of Indian wound treatments. Also, many early American physicians touted their apprenticeships to Indian herbalists.

Of course, Indian healers also had their critics, mostly among university-trained physicians. Philadelphia doctor Benjamin Rush (1745–1813), a signer of the Declaration of Independence, declared, "We have no discoveries in the materia medica . . . from the Indians. It would be a reproach to our schools of physic if modern physicians were not more successful than Indians."

How wrong Dr. Rush was. The Indians introduced white settlers to many valuable healing herbs, such as black cohosh, black haw, boneset, cascara sagrada, echinacea, chaparral, goldenseal, lobelia, Oregon grape, sarsaparilla, slippery elm, wild cherry, and witch hazel.

Healing Herbs in Early America

In their "kitchen gardens," American colonists grew both culinary and medicinal herbs, including balm, basil, caraway, chamomile, comfrey, dill, fennel, garlic, hyssop, lavender, licorice, marjoram, mints, mustard, parsley, rosemary, rue, savory, saffron, shallots, sage, tarragon, and thyme.

Thomas Jefferson was a typical herb grower. His 1,000-square-foot garden at Monticello contained 26 herbs. As president, while negotiating the Louisiana Purchase from the French, he went to great lengths to obtain some French tarragon for his garden.

Herbs were also prized imports. In addition to Chinese tea, black pepper was very popular. New England shipping magnate Elias Hasskett Derby, one of early America's first homegrown millionaires, made much of his money importing black pepper from Sumatra.

Herbs were also a major colonial export. Furs, tobacco, and cotton generated the most money, but pound for pound, nothing beat ginseng, the herb prized in Asia as the ultimate tonic.

French Jesuits began shipping Canadian ginseng to China in the early 1700s, where it brought the then-astounding price of $5 a pound. By the 1740s, news of the unassuming plant's value in the Orient spread south to the 13 colonies. Shipping agents bought it for $1 a pound, more than the wholesale value of the rarest furs. Foragers scoured the countryside, and frontier scouts, surveyors, and trappers collected ginseng as a sideline to their other work.

By the 1770s, rapacious collection had wiped out ginseng east of the Appalachians, forcing collectors into the western wilderness. The search for ginseng played a key role in the exploration of western Pennsylvania, West Virginia, Kentucky, and Tennessee. One noted ginseng collector was Daniel Boone, who, according to one account, lost 12 tons of wild ginseng when his boat capsized in the Ohio River.

The American Revolution gave the new nation not only its independence but also its first herbal, *Materia Medica Americana* (1787), by Dr. Johann David Schopf (1752–1800). Ironically, Dr. Schopf came to America in 1777 as a doctor for the Hessian mercenaries who fought for the British. After the war, he stayed long enough to compile his book on medicinal plants.

America's first resident medical botanist was Constantine S. Rafinesque (1784–1841). Born in Europe, he came to the United States as a young man and studied the herbs of the Mississippi Valley with Native American healers. In 1819, Rafinesque became a professor of botany at a college in Kentucky, where he wrote *Medical Flora* (1828).

Rafinesque coined the term *Eclectic* to describe the kind of medicine that he advocated— a combination of European, Asian, Indian, and slave herbalism. Shortly after his death, 19th-century America's most scientific herbalists decided to call themselves the Eclectics.

The Shakers: America's Premier Healing Herb Growers

Today, most Americans associate the word *Shaker* with quality furniture. Throughout the 19th century, however, the Shakers were better known for the quality of their medicinal herbs.

An English Quaker, Ann Lee, founded the sect in Manchester, England, in the early 1770s. She believed in worshiping God with singing and dancing called shaking, hence the name Shaking Quakers, then Shakers. Not surprisingly, Lee was imprisoned for a time as a witch.

In 1774, Lee and eight Shakers arrived in New York and founded their first community near Albany. The Shakers practiced strict pacifism as well as gender equality and segregation. Marriage and sex were banned. Member families were broken up. Meals were eaten in silence.

Eventually, the Shakers established 24 communities, from Maine to Indiana to Florida. Eight lasted through World War I. One still exists: Sabbathday Lake in New Gloucester, Maine.

Ann Lee's motto was "Hands to work, hearts to God." Her industrious followers launched the American medicinal herb industry in 1799, first collecting healing herbs from the wild, then growing them. The herb business prospered, and in 1824, the Sabbathday Lake community built a large herb building for drying and processing. It still stands today.

The Shakers sold their herbs through a nationally distributed catalog. The first one (1831) was headlined: "Why send to Europe's bloody shore for plants that grow by our own door?" It offered 142 herbs, roots, barks, and seeds, including angelica, basil, bayberry, belladonna, black and blue cohosh, boneset, cannabis (marijuana), catnip, chamomile, coltsfoot, comfrey, elecampane, gentian, hop, hyssop, jimson weed, juniper, lady's slipper, licorice, lobelia, marshmallow, mullein, motherwort, nux vomica, opium poppy, pennyroyal, peppermint, rosemary, saffron, senna, slippery elm, valerian, walnut, white oak, and wild cherry. The Shakers also sold a few culinary "sweet herbs": sage, marjoram, savory, and thyme.

Unlike Rome's *herbarii*, the Shakers developed a reputation for honesty and herbal purity. In 1851, Rafinesque said that they had "the best medicinal gardens in the U.S. They cultivate a great variety and sell them cheap, fresh, and genuine."

Pacifism did not prevent the Shakers from selling medicinal herbs to the Union Army during the Civil War. They supplied much of the Union's opium. After the war, the Shakers sold medicinal herbs directly to hospitals and the embryonic pharmaceutical industry.

The Shakers also invented the modern pill. Before pills, powdered herbs were sold loose in envelopes, which were inconvenient to ship. Shaker craftsmen drilled holes in simple wood frames to create the first pill molds. The herbalists poured in measured amounts of herbal powders, then hammered pegs into the holes to press the powders into pills.

When patent medicines became popular after the Civil War, the Shakers marketed several. Their biggest seller was Dr Corbett's Shaker Sarsaparilla Syrup, with sarsaparilla, dandelion, black cohosh, yellow dock, juniper, and several other herbs. The Shakers touted it for arthritis; insomnia; syphilis; anxiety; digestive and female complaints; and diseases of the blood, kidneys, liver, heart, and lungs. Two other popular items were Pain King, with opium, and Tamar Laxative, with dried prunes and senna.

The Shaker herb business died after World War II, but the Sabbathday Lake community revived it in the 1960s. The community's herb garden, herb building, and museum are open to the public.

Thomson's Botanic Medicine

Early America's leading herbalist was Samuel Thomson (1760–1843). Born in Alstead, New Hampshire, he studied with a midwife and Indian healers.

Around 1800, Thomson's daughter became seriously ill. Unsure of his skills, he called a physician, who pronounced her incurable. Then, as the story goes, Thomson cured her with herbs and hot baths. Soon after, he declared himself a "doctor."

Thomson detested the regular physicians of his day, who relied on bloodletting, violent laxatives (cathartics), and mercury. These treatments were called heroic medicine, but the heroism was entirely on the part of the patients.

Consider the case of George Washington. One day in 1799, the elderly but generally healthy father of our country developed a sore throat with a fever and chills. Chances are, he had strep throat or some other minor infection, which probably would have cleared up with rest, hot liquids, and herbal antibiotics such as garlic, onion, and goldenseal.

Instead, Washington's heroic physicians bled him of 4 pints of blood, leaving him anemic and weak. Then they gave him cathartics and mercury. He was dead within 24 hours.

Thomson developed a medical system based on herbs and hot baths, inspired by European herbalism and mineral baths and Indian herbalism and sweat lodges. His favorite herb was lobelia or Indian tobacco, which in large amounts causes vomiting, hence its names emetic herb and puke weed.

In 1809, Thomson was arrested for murder after allegedly administering a fatal dose of lobelia. He was acquitted due to a lack of evidence that lobelia was poisonous.

Samuel Thomson may not have been the nation's greatest herbalist, but he was our first medical marketing genius. In 1813, he obtained a patent for Thomson's Improved System of Botanic Practice of Medicine, which allowed him to sell his Indian-inspired herbalism nationwide while still retaining its ownership. Thomson sold "family rights" to his medical system for $20. Starting in 1822, he charged another $2 for his book, *The New Guide to Health, or the Botanic Family Physician.*

Thomson's motto was "Every man his own physician," but most of his "family rights" were purchased by women. Many of them welcomed the opportunity to add some semblance of legitimacy to the word-of-mouth herbalism that they had learned from their mothers and other women.

In 1839, at the height of his popularity, Thomson claimed 3 million adherents. This was no doubt an exaggeration, but Thomsonian herbalism was very popular. Thomson boasted that half of Ohio practiced his herbal healing. His critics said it was only one-third.

Initially, Thomsonian herbalists used 65 herbs, all available from the Shakers. Thomson soon realized that he could make more money by selling prepackaged herbal formulas. He organized his family members into Friendly Botanic Societies, cooperatives that bought his formulas and distributed them around the country. Because Thomson's formulas were part of his patented medical system, they became known as patent medicines.

As time passed, patent medicines became a major industry. Some were quality products, but many were worthless concoctions of alcohol, opium, and cocaine that were sold by hucksters whose outrageous claims eventually spurred Congress to create the Food and Drug Administration (FDA).

After Thomson's death in 1843, his medical system fell from fashion. Some practitioners preserved it. One was Dr. John Kellogg of Battle Creek, Michigan, who invented the nation's first health food, the cornflake, and founded Kellogg's cereal company. For the most part, though, Thomsonian medicine was replaced by homeopathy and Eclectic herbalism.

Homeopathy: Herbal Microdoses

From 1830 through World War I, the main competition for regular American physicians came from homeopathy, the herbally inclined medical system created by a disillusioned German physician, Dr. Samuel Hahnemann (1755–1843). Trained in heroic medicine, Dr. Hahnemann decided that bloodletting, cathartics, and mercury did more harm than good.

Dr. Hahnemann did not reject all heroic treatments. On the contrary, he was impressed with several. One was cinchona bark, the antimalarial. Another was the cowpox inoculation, initiated by Edward Jenner in 1796. It was the first effective preventive for another age-old scourge, smallpox.

In healthy people, both of these treatments produce low-level symptoms of the diseases that they are used to prevent. Dr, Hahnemann called the phenomenon homeopathy, from the Greek for "treatment by similars."

Dr. Hahnemann tested hundreds of herbs and other substances on himself, carefully cataloging their effects. Eventually, he began using them to treat illnesses with similar symptoms. He enjoyed considerable success, and his approach was less drastic than heroic medicine's. Not surprisingly, he attracted a large following.

Homeopathy came to the United States in the 1830s. It quickly won many supporters who were fed up with heroic medicine, including Mark Twain, Daniel Webster, and John D. Rockefeller. Homeopaths popularized several drugs that are used today, including ergot derivatives for migraines and nitroglycerin for the chest pain of angina.

By the early 20th century, however, homeopathy fell from U.S. medical fashion. One reason was the decline of heroic medicine. As regular physicians stopped opening veins and using mercury, their critics had less to criticize. Another reason was the unrelenting hostility of the American Medical Association (AMA). Around 1900, an estimated 25 percent of regular physicians also prescribed some homeopathic medicines. The AMA decreed that any physician caught using homeopathy would be drummed out of the organization.

The major reason for homeopathy's decline, though, was the Law of Potentization, Dr. Hahnemann's assertion that his medicines grew stronger as they became more dilute. The Law of Potentization violated Paracelsus's dose-response relationship, now a cornerstone of pharmacology. Critics charge that some medicines considered "extremely powerful" by homeopaths are so dilute that they don't contain a single molecule of the active ingredient.

As a result, American scientists dismissed homeopathy—and its largely herbal medicines—as nonsense. The practice just about died out in this country.

Homeopaths can't explain the Law of Potentization, but they insist that more than 150 years of clinical experience show that it works. They have a point. In recent years, rigorous scientific trials have found that homeopathic medicines (most of them herbal) help to treat colds, flu, hay fever, asthma, fibromyalgia, mosquito bites, rheumatoid arthritis, and infectious diarrhea.

In 1991, nonhomeopathic Dutch epidemiologists at the University of Maastricht published an analysis of 105 studies of homeopathic medicines from 1966 to 1990, most taken from French and German medical journals not usually translated into English. Of the 105 studies, 81 showed positive benefits from homeopathic treatment, while 24 showed no benefit. Some of the studies involved few subjects, however, and most were not double-blind, meaning that researcher bias may have played a role in the results.

Because of those possibilities, the Dutch investigators selected the 21 most scientifically rigorous studies and analyzed the results. Fifteen (71 percent) showed significant benefits from homeopathic treatment. While many questions remain about how homeopathy works, the researchers concluded that "the evidence presented in this review would probably be sufficient for establishing homeopathy as a regular treatment for certain conditions."

Since its founding, homeopathy has been popular in Europe. Today, the physician to the British royal family is a homeopath. Surveys show that many British, French, and German M.D.'s prescribe some homeopathic medicines in their practices.

During the last 25 years, America has witnessed a modest homeopathic renaissance. Today, about 9 percent of U.S. doctors—some 5,000 M.D.'s—incorporate homeopathic medicines into their practices. Several thousand other health professionals, including dentists, podiatrists, veterinarians, nurses, and chiropractors, use homeopathy as well.

A 1990 study by Harvard researchers suggested that more than 2.5 million Americans have tried homeopathy. Sales of homeopathic medicines now total more than $250 million a year, thanks in part to the fact that they are carried by major drugstore chains. What's more, several celebrities—including singer Tina Turner, hairstylist Vidal Sassoon, musicians Yehudi Menuhin and Dizzy Gillespie, and actors Jane Fonda, Cher, Angelica Huston, and Elizabeth Taylor— have gone public with their support for homeopathy.

The Eclectics: America's Scientific Herbalists

Despite the regular physicians' reliance on bloodletting, cathartics, and mercury, most 19th-century medicines were herbal. In 1820, two-thirds of the treatments in the *U.S. Pharmacopoeia* were botanical. In 1880, the figure was almost three-quarters.

In the 1820s, a group of anti-heroic practitioners—Thomsonians, Indian-trained herbalists, and disillusioned regulars—created the Reformed Medical Society to promote non-heroic, largely herbal healing. In 1830, the society met in New York to found a Reformed medical school. The reformers were mostly Easterners, but the East's cities were strongholds of regular medicine.

The Reformers decided to locate their school on the free-thinking western frontier, then located at the Mississippi River. Thomsonian medicine was very popular in Ohio, so the reformers established their school in Cincinnati. They adopted Rafinesque's term *Eclectic* to describe their herb-based approach, which combined European, Asian, Indian, and slave herbalism. They called their school the Eclectic Medical Institute.

The institute was the nation's first medical school to admit women, many of whom were Thomsonian herbalists interested in more training. In 1877, however, the Eclectics "yielded to the prejudices of the profession," according to Eclectic historian Henry Felter, and barred women.

The Eclectics were scientific herbalists. They experimented with herbs, performing chemical analyses and extracting active constituents. They published their findings in the scientific journals of the day and were prominent in the early pharmaceutical industry.

The two most important Eclectics were John King and John Uri Lloyd, both of whom taught at the medical institute. King (1813–1893) was a botanical pharmacologist who introduced physicians to podophyllin, a plant resin that's still used today to treat warts. In 1855, he published the first edition of his *King's American Dispensatory*, 19th-century America's most comprehensive scientific herbal. The posthumous 18th edition (1898) remains in print today.

Lloyd (1849–1936) began his career at age 14 as a Cincinnati pharmacist's apprentice. He loved pharmacy so much that he brought his brothers, Nelson Ashley Lloyd (1851–1925) and Curtis Gates Lloyd (1859–1926), into the field. Eventually, they established Lloyd Brothers Pharmacists, Inc.

John Lloyd specialized in plant chemistry and developed most of the company's products. He was also one of the first presidents of the American Pharmaceutical Association (1887–1888). In his spare time, he wrote eight novels.

Nelson Lloyd managed the business side of Lloyd Brothers. His other love was baseball. He owned the Cincinnati team that eventually became the Reds, and later, he invested in the New York Giants.

Curtis Lloyd specialized in mushrooms. He also managed the brothers' large collection of botany books.

By 1864, the collection had outgrown the brothers' homes, so they established the Lloyd Library. Today, the library houses the world's largest private collection of botanical information: 300,000 books and pamphlets as well as 500 journals. For years, the Lloyd Library also published a botanical journal, *Lloydia*, now called the *Journal of Natural Products*. The Lloyd Library in Cincinnati is open to the public.

The years 1880 to 1900 marked the heyday of Eclectic medicine. Its practitioners numbered about 8,000. But Eclectic popularity declined in the 20th century, as herbal medicines were largely replaced by pharmaceutical drugs. The medical institute graduated its last class in 1939, and Eclectic medicine's scientific herbalism almost died.

Almost, but not quite. A handful of Eclectic-inspired naturopaths hung on, particularly in the Pacific Northwest. Among them was John Bastyr, N.D. (1912–1995), of Seattle. He was affiliated with the National College of Naturopathic Medicine in Portland, Oregon, the sole surviving naturopathic medical school.

In 1978, a group of Bastyr's former students founded the John Bastyr College of Naturopathic Medicine in Seattle, now Bastyr University in nearby Kenmore. Since then, three other naturopathic medical schools have been established: the Southwest College of Naturopathic Medicine in Scottsdale, Arizona; the College of Naturopathic Medicine at the University of Bridgeport, Connecticut; and the Canadian College of Naturopathic Medicine in Etobicoke, Ontario.

Naturopaths are currently licensed to practice in 11 states (Alaska, Arizona, Connecticut, Hawaii, Maine, Montana, New Hampshire, Oregon, Utah, Vermont, and Washington) and five Canadian provinces (Alberta, British Columbia, Manitoba, Ontario, and Saskatchewan). Elsewhere, naturopaths practice under other medical credentials, typically as acupuncturists, chiropractors, or clinical nutritionists.

To be admitted to Bastyr University, students must complete standard, college-level premedical requirements. The first 2 years at Bastyr combine a mainstream medical education—courses in anatomy, physiology, human dissection, biochemistry, pathology, microbiology, pharmacology, public health, and physical examination and diagnosis—with courses on naturopathic philosophy, clinical nutrition, homeopathy, and Western, Chinese, and Ayurvedic herbal medicine.

Third- and fourth-year students apprentice with mentor naturopaths, often at Bastyr's clinic in Seattle, which treats more than 25,000 patients a year. At first glance, the clinic looks like a mainstream medical facility. Closer examination reveals that its large in-house pharmacy stocks very few pharmaceuticals and mostly herbal preparations, homeopathic medicines, and nutritional supplements.

Recently, the King County Council, which governs Seattle, awarded a landmark contract to Bastyr to open a similar facility for indigent local residents. It will be the nation's first publicly funded naturopathic clinic.

The Collapse of Professional Herbal Medicine

In 1805, a German chemist extracted the first drug from an herbal source, morphine from the opium poppy. In 1820, another German chemist achieved another first, the synthesis of an organic compound (urea) from inorganic chemicals. Modern pharmacology was born.

Early pharmacologists developed drugs largely by modifying chemicals extracted from medicinal plants. In addition to morphine, they isolated aspirin from willow bark, quinine from cinchona, caffeine from coffee, menthol from peppermint, and ephedrine (a decongestant) from Chinese ephedra, among many others.

After the Civil War, aspiring American doctors had two basic choices for medical education: apprenticeship to practicing physicians or training at medical schools in the United States or Germany. Compared with the programs in the United States, a German medical education was more scientific and rigorous and took longer, and the medical schools were affiliated with hospitals, where intensive clinical training took place.

German-trained American doctors were harsh critics of U.S. medical education. They urged medical schools to reorganize along German lines. Harvard was one of the first to do so (in 1870), after university president Charles Eliot wrote, "The ignorance and incompetency of the average graduate of American medical schools . . . is horrible to contemplate."

In 1873, a $7 million bequest led to the creation of a German-style medical school and hospital in Baltimore, Johns Hopkins University. When it opened in 1893, Johns Hopkins took the unprecedented step of refusing to admit medical students without college degrees. Harvard quickly followed in making medical training a graduate program.

Other medical schools adopted the Har-

vard–Johns Hopkins model. They dropped botany in favor of pharmacology. Heroic measures fell from fashion, but so did herbal preparations, replaced by the drugs of the new pharmaceutical industry.

Laboratories and teaching hospitals were costly, so financing became critical. Harvard, Johns Hopkins, and other well-endowed medical schools spent enormous sums on their facilities. More modestly endowed homeopathic and Eclectic schools could not keep up. As a result, students trained under the Harvard–Johns Hopkins model were considered better doctors, and state licensing boards began requiring the Harvard–Johns Hopkins curriculum. The other medical schools began to close.

Then the influential Carnegie Foundation commissioned Abraham Flexner to survey the quality of the nation's medical schools. His report, released in 1910, praised the Harvard–Johns Hopkins model and condemned all others. Carnegie and other wealthy foundations supported the Harvard–Johns Hopkins-type schools and no others.

By 1940, every surviving U.S. medical school offered only graduate training on the Harvard–Johns Hopkins model. None provided training in herbal healing.

Hoxsey's Herbal Cancer Treatment

The period from 1920 though the 1960s might be called the lost decades of American herbal healing. U.S. medical schools ignored herbs. Pharmaceutical pills and capsules replaced tinctures in the nation's pharmacies. Even many culinary herbs fell from popularity.

Nevertheless, herbal healing didn't die. It

simply reverted to what it had been for most of its history: folk medicine practiced mostly by women who grew and gathered their own herbs and prescribed them as the classic herbals recommended.

A few diehards continued to promote herbal healing. Dr. Benedict Lust (1869–1945), the father of modern naturopathy, came to the United States from Germany in 1895. He opened the nation's first health food store and established sanitariums in New Jersey and Florida based on healing baths and herbal medicines. His nephew, John Lust, wrote an influential herbal, *The Herb Book.*

Jethro Kloss (1863–1946), a sanitarium manager and health food pioneer, published *Back to Eden* in 1939. Subtitled "A Story of the Restoration to be Found in Herb, Root, and Bark," the book has been in print ever since.

In his youth, John Christopher (1909–1983) used herbs to cure himself of rheumatoid arthritis. During the 1940s and 1950s, his herb formulas resulted in his arrest many times for "practicing medicine without a license."

In England, C. F. (Hilda) Leyel (?–1957) almost single-handedly revived British herbalism when she opened the first of her Culpeper shops in 1927. In 1940, she successfully lobbied Parliament not to repeat Henry VIII's mistake of outlawing herbal medicine.

The most flamboyant and controversial herbalist of the mid-20th century, however, was Harry Hoxsey (1901–1974), who loudly proclaimed that his herbal formula cured cancer. A former Appalachian coal miner, Hoxsey graduated from high school with a correspondence diploma and had no formal medical training. He attributed his Hoxsey Cancer Formula to his great-grandfather, who, he claimed, had witnessed a cancer-stricken horse's recovery after eating a combination of herbs.

Hoxsey started selling the family formula in the 1930s. By the 1950s, his Dallas clinic was the world's largest privately owned cancer center, with branches in 17 states.

Hoxsey's claims outraged Texas medical authorities, and a Dallas prosecutor arrested him for fraud more than 100 times in the 1930s. The Hoxsey formula didn't work for everyone, but the prosecutor could not find any patients who felt that they had been defrauded. What's more, Hoxsey presented hundreds who swore that his formula had cured their cancers.

The Texas courts ruled in favor of the cancer maverick. Then the prosecutor's brother developed cancer and secretly took the Hoxsey formula. When he recovered, Hoxsey's former prosecutor became his devoted defense attorney.

Hoxsey was also attacked by the AMA. He fought back in court and—after AMA officials conceded that the Hoxsey Formula had merit as a treatment for skin cancer—was the first person ever to win a libel suit against the organization. The FDA eventually closed Hoxsey's clinics for violating federal drug-labeling regulations. His herbal ingredients were not FDA-approved cancer treatments.

Ironically, Hoxsey died of prostate cancer. He took his formula, but it didn't work for him.

The Hoxsey formula is available today at the Bio-Medical Center in Tijuana, Mexico. Studies have found that nine of the formula's herbal ingredients have anti-tumor action: barberry, buckthorn, burdock, cascara sagrada, red clover, licorice, poke, prickly ash, and bloodroot. ✳

The Herbal Renaissance

Starting in the late 1960s, many Americans began changing their attitudes about health and healing. They decided to invest their energy in preventing illness rather than in treating it after the fact.

One step in that direction was a retreat from salt as the nation's main seasoning because of research linking it to high blood pressure, heart disease, and stroke. Many Americans retired their salt shakers and began rediscovering culinary herbs and spices. Many also rediscovered the therapeutic benefits of these plants. By the late 1990s, medicinal herb sales reached more than $3 billion a year. The booming interest in herbal healing has involved the convergence of several trends.

Growing interest in self-care. Mainstream medicine has produced miracles, but it has also become impersonal and often prohibitively expensive. To save time and money and limit their dependence on doctors, many Americans have turned to prevention and self-care. Healing herbs fit neatly into lifestyles focused on sound nutrition, fitness, and stress management.

Expanding enthusiasm for the alternative healing arts. Homeopathy, naturopathy, and Chinese and Ayurvedic medicine have become increasingly popular in recent years. These healing arts make extensive use of herbal medicines.

Backlash against advanced technology. The very wizardry of high technology creates a yearning for more down-to-earth approaches to human problems. When there's a choice, many Americans prefer healing herbs to the pharmaceuticals often derived from them.

Greater environmental awareness. As destruction of tropical rainforests has become a worldwide political issue, interest has grown in rainforest plants, some of which are herbal medicines and many of which have not been screened for potential medicinal uses. The National Cancer Institute and government agencies around the world have launched testing programs, hoping to identify the therapeutic properties of these plants and others threatened with habitat destruction.

Advocacy by the United Nations. A 1974 World Health Organization report concluded that adequate worldwide health care could not be achieved unless nonindustrialized nations were encouraged to nurture traditional herbal healing. Since then, the United Nations has encouraged the use of traditional medicine alongside Western medicine.

Increasing mainstream medical acceptance. From the 1960s through the 1980s, no mainstream medical schools taught courses on alternative medicine. Today, about 80 do, including Harvard, Johns Hopkins, and Stanford.

Until the 1990s, the only coverage given to herbal medicine by mainstream medical journals was warnings—often overblown—about the alleged dire risks of using herbs. Today, leading journals—including the *Journal of the American Medical Association*, the *New England Journal of Medicine*, and the *British Medical Journal*—publish articles demonstrating the benefits of healing herbs.

What's more, mainstream doctors have become increasingly willing to recommend herbs for some conditions. Some suggest echinacea for colds, ginger for motion sickness, and St. John's wort for depression.

The FDA vs. Healing Herbs

Unfortunately, the federal agency that regulates medicinal herbs, the FDA, has been very slow to embrace the herbal renaissance. Critics of herbs are quick to cry "hucksterism" when herb marketers sell their products as dietary supplements with vague labeling. This sorry state of affairs is a direct result of current (2000) FDA regulations.

Back in the 19th century, patent medicines laced with alcohol, cocaine, and even heroin raised cries for national drug regulation. But it took *The Jungle*, Upton Sinclair's exposé of the meat-packing industry, to finally convince Congress to prohibit the adulteration and mislabeling of foods and drugs.

Congress established the FDA in 1928, but the agency had little authority. Then in 1937, an antibiotic, elixir of sulfanilamide, killed 107 people because it contained a toxic ingredient. The following year, Congress passed the Food, Drug, and Cosmetic Act, which led to the first U.S. drug regulations.

The FDA remained pretty lax about enforcement until 1959. That's when about 8,000 European babies were born with terrible birth defects because their mothers had taken Thalidomide, an over-the-counter sedative, while pregnant. Three years later, spurred by the Thalidomide scandal, Congress directed the FDA to tighten its drug safety standards.

The agency declared that pharmaceutical companies had to demonstrate their drugs' safety and effectiveness in elaborate studies. The tests required by the agency were very expensive—millions of dollars per drug in the 1960s and, by some estimates, hundreds of millions today. The original FDA ruling made no distinction between new drugs and drugs already on the market.

The makers of over-the-counter (OTC) pharmaceuticals screamed that the FDA had no right to require costly testing of drugs that had been used safely for years. As a compromise, the agency appointed panels of physicians, pharmacists, and pharmacologists to review the safety and effectiveness of OTC ingredients. These panels wrote reports, called monographs, that would serve as the basis for grandfathering approval of drugs determined to be safe and effective. The FDA began appointing OTC Review Panels in 1972. The final monographs were completed by 1985.

When the OTC review process began, more than 100 herbal medicines were listed as safe and effective in the *U.S. Pharmacopoeia*, a standard drug reference. They deserved to be approved as OTC medicines. Unfortunately, the OTC Review Panels did not undertake a comprehensive review of the medical literature. The only information examined by the panels was what OTC manufacturers submitted in support of products that they wanted to keep on pharmacy shelves.

By the end of the review process, hundreds of medicines had been incorporated into the OTC monographs, including about two dozen herbs. Among these were the active ingredients in most OTC laxatives (senna, psyllium seed, and cascara sagrada), and a few decongestants (peppermint oil, eucalyptus oil, and two ingredients derived from Chinese ephedra).

The approved herbs represented only a tiny fraction of the hundreds of botanical medicines that had extensive historical and clinical evidence of safety and efficacy. For example, before World War II, U.S. pharmacies carried several valerian-based sleep aids. By the time of the

OTC review process, the drug companies had dropped valerian in favor of sedative antihistamines such as diphenhydramine (Benadryl). As a result, no valerian products were presented to the OTC Review Panel, and none were approved. Dozens of other herbs were also ignored by the panels.

Why didn't medicinal herb companies present their products to the OTC Review Panels? There were several reasons:

• During the 1970s and early 1980s, botanical medicine was just beginning to come back from its lowest ebb in U.S. history. The few herb companies in existence were, by and large, mom-and-pop enterprises run by herbalists whose marketing efforts consisted mainly of brewing medicinal teas for friends and selling them at local health food stores. Many of these entrepreneurs had no idea that the OTC review process was even taking place, let alone how to participate. When they found out, it was too late.

• At the time, many herbalists felt uncomfortable with the word *drug*. During the 1970s, most herbalists saw their products as foods, not drugs, despite the fact that their teas and tinctures were used for pharmacological, not nutritive, purposes. A few herbalists tried to organize participation in the OTC review process, but their efforts largely fell on deaf ears.

• Finally, to herbalists, the OTC Review Panels did not look sympathetic. They were composed of mainstream health professionals who were largely unfamiliar with herbs. Except for the few herbs that were approved, the OTC Review Panels basically ignored medicinal plants.

Once the OTC review process was completed in 1985, it was closed. Any drug or herb that was not already approved had to undergo the expensive and time-consuming tests that the FDA required of new drugs.

When a new drug wins approval, the company that owns it gets a patent, the exclusive right to market that medication for many years and recoup its investment. But who's going to spend millions to prove, for example, that garlic lowers cholesterol or that valerian is an effective sleep aid? These claims are true, demonstrated in many well-designed studies, but since no herb company can patent garlic or valerian, there's no way to recoup the huge investment in the approval process.

FDA regulations have left healing herbs in limbo. Many herbs have been used for thousands of years, but to be approved as drugs, they must be tested as though they were brand-new compounds. This makes no sense economically because they can't be patented. Thus, the vast majority of medicinal herbs are sold as dietary supplements, a designation several rungs down the regulatory ladder.

The catch is that dietary supplements cannot make medicinal claims. That's why product labels are vague about the herbs' effects.

In 1994, Congress passed the Dietary Supplement Health and Education Act (DSHEA), which directed the FDA to consider petitions that would allow herbs (and vitamin and mineral supplements) to make medicinal claims. To date, a few claims have been approved, notably that soy protein helps lower cholesterol. But the FDA has declined many requests by people in the herb industry to reopen the OTC review process to accommodate healing herbs.

That's what Germany has done. Herbal medicine is considerably more mainstream there than in the United States. Like our own

FDA, the German government requires pre-approval safety and efficacy testing for all newly synthesized pharmaceuticals. However, it does not hold herbs, which the Germans call traditional medicines, to quite so high a standard.

In 1978, the counterpart of the FDA in the former West Germany convened an expert panel, Commission E, to study the extensive scientific literature for about 650 herbs. In a process quite similar to the FDA's earlier OTC review, the commission published monographs declaring several hundred herbs safe and effective for dozens of ailments. The commission also recommended dosages and warned of possible side effects.

German herb companies are allowed to make medicinal claims in line with the Commission E monographs as long as they market unadulterated, properly labeled herbs and adhere to the commission's dose recommendations. Currently, Commission E monographs stand as the world's most authoritative government-sponsored, expert-developed information on medicinal herbs' benefits, dosages, and side effects.

In this country, the National Institutes of Health's Office of Complementary and Alternative Medicine (OCAM) recently sponsored meetings between officials of the FDA and advocates of herbal medicine. The dialogue focused on the possibility of reopening the OTC review process with an American panel similar to Commission E. Some FDA officials support the idea, but at this time, the agency has taken no action.

It would clearly serve the public interest for the FDA to embrace an herbal medicine regulatory model similar to Commission E. According to a national survey conducted for *Prevention* magazine, during 1998 and 1999, 49 percent of American adults used an herbal medicine. Another 24 percent called themselves regular users.

Without clear labeling to specify benefits, side effects, and recommended dosage—labeling that the FDA currently prohibits for most medicinal herbs—many Americans remain confused about how best to use herbal remedies. This consumer information is essential as herbs become increasingly popular in the 21st century.

CHAPTER 2

Tempest in a Teapot

ARE HEALING HERBS SAFE?

Before you take anyone's advice about using medicinal herbs, ask the person, "Are healing herbs safe?" If the answer is a blanket "Yes," you'd best go to someone else for information.

The fact is, some of the most potent poisons known to humanity are herbal. One example is poison hemlock, which looks just like wild parsley. This is why you should never, ever pick parsley in the wild. Another example is the amanita mushroom (also called the death cap), which is why you should never, ever forage for mushrooms in the wild unless you're certain that you can identify them correctly.

So are herbal medicines safe? Here's the correct answer: Most popular medicinal herbs, including all the herbs discussed in this book, are reasonably safe for most people most of the time when taken in recommended amounts. But medicinal herbs contain pharmacologically active compounds that have drug effects on the body, and all drugs have the potential to cause

harm—allergic reactions, side effects, possible fetal injury, and interactions with other herbs and drugs.

Overall, herbs are safer than pharmaceuticals, but they can still cause harm, and anyone who uses them should do so cautiously and responsibly.

Herbs in the Headlines

A number of news reports about herb hazards have generated headlines.

• In February 2000, the British medical journal *Lancet* published a report by National Institutes of Health researchers advising people who are HIV-positive not to take the popular herbal antidepressant St. John's wort if they are also using protease inhibitors, currently the most beneficial AIDS medications. The herb reduces blood levels of protease inhibitors and may compromise the drugs' effectiveness.

• In the same issue of *Lancet*, Swiss scientists warned that people with transplanted organs who take the standard antirejection drug cyclosporine should also avoid St. John's wort. The herb can interfere with cyclosporine, just as it may with protease inhibitors.

• Also in 2000, surgeons raised a red flag about garlic, which has potent antibiotic and cholesterol-lowering effects when taken in medicinal amounts. Garlic is also a natural anticoagulant, meaning that it interferes with blood clotting. For people at risk for heart attack, this can be a benefit because garlic helps prevent the blood clots that trigger heart attacks. If taken within a week or so before surgery, however, garlic can contribute to bleeding complications. The surgeons exhorted garlic users to discontinue use of the herb 2 weeks before having elective surgery.

• Chinese ephedra (ma huang) has also been tarred as dangerous. In the low doses that responsible herbalists recommend, ma huang opens the bronchial passages, helping to treat asthma as well as congestion caused by colds and flu. But Chinese ephedra is also a powerful stimulant that some people have taken in enormous overdoses to obtain an amphetamine-like high. At such doses, the herb can cause heart problems and even death. The FDA estimates that between 1993 and 2000, up to 30 young, healthy thrill seekers died from ephedra overdoses.

• Or how about senna, the herbal laxative? The FDA has documented abdominal cramps, bloody stool, and even potentially serious electrolyte imbalances from regular use of unusually high doses of senna.

There's no question about it: Herbal medicines can cause problems. That's why this book contains extensive information on safety and side effects for every herb discussed. By any measure of drug safety, however, pharmaceuticals cause much more harm.

Around the same time that the above reports of problems with medicinal herbs were published, the following reports about pharmaceuticals also appeared.

• According to a study in the February 2, 2000, issue of the *Journal of the American Medical Association*, the erectile dysfunction pill sildenafil (Viagra) contributed to the deaths of 564 men from the time it was introduced in early 1998 through mid-1999. When taken at the same time as nitrate medications—notably nitroglycerin, a treatment for angina—Viagra can cause a sudden, potentially fatal drop in blood pressure. At this time, the FDA has not pulled Viagra from pharmacy shelves, but it has required a new warning label cautioning against using it while taking nitrate drugs.

• In March 2000, the FDA ordered the withdrawal of the heartburn medication cisapride (Propulsid) because it had been linked to 80 deaths.

• In March 1999, the diabetes medication troglitazone (Rezulin) was withdrawn because it had been linked to an estimated 400 cases of liver failure, including 28 documented deaths and 7 cases where liver transplants were necessary.

• According to a report from the American Association of Poison Control Centers, pain relievers, cough and cold preparations, antibiotics, sedatives, and antidepressants accounted for more than 480,000 poisonings (both accidental overdoses and intentional suicide attempts) in 1996. Among the substances listed in each category, *none* were medicinal herbs. In fact, the most hazardous plants turned out to be houseplants, because infants and toddlers sometimes munched on them and became ill.

• For a report published in the April 15, 1998, edition of the *Journal of the American Medical Association*, researchers at the University of Toronto combed through 30 years of medical literature for reports of drug side effects among hospital patients. Extrapolating from the most scientifically rigorous 39 studies, the researchers estimated that drug side effects kill an astonishing 106,000 U.S. hospital patients a year and cause 2.2 million serious but nonfatal medical problems. In other words, adverse reactions to pharmaceuticals rank as this country's fourth leading cause of death, accounting for more fatalities than AIDS, suicide, and homicide combined. These side effects did not result from medical errors. They occurred when drugs were administered in accordance with FDA dosage guidelines.

Clearly, pharmaceuticals have safety issues of their own. But which are more hazardous, pharmaceuticals or herbal medicines? Conventional medications win that contest hands down.

Even the regrettable death toll from the allegedly most hazardous herb, Chinese ephedra, is dwarfed by the problems caused by the pharmaceuticals mentioned above. What's more, a July 1999 report by the General Accounting Office, the investigative arm of Congress, called the FDA's Chinese ephedra statistics "questionable." It's possible that the herb has not caused as many problems as the FDA alleged.

Of course, many more Americans take drugs than use herbs. From a cost-benefit per-

spective, it's reasonable to prescribe potentially hazardous drugs to treat serious conditions. The point here is not to condemn pharmaceuticals but rather to point out that despite a few problems, herbal medicines are not major public health hazards.

A Double Standard

Herbal medicines are the unfortunate victims of a double standard. Doctors and the public generally believe that pharmaceuticals are more trustworthy than herbs because the former are more tightly regulated by the FDA (regulatory issues are discussed in chapter 1). In many cases, though, the FDA's supposedly tight pharmaceutical regulations deliver little more than the illusion of safety. The situations with cisapride and troglitazone are good examples of that.

The FDA requires pharmaceutical companies to conduct clinical trials to demonstrate the safety and effectiveness of new drugs, but most of these trials involve only a few thousand people. What about side effects that affect only 1 person in 10,000 or 50,000 or 1 million? They don't show up until the drug has become widely used.

Post-approval discoveries of potentially serious side effects are not limited to just cisapride and troglitazone. Within 5 years of approval, an estimated 50 percent of pharmaceuticals have their labels revised to include side effects— some potentially serious—that were discovered after the drugs were released.

Herbal medicines may not be as tightly regulated as pharmaceuticals, but they usually have much longer histories of use: decades, centuries, even millennia. They have withstood the test of time. Every now and then, an age-old herb turns out to pose a new hazard: The potentially liver-damaging pyrrolizidine alkaloids in comfrey are one example. But such findings are rare compared with the unanticipated side effects that come to light in recently approved pharmaceuticals.

Another aspect of the double standard surrounding herbal safety has to do with the mass media. Because herbal medicines are less familiar than pharmaceuticals to the vast majority of experts to whom the media turn for health information, these authorities tend to be anxious about herb safety and overstate herb hazards. Because these same authorities are much more familiar with pharmaceuticals, however, they tend to understate drug hazards.

That's why reports of relatively minor herb hazards tend to generate big headlines and persist in the media. By comparison, reports of drug hazards—for example, the fact that pharmaceuticals are the nation's fourth leading cause of death—make headlines for a day and then are largely forgotten.

Of course, as more people with a greater variety of medical conditions begin using healing herbs, especially in combination with pharmaceuticals, some new problems are bound to turn up. The interactions between St. John's wort and protease inhibitors and cyclosporine are good examples. Herbs should always be used cautiously, especially by people who are taking other medications for chronic conditions. By and large, however, herbal medicines are gentler and safer than pharmaceuticals.

The Issue of Dose Control

Some critics of herbal medicine contend that herbs are hazardous because typical preparation directions—1 to 2 teaspoons of dried herb per cup of boiling water, steeped for 10 to 20 minutes—yield infusions with highly variable doses of the medicinally active compounds. In contrast, when people take pharmaceuticals, they know precisely how much of the active ingredients they're getting.

The critics have a point. Herb potency depends on plant genetics, growing conditions, maturity at harvest, time in storage, the possibility of adulteration, and preparation method. A cup of instant coffee contains about 65 milligrams of caffeine. Cappuccino drinks may contain more than 300.

On the other hand, you need look no further than the statistics on suicide to know that precise dose control is no guarantee that pharmaceuticals will be used safely. In addition, drug effects depend on body weight. A standard dose of a pharmaceutical taken by a person who weighs 120 pounds has a greater effect than the same dose ingested by someone who weighs 200 pounds. Finally, individuals vary. Different people often have very different reactions to the same drugs.

How do you react to drugs? For headache, the standard adult aspirin dose is two tablets every 4 hours. Through experience, some people learn that one tablet provides sufficient relief, while others must take three.

In general, healing herbs cause fewer side effects than pharmaceuticals. Pharmaceuticals tend to be highly concentrated, and pills and capsules have little taste, factors that make taking an overdose easier. The active constituents in herbs are typically less concentrated, and most herbs taste bitter, both of which are qualities that help discourage overdose. Nonetheless, anyone who uses healing herbs must strive for good dose control.

The doses recommended in this book represent a consensus of the opinions found in both traditional herbals and scientific references. In the few cases where sources disagreed significantly, this book recommends the smaller amount, in the belief that it's best to err on the side of caution.

These days, an increasing number of herbal medicines are available as standardized extracts. This means that the plants were grown from seeds or clones known to produce a certain concentration of the pharmacologically active compounds. Then the plants were harvested, stored, and prepared under controlled conditions to produce dose uniformity.

Standardized extracts are not quite as dose-controlled as laboratory-synthesized pharmaceuticals, but they're considerably more dose-controlled than bulk herbs. When you buy commercial preparations, be sure to choose standardized extracts whenever possible.

How to Use Herbs Safely

Fortunately, you don't need to be a master herbalist or an M.D. or Ph.D. to use herbal medicines safely. All you need is a little information.

Before you take any herb, read up on it. Don't just listen to friends and neighbors. Each herb profile in this book contains extensive information on safety and side effects. Take any warnings seriously. When in doubt about the appropriateness of any herb for your particular medical condition or medical history, don't use it.

Don't take herb identity for granted. Look for products that identify herbs by their Latin binomial names—that is, genus and species. For example, garlic's binomial name is *Allium sativum*.

Stick with the recommended dosage, and never exceed it. Some people assume that if a little herb is good, more must be better. Wrong. Herbal dosage recommendations are based on scientific research and, often, centuries of clinical experience. Don't put yourself at risk by taking more than is suggested. As a general rule, whenever you use a commercial preparation (such as tea, a tincture, pills, or capsules), follow the label directions carefully.

Respect your individuality. Individuals vary. You may be allergic to one or more herbs or develop other unusual reactions. When you take herbal medicines, stay alert for adverse reactions such as abdominal upset, diarrhea, headache, itching, rash—anything out of the ordinary. If you notice any unusual symptoms that appear to be linked to the medicinal herb, stop taking it and discuss your reaction(s) with your doctor.

Who is most sensitive to healing herbs? Generally, people who have hay fever, those with illnesses often linked to allergies (such as asthma and eczema), and those who have had hives or experienced a serious allergic reaction called anaphylaxis.

It's extremely unlikely that medicinal herbs will cause anaphylaxis, but it's still remotely possible. The main symptom is difficulty breathing. If you develop any trouble breathing, call your emergency medical number immediately and tell the operator that you're having suspected anaphylaxis. Then give your address and phone number and do what the operator says. Paramedics should respond, as anaphylaxis can be fatal.

Be aware of your reactions. Even if you're not allergic, you may still be unusually sensitive to one or more medicinal herbs. Doctors refer to this as an idiopathic reaction. In medical lingo, *idiopathic* means "for unknown reasons"—in other words, just one of those things. Out of the blue, you may react badly to an herb that's generally considered safe. It happens.

Pay attention to your body. If things go awry and you suspect that an herb is to blame, stop taking it and consult your physician.

If you're over age 65, start with a low dose. As people grow older, they become more sensitive to drug effects, so a low dose might suffice. In addition, older people often take other medications. Starting with a low dose of medicinal herbs reduces the risk of adverse herb-drug interactions. You can always increase the dose later.

If you're pregnant or nursing, use herbs with caution. With a few exceptions, such as raspberry, women who are pregnant or nursing should not take medicinal amounts of healing herbs. Herbs that cause no problems for adults may harm the unborn and newborns. Moms-to-be and nursing moms who wish to try any herbal medicine should do so only with the consent and supervision of their professional health care providers.

Don't give healing herbs to children under age 2. While some herbalists contend that herbal medicines are okay for children 6 months and older, this book takes a more conservative position. As gentle as most herbs are, they're not appropriate for the very young. The few exceptions include cinnamon, chamomile, cranberry, dill water, and ginger—and even these need to be given cautiously.

When administering an herb to a child, dilute the remedy in accordance with the child's weight. Standard herb doses are appropriate for a 150-pound person. A child who weighs 50 pounds should get one-third of the adult dose.

Be wary of interactions. Exercise caution when adding herbs to your self-care regimen, especially if you're already taking pharmaceuticals or other herbs for any chronic condition. Do not duplicate a drug's effects with herbs.

If you're already taking an antidepressant drug, for example, don't use the herbal antidepressant St. John's wort without your doctor's approval. If you're taking a pharmaceutical blood thinner (anticoagulant) such as aspirin, don't add garlic to your treatment plan. If you're already taking a tranquilizer or an anti-anxiety medication, steer clear of kava, an herbal tranquilizer.

Think twice before jumping on an herb's bandwagon. Be extra careful when taking a newly popular herb or an old herb with a new use. In the mid-1990s, when the age-old herb St. John's wort was shown to have an important new benefit as an antidepressant, it flew off the shelves of health food stores. As the number of users jumped into the millions, rare side effects that strike only one person in a million suddenly began showing up.

That's why St. John's wort's interactions with protease inhibitors and cyclosporine, mentioned earlier, have just been identified. Until St. John's wort became popular, too few people took it for these problems to be noticed.

Be prudent when using herb oils. Aromatic herbs' essential or volatile oils are highly concentrated, and amounts that seem small may cause serious harm. As little as a teaspoon of pennyroyal oil can cause death, for example.

Many herbal oils are available commercially. They are best used topically. If you ingest any, take only a drop or two at a time. Keep herbal oils well out of the reach of children.

Pay attention to any symptoms of toxicity. If you develop stomach upset, nausea, diarrhea, or headache within an hour or two of using any healing herb, stop taking it and see if your symptoms subside. When in doubt, call your local Poison Control Center or your physician or pharmacist. If you experience a severe reaction, call your doctor immediately.

Keep your physician informed. In any medical consultation, tell the doctor which herbs you take and why. Forthrightness helps prevent potentially harmful herb-drug interactions.

Discontinue herbs before surgery. If you're scheduled for surgery, stop taking anticoagulant herbs at least 2 weeks beforehand. Anticoagulant herbs include evening primrose oil, garlic, ginger, turmeric, and white willow.

Potentially Problematic Herbs

Some popular herbs are more likely than others to cause problems. Consumers should become familiar with these herbs and exercise extra caution when taking them.

Stimulants. Stimulants are the herbs most likely to cause trouble. As mentioned earlier, large doses of Chinese ephedra can cause amphetamine-like effects and potentially fatal heart problems. Unusually large doses of other herbal stimulants can also cause problems.

Herbs with stimulant action include ginseng and all those that contain caffeine: coffee, tea, cocoa (chocolate), maté, and kola. Don't exceed the recommended doses; in the case of the herbs that contain caffeine, don't take more than what you're used to.

In addition, don't take two or more stimulant herbs at the same time. The effects are cumulative.

Laxatives. Aloe, buckthorn, cascara sagrada, and senna all contain potent laxative compounds called anthraquinones. Even in recommended doses, these herbs may cause violent purging and abdominal distress. In larger doses, they cause bloody diarrhea and a host of other problems.

Chemical laxatives—both herbal and pharmaceutical—should be last-resort treatments for constipation. First, increase your intake of dietary fiber by eating more plant foods, drink more fluids, and get more exercise. If that doesn't work, try a fiber supplement. Switch to a bran cereal for breakfast, or try the fiber-rich herb psyllium, conveniently available in products such as Metamucil. If that doesn't provide sufficient relief, try a chemical laxative such as senna—but if you need to use it more than once a week, consult your doctor.

Tranquilizers and sedatives. Just as overstimulation can be hazardous, so can oversedation. The herbal tranquilizers and sedatives include valerian, catnip, chamomile, hop, kava, lavender, lemon balm, and passionflower. Beware of using more than one of these herbs at a time as a medicinal—that is, in infusions steeped for longer than a minute or two. Don't take any of these herbs with alcohol, which is a very potent tranquilizer-sedative, and don't combine them with pharmaceutical tranquilizers or sedatives.

Undoubtedly, more herbs-can-be-hazardous headlines will appear in the future, as more people use herbal medicines more frequently, for more ailments, and in combination with more drugs. And unfortunately, some people are likely to suffer harm. By following the advice in this chapter and in the individual herb entries, you should be able to avoid most problems.

CHAPTER 3

Storing and Preparing Healing Herbs

GETTING THE MOST FROM NATURE'S MEDICINES

When you're accustomed to snapping open a plastic bottle and popping some pills or capsules into your mouth, the prospect of dealing with dried plant material can be a little daunting. Don't let it intimidate you.

Preparing healing herbs is not difficult. If you buy prepackaged commercial products (preferably standardized extracts), the preparation process is rarely more complicated than making a cup of tea. Simply follow the label directions.

On the other hand, you may enjoy growing and preparing your own herbs. With that in mind, here's what you need to know.

Directions for Drying

Culinary herbs that also have medicinal applications, such as peppermint, rosemary, and ginger, can be used fresh. But the convention among herbalists is to start with dried plant material, which is easier to store and doesn't rot or spoil as easily.

Traditionally, most herbs were simply tied in bunches and hung in a warm, dry, shady place until they crumbled easily. Roots were washed, split, and spread in a single layer on a clean tray. These drying methods are still used today. In fact, some herb shops sell herbs in dried bunches.

Traditional drying has two disadvantages, however: It often requires more room than foragers or gardeners have, and it takes time—a few days to a few weeks for many leaves, stems, and flowers, and sometimes many months for barks or roots. To preserve the volatile aromatic oils in many herbs, the faster the drying time, the better. That's why most commercial herb producers use special equipment for drying herbs.

An easy way to dry herbs at home is to place them on a baking sheet or a piece of clean window screen in a 95°F oven. Oven drying is convenient and inexpensive, but it has two drawbacks. First, if you harvest herbs in the heat of summer, the last thing you want to do is turn on your oven. Second, many ovens don't heat evenly, so some plant material may char while some remains too moist.

Another approach is to purchase a small produce dryer, a tabletop appliance with built-in removable trays that uses a hot-air fan to dry not only herbs but also other garden produce. Ask a local nursery, check garden catalogs, or contact the Gardener's Supply Catalog, 128 Intervale Road, Burlington, VT 05401.

Power for Powdering

Once herbs are dry, herbalists usually reduce them to powder, the form that's most convenient to use. Traditional herbalists made their powders with mortars and pestles, a method that still works well for those who process only small amounts of herbs.

A more modern approach is to use a small electric coffee grinder (carefully cleaned to remove all traces of coffee). For gardeners who produce large amounts of herbs, larger grinders are available.

Setup for Storing

This may come as a shock to those who store their kitchen spices in clear glass jars, but light is one of the two biggest destroyers of herb flavor and medicinal potency. The other is oxygen.

To best preserve herbs' medicinal constituents, store them in opaque glass or ceramic containers. Fill containers to the top to limit the amount of oxygen in them. As you use your herbs, add cotton wadding to prevent oxygen from seeping inside.

When stored carefully, aromatic herbs such as sage, rosemary, and thyme can remain potent for more than a year. Nonaromatic herbs such as alfalfa and uva-ursi last considerably longer.

Moisture is another herb killer. If your herbs get wet, redry them quickly to prevent the growth of mold.

Insects also take their toll. Drying kills many pests, but watch for signs of infestation. When not using your herbs, keep the containers closed tight.

Procedures for Preparation

Healing herbs are typically used as infusions, decoctions, tinctures, capsules, ointments, and compresses. They may also be added to baths.

How to Make an Infusion

Infusions are hot-water extracts made from herbs with medicinal constituents in their flowers, leaves, and stems. Some herbalists use the terms *infusion* and *tea* interchangeably, but the two are quite different. Infusions are prepared like teas, but they are steeped longer so they become considerably stronger.

The standard traditional infusion recipe calls for ½ to 1 ounce of dried herb steeped in a pint of boiling water for 10 to 20 minutes, then strained. But infusions do not have long shelf lives and should be made as needed. So modern herbalists generally recommend 1 to 2 rounded teaspoons of dried herb per cup of boiling water and steeped for the same amount of time.

Of course, after 20 minutes, infusions are no longer hot. They may be drunk at room temperature or reheated. A handy way to reheat them is in a microwave.

You can use fresh herbs instead of dried to make an infusion. Simply double the amount of herb. (Fresh herbs contain more moisture, which makes them bulkier, so you need more of them.)

Making infusions can be as therapeutic as drinking them. While your infusion is steeping, inhale the warm, steamy vapors. They can act as a nasal decongestant and may help relieve the discomfort of colds, flu, cough, bronchitis, and allergies. As you inhale the vapors, close your eyes and visualize your immune system attacking your illness and making you well. Studies show that such meditative visualizations stimulate the immune system to more effectively fight many diseases.

Some herbal infusions, such as chamomile, ginger, and peppermint, are quite tasty. But others are unpalatably bitter. This is nature's way of discouraging overdose, but if you can't get your medicine down, it can't do any good. To make bitter infusions more palatable, add sugar, honey, or lemon, or mix them with herbal beverage blends or fruit juice. If you still can't stomach an infusion, try a different preparation.

How to Make a Decoction

Similar to infusions, decoctions are extracts made from roots and barks. Compared with flowers, leaves, and stems, roots and barks give up their active compounds less readily. So instead of steeping, you bring the water to a boil, reduce the heat and gently simmer the dried herb material for 10 to 20 minutes, then strain.

How to Make a Tincture

Tinctures are extracts made with alcohol instead of water. They are highly concentrated, so they're more portable than infusions or decoctions or even the herbs themselves. They also remain potent longer—up to several years.

To make tinctures, commercial manufacturers typically use pure grain alcohol, which is 198 proof. But home tincture makers can use 100 proof vodka or brandy. Vodka is less expensive.

The standard tincture recipe calls for 1 ounce of powdered dried herb steeped in 5 ounces of distilled spirits for 6 weeks. Here are some tips for tincture making.

• Seal tincture containers tightly.
• Despite sealing, some containers may ooze. Don't store developing tinctures on valuable furniture.
• Label each tincture with the herb used and the date you put it up to steep. That way, you'll know when 6 weeks have passed.
• Shake each mixture every few days to encourage alcohol uptake of the herb's medicinal constituents.
• Keep tinctures out of direct sunlight.
• If possible, use brown glass containers to minimize light damage.
• Don't be surprised if a tincture changes color as it develops. It happens.
• As the liquid level in a developing tincture goes down, top it off with more distilled spirits.
• After 6 weeks, strain out the plant material, if you wish. Many herbalists recommend doing this, but it's not necessary.
• Store tinctures in a cool place.
• Keep tinctures out of the reach of children. They are quite potent, and a small amount might trigger a harmful reaction.

People who do not drink alcohol can make tinctures using warm (but not boiled) vinegar.

Herbalists recommend wine or apple cider vinegar, not white vinegar. The directions are the same as for alcohol tinctures.

Using Capsules

Powdered herbs can also be packed inside standard pharmaceutical gelatin capsules. Capsules are a convenient way to carry healing herbs while you travel or to take herbs that taste unpleasant. Many herb supply catalogs offer empty capsules and capsule-packing devices.

Capsules come in different sizes. The "00" size is standard. If you make capsules, measure how much powdered herb fits into the capsules you're using so you won't exceed the dosage recommended in this book.

Store capsules away from light and out of the reach of children.

External Preparations: Ointments, Compresses, and Baths

You can make your own herbal ointment by adding 1 to 2 teaspoons of tincture per ounce of commercial skin lotion.

For compresses to treat cuts, burns, and other skin problems, dip a clean cloth in a cool infusion or decoction and drape it over the affected area for 20 minutes. Repeat as needed.

To make baths more relaxing, fill a cloth bag with a few handfuls of aromatic herbs, then allow water to run over it. For additional aroma, leave the herb bag in the water as you bathe.

CHAPTER 4

How to Obtain Healing Herbs

THE BEST SOURCES ARE CLOSE AT HAND

There are three ways to obtain healing herbs: Gather them, grow them, or buy them.

Gathering Your Own

If you enjoy long walks in meadows and forests, gathering herbs can be great fun. Of course, not all healing herbs grow in the United States, but many do.

To go "herbing," you need a good field guide. One of the best is *A Field Guide to Medicinal Plants: Eastern and Central North America*, written by noted herbalists Steven Foster and James A. Duke, Ph.D. It's part of the Peterson Field Guides series. The book discusses more than 500 healing herbs and includes 500 pen-and-ink drawings and 200 color photos. Although it focuses on the United States east of the Rocky Mountains, it contains many herbs that grow throughout the West. Any bookstore can order it for you.

Some herbs, such as dandelion, are easy to recognize and safe to pick. In fact, with dandelion, your neighbors will probably thank you for pulling it out of their lawns. But other herbs, particularly ginseng, are more difficult to find.

Some healing herbs—including blackberry, raspberry, nettle, and rose—have thorns. Wear gloves, long pants, and long sleeves to gather these favorites.

Other herbs, such as angelica root and cascara sagrada bark, are safe to ingest when dried but hazardous when fresh.

In a few herbs, the medicinal parts are safe but other parts cause problems. Blue cohosh is a good example. Its medicinal root is safe when used properly, but its berries are poisonous. Likewise, rhubarb's medicinal root can be used safely, but its leaf blades are poisonous.

Finally, a few poisonous plants resemble healing herbs. Three poisonous species of hemlock look like parsley. Some herb gatherers have died because they mistook poison hemlock—

also known as fool's parsley—for the familiar garnish. Never ingest any wild parsley.

If you stalk the wild healers, dress appropriately, read up on the herbs in chapter 5 to see if they're safe or problematic, and use a good field guide. Most important, when in doubt about any plant's identity, don't ingest it.

Growing Your Own

The herb entries in chapter 5 contain directions for cultivating the healing herbs that grow in the United States. To get started, you'll still need cuttings, seeds, or root divisions.

Cuttings can be difficult to obtain. You have to know an herb gardener. But cuttings are rarely necessary. Most nurseries carry quite a few culinary herb seeds. Standard seed catalogs usually contain dozens of herbs as well. Most nurseries also carry herb seedlings. If you don't see the herbs you want, ask if your nursery can obtain them for you.

For the committed herb gardener, nothing compares with the specialty catalogs published by many of the nation's hundreds of commercial herb growers. Most charge a small fee for the catalog. Here are some of the best mail-order companies.

• Companion Plants features more than 300 varieties of plants and 100 varieties of seeds. Write to 7247 North Coolville Ridge Road, Athens, OH 45701, or visit the Web site at www.companionplants.com.
• The Rosemary House offers more than 100 varieties of plants and 200 varieties of seeds. Its address is 120 South Market Street, Mechanicsburg, PA 17055.

• Mountain Rose Herbs sells more than 100 varieties of herbs, seeds, herbalist supplies, and other herbal products. Write to 29181 High Street, North San Juan, CA 95960, or try the Web site at http://mountainroseherbs.com.
• Sandy Mush Herb Nursery features more than 1,000 herbs and other plants. Contact the nursery at 316 Surrett Cove Road, Leicester, NC 28748.
• The International Herb Association (IHA) provides an enormous number of services to herb growers. It publishes a member directory and newsletter and sponsors conferences. Membership cost varies from $25 to $200 per year. The mailing address is 910 Charles Street, Fredericksburg, VA 22401; the Web address is www.iherb.org.

You Can Always Buy

Supermarkets now carry many herbal beverage teas, some of which can be brewed into medicinal infusions. For a better selection, try a health food store. Most carry dozens of bulk herbs, medicinal herb blends, tinctures, oils, and tablets.

Bulk herbs, tinctures, oils, and tablets can also be purchased by mail. Many of the gardeners' resources listed above sell dried herbs and herb preparations. In addition, the following catalog companies offer large selections.

• Jean's Greens features more than 200 varieties of organic and wildcrafted herbs, along with other herbal products. Write to 119 Sulphur Spring Road, Norway, NY 13416, or log on to www.jeansgreens.com.
• Wild Weeds offers more than 100 herbs and herbal products. The mailing address is 1302

Camp Weott Road, Ferndale, CA 95536; the Web address is www.wildweeds.com.

• Monterey Bay Spice Company sells more than 500 herbs and spices. Contact the company at 719 Swift Street, #106, Santa Cruz, CA 95060, or www.herbco.com.

• HerbPharm features more than 250 herb products. Write to P.O. Box 116, Williams, OR 97544.

Noteworthy Herb Publications

Another way to find herbs—and to learn more about them—is to read the herb press. Recommended publications include the following.

• *HerbalGram* is the quarterly magazine of the American Botanical Council and the Herb Research Foundation. It's an excellent, authoritative source of the latest herb research, with an emphasis on herbal healing. To order it, contact the American Botanical Council, P.O. Box 144345, Austin, TX 78714, or log on to www.herbalgram.org.

• *The Herb Quarterly* is a wonderful magazine with a broad scope, including herb gardening, cookery, crafts, history, and medicine. To subscribe, write to P.O. Box 689, San Anselmo, CA 94979, or log on to www.herbquarterly.com.

• *Herbs for Health* is a beautiful magazine filled with accessible, highly authoritative information about using medicinal herbs. For a subscription, write to 201 East Fourth Street, Loveland, CO 80537, or visit the Web site at www.discoverherbs.com.

PART II

He causeth the grass to grow for the cattle and herbs for the service of humanity.

—Psalm 104:14

CHAPTER 5

100 Healing Herbs

THE CREAM OF THE HERBAL CROP

This chapter features profiles of 100 of the world's widely used medicinal plants. Why these 100? There are several reasons.

They're available. The selected herbs are generally Western in origin, from the Egyptian, European, and Native American healing traditions. Some of the more familiar Asian herbs have also been included, such as cinnamon, ginger, ginseng, rhubarb, and tea. Plants unique to Chinese herbalism have been omitted, however, despite their medical effectiveness, because they're not widely available in the United States.

They're useful. All of the selected herbs have practical applications for everyday health concerns.

They're reasonably safe. The selected herbs should not cause serious side effects or other problems when used as recommended. Each profile provides detailed information on dosage limits, precautions, and potential haz-

ards. (See chapter 2 for a general discussion of herb safety.)

They're often in kitchen spice racks. Centuries ago, all of the herbs and spices used in cooking today were prized mainly for their food preservation and healing powers. Few people realize that they have fully stocked pharmacies right in their own kitchens.

They're fascinating. The Pied Piper was as much an herbalist as a musician (see page 402). The makers of Bayer were originally skeptical of aspirin (see page 411). A 19th-century battle over abortion popularized a modern remedy for menstrual cramps (see page 91). And cowboys who drank sarsaparilla were less interested in refreshment than in preventing venereal diseases (see page 359).

They're popular. Every year, *Whole Foods Magazine*, the health food industry trade journal, ranks medicinal herbs by popularity based on sales. All of the top-rated herbs are represented here.

Alfalfa

Family: Leguminosae; other members include beans and peas

Genus and species: *Medicago sativa*

Also known as: Chilean clover, buffalo grass, and lucerne (in Britain)

Parts used: Leaves

Farmers have long prized the alfalfa plant as animal forage, and in the past 20 years, people who graze on salads have come to appreciate the herb's sprouts as well. But it's the leaves that may contain the real healing power: They may help reduce cholesterol and help prevent heart disease and some strokes.

Healing History

What's good for cattle is good for you, too, or so the ancient Chinese thought. Their animals ate alfalfa so enthusiastically that the Chinese began preparing the herb's tender young leaves as a vegetable. Soon, traditional Chinese physicians were using the plant to stimulate appetite and to treat digestive problems, particularly ulcers.

Ancient India's traditional Ayurvedic physicians also used alfalfa to treat ulcers, and they prescribed it for arthritis pain and fluid retention as well. Ancient Arabs fed their horses alfalfa, believing that it made the animals swift and strong. They called it *al-fac-facah*, or "father of all foods." The Spanish changed the name to alfalfa.

Spain introduced alfalfa into the Americas, where it became a popular forage crop, particularly in the Great Plains. Like the ancient Chinese, the pioneers believed that what was good for their cattle was good for themselves, so they used alfalfa to treat arthritis, boils, cancer, scurvy, and urinary and bowel problems. Pioneer women used it to bring on menstruation.

After the Civil War, alfalfa fell out of favor as a healing herb. It wasn't until the 1970s that it returned to popularity via the salad bowl.

Therapeutic Uses

Most of alfalfa's traditional therapeutic uses have long been disproved. Modern scientists may have discovered a potential healing benefit that our ancestors never dreamed of, however: Alfalfa as an agent in the war against heart disease, stroke, and cancer, the nation's top three killers.

Heart disease and stroke. Animal studies show that alfalfa leaves help reduce blood cholesterol levels and plaque deposits on artery walls. High cholesterol levels and plaque deposits lead to heart disease and most strokes. Alfalfa sprouts produce a similar, but less significant, effect.

Of course, results in animals don't necessarily apply to people, but one case study published in the British medical journal *Lancet* documented substantial cholesterol reduction in a man who ate large amounts of alfalfa.

Cancer. One study suggests that alfalfa helps neutralize cancer-causing substances in the intestine. Another, published in the *Journal of the National Cancer Institute*, shows that the herb binds carcinogens in the colon and helps speed their elimination.

Women's health concerns. Alfalfa seeds contain two chemicals, stachydrine and homostachydrine, that promote menstruation. They can also cause miscarriage, which is why pregnant women should not eat alfalfa seeds (see "The Safety Factor" on page 58). Nor should women consider the herb a reliable contraceptive.

Bad breath. Alfalfa is a source of chlorophyll, the active ingredient in most commercial breath fresheners. Sip an alfalfa infusion if you're concerned about bad breath.

Intriguing Possibility

In laboratory studies, alfalfa helps fight disease-causing fungi. One day, it may be used to treat fungal infections.

Medicinal Myths

While many contemporary herbalists still espouse the age-old view that alfalfa treats ulcers, they may have to eat their words. Scientific research has found no support for this traditional use of the herb.

Herbalists also recommend alfalfa for bowel problems and as a diuretic to treat fluid retention. Unfortunately, these traditional uses have not held up under scientific scrutiny either.

Although some supplement manufacturers promote alfalfa tablets as a treatment for asthma and hay fever, a study published in the *Journal of the American Medical Association* shows that these claims have no merit. Alfalfa contains neither bronchodilators, which arrest an asthma attack, nor antihistamines, which relieve hay fever.

Rx Recommendations

Save alfalfa sprouts to dress up your salads; it's the leaves that are used in herbal healing. Alfalfa leaf tablets and capsules are available in health food stores or wherever herbal supplements are sold. Take them according to package directions.

When using the bulk herb, prepare medicinal infusions with 1 to 2 teaspoons of dried leaves per cup of boiling water and steep for 10 to 20 minutes. Enjoy up to 3 cups a day to take advantage of alfalfa's cholesterol-reducing potential. The infusion has a haylike aroma and tastes like chamomile, with a slightly bitter aftertaste.

Do not give medicinal infusions of the leaves to children under age 2. For older children and people over 65, start with low-strength preparations and increase the strength if necessary.

The Safety Factor

No one should ever eat alfalfa seeds. They contain relatively high levels of the toxic amino acid canavanine. Over time, eating large quantities of seeds may introduce enough canavanine into the body to cause the reversible blood disorder pancytopenia, according to a report in *Lancet*. This condition impairs blood platelets, which are necessary for clotting, and white blood cells, which fight infection.

The canavanine in alfalfa seeds has also been linked to systemic lupus erythematosus, a serious inflammatory disease that can attack many organs, particularly the kidneys. Alfalfa seeds have reactivated the disease in some people who were in remission, according to a report published in the *New England Journal of Medicine*. Another study shows that the seeds actually induce lupus in monkeys.

Alfalfa also contains saponins, chemicals that may destroy red blood cells and—at least theoretically—cause anemia. Because of this, some herb critics warn against ingesting alfalfa (and the many other healing herbs that contain saponins) in any form. Such dire warnings seem unjustified. For adults who are not pregnant or nursing and do not have blood disorders, alfalfa is considered safe in the amounts typically recommended. There have been no reports of healthy people developing anemia from using recommended amounts of healing herbs containing saponins, but if you have anemia, check with your doctor before using alfalfa.

Wise-Use Guidelines

Alfalfa leaf is on the FDA list of herbs generally regarded as safe. Still, you should use it in medicinal amounts only in consultation with your doctor. If it causes minor discomfort, such as stomach upset or diarrhea, reduce the dosage or stop using it altogether. Let your doctor know if you experience unpleasant effects or if the symptoms for which you are using the herb do not improve significantly within 2 weeks.

Growing Information

If you can't find alfalfa leaf tablets or capsules in your local health food store, it's a snap to grow your own supply of the herb. The plant is a deep-rooting, bushy perennial that grows to 3 feet and resembles tall clover. The leaves are divided into three leaflets. The herb's lavender, pale blue, or yellow flowers bloom from May through October, depending on location.

Alfalfa grows best in loamy soil. It tolerates clay but not sand, which lacks sufficient nutrients. Seeds are usually sown in autumn in rows 18 inches apart. Prepare the soil with manure and rock phosphate. Young plants require regular watering, but once established, they become fairly drought tolerant. Harvest plants when they bloom by cutting them back to within 3 inches of the ground, then hang them to dry. When dry, pick off the leaves.

Aloe

Family: Liliaceae; other members include lily, tulip, garlic, and onion

Genus and species: *Aloe vera* and an estimated 500 other species

Also known as: Cape, Barbados, Curaiao, Socotrine, and Zanzibar aloe

Parts used: Leaves (gel and juice, or latex)

Every kitchen should have a potted aloe on the windowsill. That way, when minor burns, scalds, or cuts occur, it's easy to cut off one of the plant's thick, fleshy leaves and scoop the clear gel onto the injury. Aloe gel dries into a natural bandage. It also promotes wound healing and helps prevent infection.

Another part of aloe, the latex (extracted from special cells on the leaf's inner skin), is a powerful laxative. It's so potent, in fact, that many authorities say it should not be taken internally.

Healing History

Our word *aloe* comes from the Arabic *alloeh*, meaning "bitter and shiny"—an apt description of the plant's wound-healing inner leaf gel. Drawings of aloe have been found in Egyptian temples dating to 3000 B.C. The Bible mentions

aloe several times, in passages such as "I have perfumed my bed with myrrh, aloes, and cinnamon" (Proverbs 7:17), but it's unlikely that biblical aloe was *Aloe vera*. In the ancient world, many bitter, resinous plants were called aloe.

Aloe has played a role in healing since the dawn of history. Egyptian medical writings from 1500 B.C. recommend it for infections and skin problems and as a laxative, uses that are supported by modern science.

Aloe is one of the few nonnarcotic plants to cause a war. When Alexander the Great conquered Egypt in 332 B.C., he heard of a plant with amazing wound-healing powers on an island off Somalia. Intent on healing his soldiers' wounds—and on denying this healer to his enemies—Alexander sent an army to seize the island and the plant, which turned out to be aloe.

The Greek physician Dioscorides recommended aloe externally for wounds, hemorrhoids, ulcers, and hair loss. The Roman naturalist Pliny prescribed it for internal use as a laxative.

Arab traders carried aloe from Spain to Asia around the 6th century. They introduced the herb to India's traditional Ayurvedic physicians, who used it to treat skin problems, intestinal worms, and menstrual discomforts. Chinese healers used it similarly.

More recently, American pioneers relied on aloe gel to treat wounds, burns, and hemorrhoids. These uses continue today.

Therapeutic Uses

Contemporary herbalists use aloe in at least one of the ways that Dioscorides suggested almost 2,000 years ago—externally, to treat wounds.

Wounds (including burns, scalds, scrapes, and sunburn). Aloe contains various compounds—bradykinase, salicylic acid, and magnesium lactate—that reduce the inflammation, swelling, and redness of wounds. They also help relieve pain and itching.

Scientific evidence of aloe's wound-healing power was first documented in 1935, when an American medical journal reported the case of a woman whose x-ray burns were successfully treated with aloe gel scooped straight from leaves cut from the plant. Since then, several studies have supported the herb's ability to stimulate healing of first- and second-degree burns as well as other minor skin conditions, including acne and poison ivy rash. When used in conjunction with standard medical care, aloe has also been shown to accelerate wound healing in people with frostbite.

Aloe works best for superficial wounds. In a study published in the *Journal of Dermatology*

and Surgical Oncology, the herb sped the healing of pimples by 3 days compared with standard medical treatment. For deep wounds, however, it actually slows healing. That was what researchers found when they studied the effect of aloe on cesarean section incisions. In the study, published in *Obstetrics and Gynecology*, the incisions not treated with aloe gel healed in 53 days, but for those treated with aloe, healing took 83 days.

As a rule of thumb, feel free to use aloe gel on wounds that don't require stitches, but don't use it to treat deep wounds that require stitches.

Infections. Aloe gel not only spurs wound healing, it also helps keep injured skin from getting infected. Several studies have found aloe to be effective against many different bacteria and fungi that can invade a wound, including *Escherichia coli* and strains of staphylococcus, streptococcus, salmonella, shigella, and candida. It also boosts the immune system, which helps the body fight infection.

Psoriasis. This skin condition, which affects some 5 million Americans, causes eruptions of red, raised skin patches that are usually topped with gray, white, or silvery scaly tissue. At Malmo University Hospital in Sweden, researchers gave 60 people with psoriasis either a medically inactive placebo cream or a cream containing 0.5 percent aloe gel. The participants were instructed to use the creams three times a day, 5 days a week for 16 weeks. Among those using the placebo cream, 7 percent experienced substantial clearing of their psoriasis skin patches. Among those using the aloe cream, that figure rose to 83 percent.

General skin care. Cleopatra massaged aloe gel into her skin to make it shine, and the herb remains a popular ingredient in skin-care products. But if you're after beautiful skin, do what the legendary beauty did: Use the fresh leaf gel. The "stabilized" (preserved) gel found in commercial skin-care products and shampoos may not provide the fresh herb's skin-enhancing benefits. If you enjoy the fragrance of aloe shampoos and skin lotions, that's fine. Just don't expect them to turn you into Cleopatra.

Intriguing Possibilities

Aloe juice and aloe-based beverages are widely available in health food stores. Their labels claim that these products are good for the digestive tract. Anecdotal reports suggest possible benefits for inflammatory bowel disease (colitis and Crohn's disease), but there is no rigorous research to support this.

Studies show that aloe may kill the fungus (*Candida albicans*) that causes vaginal yeast infections. Its possible effectiveness against the yeast fungus has led some herbalists to recommend using it to treat the infection itself. But just because it kills the fungus in laboratory tests doesn't mean that it can wipe out the infection in the human body. No scientific studies support this use, and an FDA advisory panel found insufficient evidence to recommend aloe as a yeast treatment.

In laboratory tests, a chemical in aloe called aloe-emodin has shown promise against leukemia. But National Cancer Institute scientists say that experimental preparations are still too toxic to give to people with leukemia.

Although aloe has been used in folk medicine as an external treatment for skin cancer, its effectiveness has never been studied scientifically.

European and Thai studies suggest that aloe juice reduces blood sugar (glucose) levels in experimental animals and in people with diabetes. Aloe juice may one day be used to help manage diabetes, especially in poorer countries, because it is cheaper than pharmaceutical diabetes medications.

Rx Recommendations

To help soothe wounds, including burns, scalds, scrapes, and sunburn, and to help prevent infection, select a lower (older) aloe leaf and cut off several inches. Then slice it lengthwise, scoop the gel onto the wound, and let it dry. Be sure to clean the wound properly with soap and water first. As for the injured leaf, it quickly closes its own wound. You can use the rest of it in the future.

To enjoy the cosmetic benefits of aloe, apply the leaf gel to freshly washed skin. Discontinue use if it seems to irritate your skin.

The Safety Factor

Aloe gel is safe for external use by anyone who does not develop an allergic reaction. Still, it's best used in consultation with your doctor. Tell your doctor if a wound does not heal significantly within 2 weeks or if it appears to be getting worse.

Although the gel may help heal injured skin, one case study reported eczema-like welts in a man who had used it for several years. This seems to prove that too much of a good thing may cause problems.

Commercial aloe juice may have a mild laxative effect, but stay away from laxatives containing aloe latex. The latex contains laxative compounds (anthraquinones) with such powerful purgative action that they are called cathartics. Other laxative herbs, such as senna, rhubarb, buckthorn, and cascara sagrada, also contain anthraquinones, but aloe's action is considered the most drastic—and least recommended—because it often causes severe intestinal cramps and diarrhea.

Although many herbalists discourage the use of aloe as a laxative, some supplement companies sell aloe laxative tablets on the strength of approval by Commission E, the expert panel that evaluates herbal medicines for the German counterpart of the FDA. If you take aloe as a laxative, never exceed the dosage recommendations on the package, and reduce the dosage or stop using the product if you develop intestinal cramps.

If you're looking for a natural laxative, your best bet is to seek other herbs with proven, but milder, effects. These include psyllium (see page 325) and cascara sagrada (see page 110).

Women who are pregnant or trying to conceive should not take aloe latex, as its cathartic nature may stimulate uterine contractions and trigger miscarriage. Nor should latex be used by nursing mothers. The latex enters mother's milk and may cause stomach cramps and violent catharsis in infants.

Aloe latex's cathartic power may also aggravate ulcers, hemorrhoids, diverticulosis, diverticulitis, colitis, Crohn's disease, or irritable bowel syndrome. Anyone with a gastrointestinal illness should not use aloe latex as a laxative.

In general, aloe latex is not recommended for any internal use.

Growing Information

Aloe is the perfect houseplant for people with brown thumbs because it requires little water and no other care. Aloe prefers sun, but it tolerates shade and doesn't mind poor soil. The only conditions this hardy succulent cannot tolerate are poor drainage and cold temperatures. Bring potted aloe indoors before the temperature falls below about 40°F.

Aloe periodically produces offshoots, which you may remove and replant when they are a few inches tall. Simply uproot or unpot the plant, work the soil gently to separate the offshoot, and return the mother plant to its bed or pot.

Angelica

Family: Umbelliferae; other members include carrot, parsley, celery, fennel, and dill

Genus and species: *Angelica archangelica* (European), *A. atropurpurea* (American), *A. sinensis* (Chinese), and other species

Also known as: Wild celery and masterwort; in China, dang gui and dong quai

Parts used: Roots, leaves, and seeds

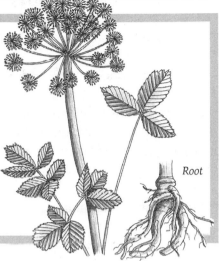

Root

Tall, striking, and attractive, angelica has played a role in magic and medicine for several thousand years. But the species used in Western and Chinese herbal medicine have always differed. So, too, have opinions of the herb's medicinal value.

In the West, European angelica has been a minor player. But in Asia, Chinese angelica, usually called dang gui, has long been considered *the* herb for gynecological complaints. This claim is controversial, but still, Western researchers may have been too quick to dismiss Chinese angelica as medically worthless.

Healing History

In Asia, where Chinese angelica has been used since the dawn of history, the herb has always been considered the premier tonic for menstrual problems, menopausal complaints, and other women's health concerns. Traditional Chinese practitioners and Indian Ayurvedic physicians still prescribe it for gynecological conditions, arthritis, abdominal pain, colds, and flu.

European angelica has been viewed as a magical herb for more than 1,000 years. European peasants made angelica leaf necklaces to protect their children from illness and witchcraft. Angelica was reputed to be the only herb that witches never used, and its presence in a woman's garden or cupboard was once considered a defense against charges of witchcraft.

During the 16th and 17th centuries, the juice from crushed angelica roots was combined with other herbs to make "Carmelite water." This medieval drink was said to cure headache, promote relaxation and long life, and protect against poisons and witches' spells.

In 1665, Europe was decimated by bubonic plague. Legend has it that a monk dreamed that he met an angel, who showed him an herb that could cure the scourge. The herb was angelica, and the monk named it in honor of the angel in his dream. The name stuck, and angelica water was incorporated into the official English plague remedy, developed by the Royal College of Physicians in London and called the King's Excellent Plague Recipe.

History provides no clear verdict on the effectiveness of the "excellent recipe," but perhaps the old monk's dream was prophetic. Bubonic plague is a bacterial disease, and modern science has discovered that certain substances isolated from angelica have some antibacterial action.

During the 17th century, European angelica became a popular treatment for colds and other respiratory ailments. Its stems are hollow, allowing air to pass through them. Under the Doctrine of Signatures—the medieval belief that an herb's physical appearance reveals its healing benefits—hollow-stemmed plants were considered beneficial for respiratory problems.

When European colonists arrived in North America, they found many Native American tribes using American angelica the same way their own healers used the European species— to treat respiratory ailments, particularly tuberculosis. Eventually, the colonists began using large doses to induce abortion. The 19th-century American Eclectic physicians, forerunners of today's naturopaths, recommended angelica for heartburn, indigestion, bronchitis, malaria, and typhoid.

Therapeutic Uses

Contrary to legend, angelica does not deliver humanity from epidemic disease, but the Chinese species of the herb has delivered a good deal of controversy. One study showed that it helped menopausal discomforts, while another found no such effect. Meanwhile, most of the traditional uses for European angelica have not stood up to scientific scrutiny all that well.

Contemporary herbalists generally recommend angelica mostly for digestive problems and to help clear mucus. These uses may have some validity.

Menopausal complaints. The study that substantiated Chinese angelica's benefits for menopausal discomforts was conducted by researchers at the National College of Naturopathic Medicine in Portland, Oregon, and Bastyr University, the naturopathic medical school in Kenmore, Washington. The researchers gave 13 menopausal women either medically inactive placebos or a Chinese herbal formula containing dang gui, licorice root, hawthorn leaf, burdock root, and wild yam root. After 3 months, the women who took the herbal formula reported significantly greater relief.

In a similar study conducted by researchers at Kaiser Permanente Medical Center in Oakland, California, 71 menopausal women were treated with Chinese angelica for 3 months. This time, however, the women showed no improvement.

Experts in Chinese herbal medicine have criticized the Kaiser Permanente study because it used only dang gui. In Chinese herbal medicine, the herb is never used alone; it's combined with other herbs in formulas, as was done in the other study.

Respiratory ailments. Score one for the Doctrine of Signatures. German researchers have determined that angelica relaxes the windpipe, suggesting that it may have some value in treating colds, flu, bronchitis, and asthma.

Digestive problems. The same German investigators found that angelica relaxes the intestines. This lends some credence to the herb's traditional use in treating digestive complaints.

Arthritis. Japanese researchers have reported that angelica has anti-inflammatory effects, so there may be something to angelica's traditional Asian use as an arthritis treatment.

Intriguing Possibilities

Preliminary research from China suggests that dang gui increases red blood cell counts, indicating that the herb may someday prove beneficial in treating anemia. This would also increase its value as a treatment for menstrual cramps because it would help the body compensate for monthly blood loss.

Asian researchers report that Chinese angelica increases the ability of blood to clot. If they're correct, that's good news for people with impaired clotting. It also means that anyone at risk for heart disease should avoid this herb. Increased clotting can lead to decreased blood flow to the heart and, in some cases, may trigger a heart attack.

The Chinese have also found that dang gui improves liver function in people with cirrhosis or chronic hepatitis. Their research is preliminary, however, and no specific recommendations can be made at this time about using angelica for liver problems.

Rx Recommendations

If you'd like to use Chinese angelica to treat gynecological problems, consult a practitioner of Chinese herbal medicine for a multi-herb formula.

Commission E, the expert panel that evaluates herbal medicines for the German counterpart of the FDA, endorses European angelica as a treatment for appetite loss, abdominal distress, and flatulence.

There are many ways to prepare this herb, depending on your personal preference. To make an infusion, use 1 teaspoon of powdered seeds or leaves per cup of boiling water. Steep for 10 to 20 minutes and strain if you wish.

For a decoction, use 1 teaspoon of powdered root per cup of water. Bring to a boil and simmer for 2 minutes. Remove from the heat, let stand for 15 minutes, and strain if you wish. Drink up to 2 cups a day. Angelica decoctions have a bitter taste.

As a homemade tincture, use ½ to 1 teaspoon up to twice a day.

When using commercial preparations, follow the package directions.

Do not give angelica to children under age 2. For older children and adults over age 65, start with low-strength preparations and increase the strength if necessary.

The Safety Factor

Angelica has never been shown to stimulate uterine contractions, but given its traditional use to induce menstruation and abortions, women who are pregnant or trying to conceive should not take medicinal amounts.

Angelica contains chemicals known as psoralens. Exposure to sunlight may cause a rash in people who have ingested psoralens, a reaction known as photosensitivity. Psoralens may also promote tumor growth, leading the authors of a report in the journal *Science* to advise against taking angelica internally.

On the other hand, an animal study showed that the angelica constituent alpha-angelica lactone has an anticancer effect. Angelica's role in human cancer, if any, remains unclear. People with a history of cancer probably should not take the herb until questions about it have been answered.

Fresh angelica roots are poisonous, but drying eliminates the hazard. Herb gardeners should be sure to dry the roots thoroughly before using them.

Finally, unless you are a confident field botanist, do not collect angelica in the wild. It's easy to confuse with water hemlock (*Cicuta maculata*), an extremely poisonous plant.

Wise-Use Guidelines

The FDA includes angelica in its list of herbs that are generally regarded as safe. For adults who are not pregnant or nursing and do not have a history of cancer, heart attack, or photosensitivity, it is considered relatively safe in the amounts typically recommended.

You should use medicinal amounts of angelica only in consultation with your doctor. If it causes minor discomfort, such as stomach upset or diarrhea, reduce the dosage or stop using it altogether. Let your doctor know if you experience any unpleasant effects or if the symptoms for which you are using the herb do not improve significantly within 2 weeks.

Growing Information

Angelica often blooms around May 8, the feast day of St. Michael the Archangel, which is the source of European angelica's species name, *archangelica*. The plant grows to 8 feet and resembles celery—hence its common name, wild celery—and is a biennial that dies after producing seeds. It grows from seeds or root divisions. Seed viability is relatively brief, only about 6 months, but refrigeration extends it up to a year. Germination may take a month. Sow angelica in the fall or spring ½ inch deep in well-prepared beds. Space plants 2 feet apart in all directions.

Angelica thrives in rich, moist, well-drained, slightly acidic soil. It prefers partial shade. Leaves may be harvested in the fall of the first year and roots during the spring or fall of the second year.

Angelica is not usually considered a culinary herb, but fresh leaves provide a zesty accent to soups and salads. It has a fragrant aroma and a warm, vaguely sweet taste reminiscent of juniper, followed by a bitter aftertaste. You can eat steamed stems with butter, and chopped stems add flavor to roast pork.

Apple

Family: Rosaceae; other members include rose, peach, almond, and strawberry

Genus and species: *Malus sylvestris* or *Pyrus malus*

Also known as: No other common names

Parts used: Fruits

An apple a day keeps the doctor away." The old rhyme is truer than ever, particularly if the doctor is a gastroenterologist, oncologist, or cardiologist. Apples help treat both diarrhea and constipation, and they may help prevent cancer, heart disease, and some types of stroke—America's top three killers.

Although few contemporary herbalists consider the apple to be an herb, it has a venerable tradition as a healing agent. So much of what the ancient herbalists believed about the therapeutic powers of this delectable fruit has been scientifically supported that it's time to let the apple resume its respected place on the herbal roster.

Healing History

The Bible never identifies the Garden of Eden's "forbidden fruit," but since ancient times, people have believed that it was an apple. Legend has it that a piece got stuck in Adam's throat; hence the term *Adam's apple.*

The "apple of discord" started the Trojan War. Snow White's coma was induced by a poisoned apple. And William Tell shot an apple off his young son's head.

Then there was early America's own apple eccentric, John "Johnny Appleseed" Chapman. This pioneer spent most of his life wandering around Pennsylvania, Ohio, and Indiana sowing apple seeds—and becoming a legend.

The ancient Egyptians, Greeks, and Romans loved apples and developed dozens of varieties, but it was ancient India's traditional Ayurvedic physicians who first prescribed them to relieve diarrhea. Applesauce is still a popular home remedy for diarrhea.

Traditional Chinese physicians have used apple bark for centuries to treat diabetes, another use that's supported by modern science.

The medieval German abbess/herbalist Hildegard of Bingen prescribed raw apples as a tonic for healthy people and cooked apples as the first treatment for any sickness.

Around the same time in England, people said, "To eat an apple before going to bed/Will make the doctor beg his bread." This evolved into our saying about an apple a day.

Not everything the English had to say about apples was so apt, however. Seventeenth-century English herbalist Nicholas Culpeper recommended apples "for hot and bilious stomachs . . . inflammations of the breast and lungs . . . [and] asthma." He also suggested boiled apples mixed with milk as a treatment for gunpowder burns.

The Americas had no native apples, but the Pilgrims brought apple seeds with them, and the fruit quickly became, well, as American as apple pie. Apples, apple bark, and apple cider soon became mainstays of American folk medicine.

Speaking of apple pie, when the poor baked pies, they used only a bottom crust. Richer bakers could afford to add a top crust—hence our description of the wealthy as "upper crust."

A century ago, American Eclectic physicians, forerunners of today's naturopaths, recommended apples in many forms: raw apples for constipation, baked or stewed apples for minor fevers, apple bark decoction for intermittent fever (malaria), and apple cider "as a refreshing drink for patients with fever."

Therapeutic Uses

Modern medical science has found that Johnny Appleseed's favorite fruit has tremendous value in healing thanks to its pulp, which is high in pectin, a soluble form of fiber.

Diarrhea. Studies show that pectin helps relieve diarrhea because intestinal bacteria transform it into a soothing, protective coating for the irritated intestinal lining. In addition, pectin adds bulk to the stool, which helps resolve diarrhea.

Some diarrhea results from bacterial infection. One study found that apple pectin is effective against several types of bacteria that are known to cause diarrhea, among them salmonella, staphylococcus, and *Escherichia coli*. In fact, pectin is the "pectate" in the over-the-counter diarrhea preparation Kaopectate.

Constipation. Physicians recommend diets high in fiber to add bulk to stool. Since pectin is a type of fiber, it can help with constipation by adding bulk and stimulating bowel contractions.

Heart disease and stroke. A diet high in fiber helps reduce blood cholesterol, a key risk factor for heart disease and some types of stroke. In the presence of fiber, the cholesterol we eat remains in the intestinal tract until it is eliminated. So if you eat a pectin-rich, high-fiber apple for dessert when you have meat and dairy products, you will enjoy some protection from their cholesterol.

In a long-term study involving 805 Dutch men, researchers discovered that those who ate the most apples experienced the fewest heart attacks. The scientists concluded that in addition to pectin, compounds in apples called flavonoids played an important protective role. Flavonoids are antioxidants that help prevent the cell damage that's at the root of the arterial narrowing that leads to heart disease.

Cancer. The American Cancer Society recommends a high-fiber diet to help prevent several forms of cancer, particularly colon cancer. Pectin binds certain cancer-causing compounds in the colon, speeding their elimination from the body, according to a study published in the *Journal of the National Cancer Institute*.

The antioxidant flavonoids in apples also help prevent the cell damage that causes many cancers.

Diabetes. Physicians also recommend a high-fiber diet to control diabetes. A study published in the *Annals of Internal Medicine* showed that apple pectin helps reduce blood sugar (glucose) levels in people with the disease.

Toxin exposure. European studies suggest that apple pectin helps eliminate lead, mercury, and other toxic heavy metals from the body. Cleansing the body of these poisons is yet another reason for people who live in polluted cities to enjoy the proverbial apple a day.

Wounds. Although pectin is the apple's major medicinal component, the fruit's leaves contain an antibiotic called phloretin. If you cut yourself out in the orchard, you can use apple leaves as immediate first-aid

Intriguing Possibility

A few studies, including one published in the *Journal of the National Cancer Institute*, hint that pectin may help keep cancer from spreading around the body (metastasizing).

Rx Recommendations

For handy first-aid for minor wounds, crush some apple leaves and apply them to the cut or scrape until you can wash and bandage it.

Eat the whole fresh fruit to enjoy a wide range of healthful benefits. Green apples tend to be tart, but they usually have more "snap." Red apples are usually sweeter but may have a mealy texture. Wash apples with soap and water before eating to eliminate any pesticide residue.

The Safety Factor

James A. Duke, Ph.D., retired USDA herbal medicine authority (and poet), sums up apple safety this way:

> *An apple a day keeps the doctor away,*
> *Or at least that's what some people say.*
> *But one man, we read,*
> *Ate a cupful of seed,*
> *And this man died.*
> *Overdosed. Cyanide.*

It's strange but true: Apple seeds contain high levels of cyanide, the powerful poison. About 1/2 cup of seeds can be deadly for the average adult, but considerably less is fatal for children and the elderly. Many parents are familiar with the stomachaches that young children develop when they eat apple cores. The few seeds in the typical core pose little risk of serious poisoning. But to be prudent, teach children not to eat apple seeds, and stay away from them yourself.

If apples cause minor discomfort, such as diarrhea or constipation, eat fewer of them or none at all. If diarrhea or constipation does not improve within a week, consult a physician.

Do not attempt to treat diabetes, high cholesterol, or colon disease solely with herbs. In such cases, apples should be used to complement professional medical care.

Growing Information

Archeologists have found evidence that humans have been enjoying apples since at least 6500 B.C. Prehistoric apples resembled today's crab apples—small, dry, and mealy. But as agriculture developed, apples became one of the world's first hybridized orchard fruits.

Today, about 300 apple varieties grow in the 50 states. Special varieties have been developed for just about every set of growing conditions in North America. Consult a nursery for the varieties best suited to your locale.

Full-size apple trees grow to about 40 feet and spread over 1,600 square feet (40 by 40). Genetic dwarf apple varieties produce delicious, full-size fruits but grow to only 6 to 12 feet and spread over less than 150 square feet (12 by 12).

Plant the rootstock in a sunny location and water regularly. Prune at planting, then annually. Different apple varieties have different fertilizer requirements and different pest problems. Consult a nursery for advice.

Astragalus

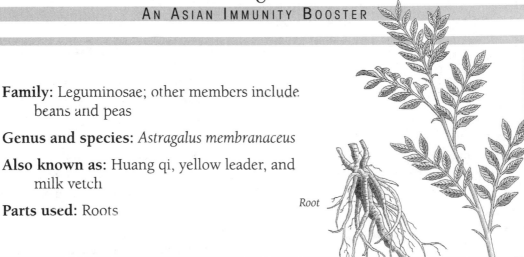

Family: Leguminosae; other members include beans and peas

Genus and species: *Astragalus membranaceus*

Also known as: Huang qi, yellow leader, and milk vetch

Parts used: Roots

Root

The Chinese refer to astragalus as huang qi, which, loosely translated, means "strengthener of qi." Qi (or *chi*) is the Chinese term for life force, vitality, stamina, disease resistance, and the ability to cope with physical and emotional stress. As a strengthener of qi, astragalus is powerful medicine.

Healing History

The medicinal use of astragalus was first recorded in China some 2,000 years ago. Modern-day practitioners of Chinese medicine believe that the herb strengthens all body systems and that it's particularly effective for treating illnesses that cause fatigue. They consider it similar to ginseng, and they prescribe it for diabetes, heart disease, and high blood pressure.

Therapeutic Uses

Western scientists have begun to study astragalus only recently, so there are still more questions than answers about the herb's effects. But research to date confirms the Chinese claims for it.

Enhanced immunity. The first Western study of astragalus took place in 1983 at the University of Texas M. D. Anderson Cancer Center in Houston. The herb improved immune function in 19 cancer patients who were being treated with immune-suppressing chemotherapy drugs.

Since then, several studies—most involving animals—have shown that astragalus, administered either orally or by injection, improves various measures of immune function. In one study, infection-fighting human T cells became significantly more vigorous after being treated with astragalus. In another, astragalus injected into mice improved the ability of their infection-fighting macrophages (a type of white blood cells) to devour bacteria, viruses, and fungi.

In a Chinese study, 10 people with viral heart infections and depressed immune systems were given daily injections of 8 grams of astragalus extract. The patients' immune system functions improved significantly.

Currently, Americans are most likely to use astragalus while taking immune-suppressing cancer chemotherapy drugs.

Liver damage. Chinese researchers exposed mice to stilbenemide, a cancer chemotherapy drug that causes liver damage as a side effect. Animals that received only the drug developed serious liver damage, while those given the drug plus an oral astragalus extract did not.

Intriguing Possibilities

Other Chinese studies suggest that astragalus improves sperm motility, reduces blood pressure, improves heart function, and enhances immune function in people infected with HIV, the virus that causes AIDS.

Rx Recommendations

When using the dried root sticks, finely chop 4 or 5 sticks and simmer them in 4 cups of boiling water for 1 hour. Drink 1 cup in the morning and 1 cup in the evening. Astragalus tastes mildly sweet, but you may prefer it blended with other beverage herbs.

Astragalus is also available in a variety of commercial preparations, including tinctures, capsules, and tablets. Follow the package directions.

The Safety Factor

Astragalus is generally considered safe when used as recommended. One laboratory test, however, found that a strong decoction caused chromosome mutations, a hint that the herb might be carcinogenic. Traditional Chinese herbalists recommend using astragalus for only a few weeks during an illness, and not routinely. This would be prudent advice if the herb's mutagenic action is confirmed.

Chinese practitioners advise against taking astragalus for acute infections; instead, they recommend reserving it to strengthen the body after it has begun to heal.

Growing Information

Astragalus is not grown in the United States. It is a perennial plant native to northern China and Mongolia that produces small yellow flowers. Its thick, carrotlike root has a tough fibrous skin with a yellowish interior, which is the medicinal part. The root has a sweetish, licorice-like taste.

In China, the root is peeled and dried, sometimes after being soaked in honey. Then it's cut into long slices that resemble ice-pop sticks. Chinese herb shops sell the sticks, but for U.S. consumers, the herb is typically powdered and sold in capsules.

Barberry

Family: Berbericlaceae; other members include May apple, mandrake, and blue cohosh

Genus and species: *Berberis vulgaris*; Oregon grape: *B. aquifolium* or *Mahonia aquifolium*

Also known as: Berberry, berberis, and jaundice berry

Part used: Root bark

Who says herbs can't compete with pharmaceutical drugs? In one study, berberine, the active constituent in barberry, proved more potent against bacteria than chloramphenicol, a powerful pharmaceutical antibiotic.

But there's a lot more to this herb than mere infection treatment. Barberry, and its close relative Oregon grape, may also stimulate the immune system, reduce blood pressure, and even shrink some tumors.

Healing History

Barberry has played a prominent role in herbal healing for more than 2,500 years. The ancient Egyptians relied on it to prevent plague, a use that was probably effective considering the herb's antibiotic action. India's traditional Ayurvedic healers prescribed barberry for dysentery,

another use that's been confirmed by modern science.

During the early Middle Ages, European herbalists were guided by the Doctrine of Signatures, the belief that a plant's physical appearance revealed its therapeutic benefits. Barberry has yellow flowers, and its roots produce a yellow dye. These features were linked to the yellowing of the skin and eyes of jaundice, a symptom of liver disease. As a result, barberry was widely used to treat liver and gallbladder ailments, earning the name jaundice berry.

In addition to treating liver and gallbladder ailments, traditional Russian healers recommended it for skin inflammations, high blood pressure, and abnormal uterine bleeding.

When colonists introduced barberry into North America, the Native Americans recognized it as a relative of the native Oregon grape, a hollylike plant that they considered a powerful healer. Many tribes adopted barberry enthusiastically and used it to treat dysentery, mouth ulcers, sore throat, wound infections, and intestinal complaints.

The 19th-century American Eclectic physicians, forerunners of today's naturopaths, prescribed barberry as a purgative and treatment for jaundice, dysentery, eye infections, cholera, fevers, and "impurities of the blood," which was a euphemism for syphilis.

Barberry was also an ingredient in the popular but highly controversial Hoxsey Cancer Formula, an alternative cancer therapy marketed from the 1930s to the 1950s by ex-coal miner Harry Hoxsey (see page 32).

Therapeutic Uses

Most present-day herbalists limit their recommendations to gargling barberry decoction for sore throat and drinking it for diarrhea and constipation. But if they were reading the medical journals, they'd be recommending it for a great deal more.

Infections. The berberine in barberry has remarkable infection-fighting properties. Studies around the world show that it kills microorganisms that cause wound infections (staphylococcus and streptococcus), diarrhea (salmonella and shigella), dysentery (*Entamoeba histolytica*), cholera (*Vibrio cholerae*), giardiasis (*Giardia lamblia*), urinary tract infections (*Escherichia coli*), and vaginal yeast infections (*Candida albicans*).

Enhanced immunity. Berberine may also fight infection by stimulating the immune system. Studies show that it activates macrophages (literally, "big eaters"), the white blood cells that devour harmful microorganisms.

Liver damage. Score one for the Doctrine of Signatures and "jaundice berry." Pakistani researchers gave laboratory animals large doses of acetaminophen to produce liver damage, as measured by significant increases in blood levels of liver enzymes. Then some of the animals were treated with a barberry preparation. Levels of liver enzymes remained abnormally high in the animals that didn't receive barberry, but in those that did, the enzymes declined, showing significant normalization of liver function. The researchers concluded, "This study provides a scientific basis for the traditional use of barberry in liver disorders."

Psoriasis. Barberry's traditional use as a treatment for skin problems was confirmed by German researchers in a 4-week study involving 82 people with psoriasis, a condition that produces red, raised, scaly skin eruptions. Each study participant was given two tubes of ointment—one with barberry extract, the other without. The tubes were marked "left" and "right," and people were instructed to apply each ointment to the respective sides of their bodies. The barberry ointment produced significantly greater shrinkage of skin eruptions.

Pinkeye. Barberry's traditional use for treating eye problems is alive and well in Germany, where a berberine preparation called Ophthiole is prescribed to treat sensitive eyes, inflamed lids, and pinkeye (conjunctivitis). Unfortunately, the product is not available in the United States. A compress made from an herbal infusion may prove helpful, however.

High blood pressure. Barberry contains chemicals that may help reduce elevated blood pressure by enlarging blood vessels. This lends support to the herb's traditional Russian use as a treatment for high blood pressure.

Intriguing Possibilities

Perhaps old Harry Hoxsey was right. One study found that barberry helps shrink some tumors. Another showed it has anti-inflammatory activity, suggesting possible value in treating arthritis. More research needs to be done in both areas before any specific recommendations can be made.

Rx Recommendations

To prepare a decoction, boil ½ teaspoon of powdered root bark in 1 cup of water for 15 to 30 minutes, then strain if you wish. Let it cool, and drink up to 1 cup a day. The taste is quite bitter, but you can mask it with honey or an herbal beverage blend.

When using commercial preparations, follow the package directions.

Do not give barberry to children under age 2. For older children and adults over age 65, start with lower-strength preparations and increase the strength if necessary.

To make a compress to treat pinkeye, soak a clean cloth in a barberry infusion.

The Safety Factor

Barberry is a powerful herb. Adults who are not pregnant or nursing may use it cautiously in consultation with a doctor. If it causes minor discomfort, such as stomach upset or diarrhea, decrease the dosage or stop using it altogether. Likewise, stop using it if it causes dizziness or faintness. Let your doctor know if you experience any unpleasant effects or if the symptoms for which you are using the herb do not improve significantly within 2 weeks.

In large doses, barberry can cause nausea, vomiting, convulsions, hazardous drops in blood pressure, and depression of heart rate and breathing. People with heart disease or chronic respiratory problems should be careful not to take large doses and should take this herb only with the knowledge and approval of their physicians.

Berberine may stimulate uterine contractions. For this reason, women who are pregnant or trying to conceive should not use it.

Growing Information

Barberry is a perennial shrub that reaches 10 feet. It has smooth gray bark, long spines, and hanging clusters of bright yellow flowers that bloom in spring.

Barberry grows easily in the Northeast and Midwest. Plant seeds in the fall in fertile, moist, well-drained soil. Germination occurs the following spring. The shrub can also be propagated from cuttings

Barberry prefers sun but tolerates shade. Prune and thin the branches in the spring after the shrub flowers. Neglected shrubs become overgrown and unhealthy, but they can be rejuvenated by fertilizing and cutting back to within a foot of the ground in late winter. In areas with cold winters, shelter the plant from the wind. Harvest the root bark in spring or fall, and dry it.

The herb's edible berries are used to make jams and jellies. The berry juice may be substituted for lemon juice.

Bayberry

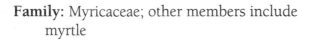

Family: Myricaceae; other members include myrtle

Genus and species: *Myrica cerifera*

Also known as: Wax myrtle, candleberry, and tallow shrub

Part used: Root bark

Before electric lights were commonplace, bayberry was highly prized as the source of a fragrant candlewax that produced considerably less smoke than tallow. Today, bayberry candles are still with us, but only as Christmas curiosities.

Healing History

In early America, bayberry trees grew throughout the East. But bayberry was used medicinally mainly in the South, where Choctaw tribes boiled the leaves and drank the decoction as a treatment for fever. Later, white settlers adopted the plant and drank bayberry wax in hot water "as a certain cure for the most violent cases of dysentery," according to a medical account from 1722.

During the early 19th century, bayberry was popularized by Samuel A. Thomson, a New England herbalist and creator of some of the first patent medicines. He touted the herb as second only to red pepper for producing "heat" within the body. Thomson recommended bayberry for colds, flu, and other infectious diseases as well as for diarrhea and fever.

Thomson's herbalism lost popularity after the Civil War, when it was replaced by the teachings of the more scientific Eclectic physicians, forerunners of today's naturopaths. They prescribed bayberry topically for bleeding gums and internally for diarrhea, dysentery, sore throat, scarlet fever, menstrual difficulties, and even typhoid.

Although bayberry has since waned in popularity, some contemporary herbalists recommend using it externally for varicose veins and internally for diarrhea, dysentery, colds, flu, bleeding gums, and sore throat. One modern herbal calls it one of the most useful herbs in botanical medicine and goes so far as to advocate treating uterine bleeding by packing the vagina with cotton soaked in bayberry tea. (Do not try this remedy; see a physician for unusual uterine bleeding.)

Therapeutic Uses

Two hundred years ago, bayberry was widely used medicinally. It's a shame that this native American herb has been all but forgotten, because science has shown that bayberry may have some real benefits in treating fever and diarrhea.

Diarrhea. Bayberry root bark contains myricitrin, an antibiotic chemical that fights a broad range of bacteria and protozoa. Myricitrin's antibiotic action supports bayberry's traditional use against diarrhea and dysentery.

Bayberry also contains astringent tannins, which add to its value in treating diarrhea.

Fever. The antibiotic myricitrin also helps reduce fever, thus lending credence to bayberry's traditional use among the Choctaws.

Intriguing Possibility

Myricitrin promotes the flow of bile, so bayberry may potentially be of value in treating liver and gallbladder ailments. As yet, however, no research demonstrates this use.

Rx Recommendations

To prepare a decoction, boil 1 teaspoon of powdered root bark in 1 pint of water for 10 to 15 minutes, then strain if you wish. Add a bit of milk and drink up to 2 cups a day of the cooled beverage. You'll find the taste bitter and astringent. A tincture might go down more easily. If you use a homemade tincture, take ½ teaspoon up to twice a day.

When using commercial preparations, follow the package directions.

Do not give bayberry to children under age 2. For older children and adults over age 65, start with a low-strength preparation and increase the strength if necessary.

The Safety Factor

Bayberry's high tannin content makes the herb of questionable value for anyone with a history of cancer. In various studies, tannins show both procancer and anticancer actions. Their cancer-promoting action has received more publicity, notably from a study published in the *Journal of the National Cancer Institute*, which showed that tannins produce malignant tumors in laboratory animals. But tannins have also been found to have an anticancer effect on some tumors in animals.

Tannins' effects on human cancer remain unclear. Small quantities have never been implicated in human tumors, but Asians who drink large quantities of tea, which contains tannins, show unusually high rates of stomach cancer. The British also love tea, but their rates of stomach cancer remain low. One reason may be that they drink their tea with milk, which neutralizes the tannins.

People with a history of cancer, particularly stomach or colon cancer, should exercise caution and not use bayberry. Others should drink no more than the recommended amounts and, for extra safety, add milk.

In large doses, bayberry root bark may cause stomach distress, nausea, and vomiting. People with chronic gastrointestinal conditions, such as colitis, should use it cautiously.

Bayberry changes the way the body uses sodium and potassium, so people who must watch their sodium/potassium balance, such as those with kidney disease, high blood pressure, or congestive heart failure, should consult their physicians before using it.

Wise-Use Guidelines

For adults who are not pregnant or nursing and do not have a history of cancer, kidney disease, high blood pressure, or congestive heart failure, bayberry root bark may be used cautiously in the amounts typically recommended.

You should use medicinal amounts of bayberry only in consultation with your doctor. If it causes minor discomfort, such as nausea or vomiting, reduce the dosage or stop using it altogether. Let your doctor know if you experience any unpleasant effects or if the symptoms for which you are using the herb do not improve significantly within 2 weeks.

Growing Information

Bayberry is native to the area from New Jersey to the Great Lakes and south to Florida and Texas. In the Southeast, it matures into an evergreen tree that reaches about 35 feet. Farther north, the plant does not grow that tall. Around the Great Lakes, mature plants rarely grow taller than 3 feet.

Bayberry has grayish bark; waxy branches; and dense, narrow, delicately toothed leaves dotted with resin glands, which produce a fragrant aroma when crushed. Yellow flowers appear in spring and produce nutlike fruits thickly covered with the wax once so highly valued in candle making.

Bayberry grows from seeds planted in spring or early fall. It prefers peaty soil under full sun but tolerates poorer, sandy soil along streams and in swampy areas. Plants require little care other than pruning. Harvest the root bark after a few years.

Bilberry

Family: Ericaceae; other members include azalea, blueberry, cranberry, and uva-ursi

Genus and species: *Vaccinium myrtillus*

Also known as: European blueberry, bogberry, and whortleberry

Parts used: Fruits

Bilberries, sometimes called European blueberries, are small blue berries that have been used in herbal medicine for at least 800 years. But it wasn't until World War II that the herb's real value was discovered—not by scientists, but by aviators.

Healing History

No one knows exactly when bilberries began to be used for healing. The first written recommendations date from the 12th century, when Hildegard of Bingen, an abbess, herbalist, and composer, recommended the berries to treat a variety of complaints, including respiratory problems.

Bilberries are astringent, meaning that they draw tissue together. Bilberry and other astringent herbs, such as tea, have been used for thousands of years to treat wounds, mouth sores, and diarrhea.

In Elizabethan England, a combination of bilberries and honey, called rob, was a popular remedy for diarrhea. Later, bilberries were typically prepared as jam, but their use for treating diarrhea continued. Over time, people who ate bilberries or the jam reported clearer vision, and folk herbalists began touting the berries for eyesight. Herbalists also recommended them to treat diabetes.

During World War II, British fliers ate bilberry jam before nighttime bombing missions. They swore that the berries prevented night blindness and sharpened their vision. After the war, researchers began studying the herb and discovered that it did indeed improve night vision and accelerate adjustment to glare.

Therapeutic Uses

Bilberries owe their color to high levels of potent antioxidant compounds called anthocyanosides. Antioxidants help prevent and reverse the cell damage inflicted by highly reactive oxygen molecules called free radicals. Scientists now agree that the damage produced by free radicals (oxidative damage) is an underlying cause of heart disease, many cancers, and other degenerative illnesses.

General disease prevention. Antioxidants—including vitamins C and E, the mineral selenium, carotenoids (including beta-carotene), and anthocyanosides—are found in plant foods. At the Jean Mayer USDA Human Nutrition Research Center on Aging at Tufts University, researchers analyzed the antioxidant content of dozens of common plant foods. Those richest in antioxidants turned out to be the dark-colored fruits and berries that contain generous amounts of anthocyanosides: blueberries, blackberries, raspberries, cherries, cranberries, red grapes, plums, raisins, and prunes.

The study did not include bilberries because they are not common in the United States, but they are about as rich in anthocyanosides as blueberries, which ranked near the top in terms of antioxidant content.

Cataracts. In the United States, cataracts are a major cause of vision impairment and blindness among older adults. The condition results from oxidative damage to the normally clear lens of the eye, which leads to the development of cloudy spots.

For reasons that remain unclear, the anthocyanosides in bilberry have unusually powerful effects on the eyes. In one Italian study, 50 people with early-stage cataracts were given bilberry extracts three times a day in combination with another antioxidant, vitamin E. The treatment stopped the progression of cataracts in 97 percent of the study participants.

Macular degeneration. The nerve-rich retina in the back of the eye plays a key role in vision. Macular degeneration involves deterioration of the macula, the most sensitive part of the retina. It's the part that's responsible for seeing what's directly in front of you (central vision) as well as fine detail.

In a European study, 31 people with various types of retinal problems, including macular degeneration, were given bilberry extract. Those with macular degeneration experienced significant vision improvement.

For another study, a South Dakota researcher recruited 10 men and women, ages 61 to 77, all with macular degeneration. He gave his volunteers a list of antioxidant-rich fruits and vegetables and asked them to eat two servings of fruit and three servings of vegetables from the list every day. He also instructed the participants to take supplements containing antioxidant vitamins and minerals plus extracts of bilberry and ginkgo (like bilberry, ginkgo is an antioxidant). One year later, all 10 people showed significant vision improvement in at least one eye.

Diabetic retinopathy. Diabetes damages all the blood vessels in the body, including the tiny capillaries in the eye that nourish the retina. When these capillaries develop diabetes-related damage, they leak blood into the eye, causing the blurred vision of retinopathy.

Bilberry's powerful antioxidants help strengthen retinal blood vessels, reducing blood leakage from the capillaries. In the European study mentioned above, people with diabetic retinopathy showed significant improvement when treated with bilberry.

Varicose veins. Varicose veins result from weakness of the biological "glue" that holds together the veins' cell structure. Once weakened, the veins stretch abnormally, allowing blood to pool in them. Varicose veins usually occur in the legs; when they affect the anal area, they're known as hemorrhoids.

Because bilberry strengthens the structure of veins, it can help treat varicose veins. When Italian researchers gave bilberry extract to 47 people with this condition, their symptoms improved significantly.

Diarrhea and mouth sores. Commission E, the expert panel that evaluates herbal medicines for the German counterpart of the FDA, endorses bilberry as a treatment for diarrhea and mouth sores—the herb's primary traditional uses.

Intriguing Possibilities

Some studies suggest that bilberry lowers blood sugar levels in people with diabetes, a finding that supports another of the herb's traditional uses. In addition, animal studies suggest that it helps prevent and treat ulcers.

Rx Recommendations

European herbalists have bred a variety of bilberry that is processed into a standardized extract containing 25 percent anthocyanosides. Check the labels of commercial preparations. In most studies that showed the herb's benefit, participants took one or two 80- to 160-milligram capsules of standardized bilberry extract three times a day. Follow the package directions.

The Safety Factor

You should use medicinal amounts of bilberry only in consultation with your doctor. The herb has no known side effects or interactions with drugs or other herbs. Still, allergic reactions are possible. If you notice any unusual symptoms, stop taking it.

Growing Information

Bilberry is a shrubby perennial that grows to about 18 inches in forested areas of Northern and Central Europe. The leaves are oval, bright green, and about 1 inch long. Red or pink bell-shaped flowers appear in spring, with blue-black or blue-purple berries forming in late summer and fall. Bilberry does not grow well in the United States and is rarely cultivated here.

Blackberry

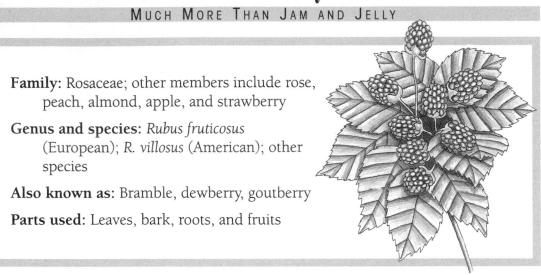

Family: Rosaceae; other members include rose, peach, almond, apple, and strawberry

Genus and species: *Rubus fruticosus* (European); *R. villosus* (American); other species

Also known as: Bramble, dewberry, goutberry

Parts used: Leaves, bark, roots, and fruits

If your acquaintance with the blackberry is confined to jam and jelly, it's time to branch out. The blackberry bush was once as highly prized for its medicinal leaves, bark, and roots as for its sweet fruit.

Until recently, however, blackberry had fallen from healing fashion. Now that's changing, based on research showing that the pigment that gives blackberries their color is a potent antioxidant with remarkable health benefits.

Healing History

The ancient Greeks relied on blackberry to treat gout. They were the only people to use the herb for this condition, but Greek medicine was so influential in Europe that well into the 18th century, the herb was called goutberry.

The ancient Chinese used the unripe berries to treat kidney problems, urinary incontinence, and impotence. The Romans chewed the leaves and bark for bleeding gums and drank a decoction for diarrhea.

Tenth-century Arab physicians considered the fruit to be an aphrodisiac (it isn't). During the Middle Ages, blackberry leaves were applied to the skin to soothe burns and scalds.

In his influential *Herbal*, 17th-century English herbalist Nicholas Culpeper described blackberry as "very binding" and good for "fevers, ulcers, putrid sores of the mouth and secret parts [genitals], spitting blood [tuberculosis], piles [hemorrhoids], stones of the kidney, too much flowing of women's courses [menstruation], and hot distempers of the head, eyes, and body."

Nineteenth-century American Eclectic physicians, forerunners of today's naturopaths, recommended a preparation made from blackberry fruit as "an excellent syrup which is of much service in dysentery, being pleasant to the taste, mitigating the sufferings of the patient, and ultimately effecting a cure." They also recommended blackberry leaves for gonorrhea, vaginal discharges, recovery from childbirth, and "cholera infantum," an old term for infant infectious diarrhea, which, in the days before antibiotics, was often fatal (and still is in many parts of the world).

Few contemporary herbalists recommended blackberry for anything beyond treating diarrhea until the mid-1990s, when scientists discovered the value of the pigment that gives the berries their dark color.

Therapeutic Uses

Contrary to the claims of Nicholas Culpeper, blackberry doesn't do much for the genitals. But the fruit and leaves of this herb help prevent and treat quite a few common ills.

Blackberries owe their healing power to high levels of anthocyanosides, compounds in the pigment that give the fruits their dark color. Anthocyanosides are potent antioxidants, helping to prevent and reverse the cell damage produced by highly reactive oxygen molecules called free radicals. Scientists now agree that the damage resulting from free radicals (oxidative damage) is the underlying cause of heart disease, many cancers, and other degenerative illnesses.

General disease prevention. Antioxidants such as vitamins C and E, the mineral selenium, carotenoids (including beta-carotene), and anthocyanosides are found only in plant foods. In a study conducted at the Jean Mayer USDA Human Nutrition Research Center on Aging at Tufts University, researchers assessed the antioxidant content of dozens of common plant foods. The scientists determined that the best sources of antioxidants are the dark-colored fruits that contain generous amounts of anthocyanosides, including blackberries, blueberries, cherries, red grapes, plums, raisins, and prunes.

Cataracts. Cataracts are a major cause of vision impairment and blindness among older Americans. The condition occurs when oxidative damage to the normally clear lens of the eye leads to the development of cloudy spots.

For reasons that scientists can't yet explain, anthocyanosides have unusually powerful effects on the eyes. Most of the research into their benefits has been performed in Europe using bilberry, a distinctly European fruit that's similar to the American blueberry and rich in the same pigment. But medicinal herb experts, including James A. Duke, Ph.D., retired USDA herbal medicine authority and author of several highly regarded herbal medicine references, agree that all fruits rich in anthocyanosides should produce similar benefits.

In one Italian study, 50 people with early stage cataracts were given bilberry extracts containing anthocyanosides three times a day, along with vitamin E, which is also an antioxidant. In 97 percent of the study participants, cataract progression stopped.

Macular degeneration. At the back of the eye is a nerve-rich structure called the retina, which plays an important role in vision. The most sensitive part of the retina, called the macula, is responsible for discerning what's directly in front of you (central vision) as well as fine detail. Macular degeneration involves deterioration of the macula, which can lead to the loss of central vision.

In a European study, 31 people with macular degeneration and various other types of retinal problems were treated with anthocyanosides in the form of bilberry extract. Those with macular degeneration showed significant vision improvement.

On this side of the Atlantic, a South Dakota researcher conducted a study involving 10 men and women between the ages of 61 and 77, all with macular degeneration. The researcher presented his volunteers with a list of antioxidant-rich fruits and vegetables, along with instructions to eat two servings of fruit and three servings of vegetables from the list every day. He also asked each person to take supplements containing antioxidant vitamins and minerals, plus bilberry (with its antioxidant anthocyanosides) and ginkgo (also an antioxidant). One year later, all 10 people showed significant vision improvement in at least one eye.

Diabetic retinopathy. Diabetes damages all of the blood vessels in the body, including the tiny capillaries in the eye that nourish the retina. The injured capillaries leak blood into the eye, setting the stage for the blurred vision of diabetic retinopathy.

With their powerful antioxidant action, anthocyanosides help strengthen retinal blood vessels, thus reducing leakage into the eye. In the European study mentioned above, the participants with diabetic retinopathy showed significant improvement when treated with anthocyanosides from bilberry.

Varicose veins. Varicose veins occur when the biological "glue" that holds together the veins' cell structure begins to weaken. This allows the veins to stretch abnormally, causing blood to pool in them. The condition can affect veins in the legs or in the anal area, where they're known as hemorrhoids.

Anthocyanosides can help treat varicose veins by strengthening their structure. In an Italian study, when 47 people received anthocyanosides (in the form of bilberry extract) for their varicose veins, they experienced significant improvement in their symptoms.

Diarrhea. Blackberry leaves contain large amounts of astringent tannins. In the digestive tract, the action of tannins helps control diarrhea and dysentery, confirming a traditional use for the herb. Commission E, the expert panel that evaluates herbal medicines for the German counterpart of the FDA, endorses blackberry leaf as a treatment for diarrhea.

Wounds. The astringent action of tannins also helps to constrict blood vessels and stop minor bleeding. This would tend to explain blackberry's traditional use as an external treatment for wounds. Blackberry thorns often cause minor cuts, so it's nice to know that first-aid is close at hand.

Mouth sores and sore throat. The astringent properties of blackberry leaf tea may help soothe mouth sores and sore throat.

Hemorrhoids. The herb's astringent nature may also help explain its traditional use as a hemorrhoid remedy.

Intriguing Possibilities

One study found that a strong infusion of blackberry leaves reduces blood sugar levels in rabbits with diabetes, hinting at the herb's possible value in diabetes management.

Research has shown that blackberry's close relative, raspberry, relaxes the uterus. Women might try blackberry for painful menstrual cramps.

Rx Recommendations

To help protect yourself against degenerative conditions such as heart disease, cancer, cataracts, and macular degeneration, eat blackberry fruit. It doesn't matter how you eat the berries—fresh, frozen, canned, or in preserves, jams, or jellies. In any form, blackberries contain generous amounts of anthocyanosides.

To treat diarrhea or soothe a sore throat, try an infusion, decoction, or tincture. To prepare an infusion, use 2 to 3 teaspoons of dried leaves per cup of boiling water. (If you prefer, you can use a handful of dried or fresh crushed berries or 1 to 2 teaspoons of dried powdered bark instead of dried leaves.) Steep for 10 to 20 minutes, strain, and add a bit of milk. Drink up to 3 cups a day.

For a decoction, use 1 teaspoon of powdered root per cup of water. Boil for 30 minutes and strain if you wish. Drink up to 1 cup a day with a bit of milk.

If you're using a homemade tincture, take up to 1 teaspoon up to twice a day.

To treat wounds or hemorrhoids, soak a clean cloth in a tincture or strong infusion and apply it externally.

When using commercial preparations, follow the package directions.

Do not give medicinal doses of blackberry leaf tea to children under age 2. For older children and adults over age 65, start with low-strength preparations and increase the strength if necessary.

The Safety Factor

Blackberries are considered safe for anyone who is not allergic to them, but questions have been raised about the tannins in medicinal preparations of blackberry leaf. In various studies, tannins show both procancer and anticancer actions. Their cancer-promoting action has attracted a lot more attention, primarily because of a study published in the *Journal of the National Cancer Institute*, which showed that tannins produce malignant tumors in laboratory animals. But tannins appear to also have an anticancer effect on some tumors in animals.

The relationship between tannins and human cancer remains unclear. In small quantities, such as the amount found in blackberry fruits, the compounds have never been proven to cause human tumors. It has been noted that Asians who drink large quantities of tea, which is high in tannins, show unusually high rates of stomach cancer. The British also love tea, but their rates of stomach cancer remain low. One reason may be that they drink their tea with milk, which neutralizes the tannins.

People with a history of cancer, particularly stomach or colon cancer, should exercise caution and not ingest blackberry leaf tea. Others should take no more than the recommended amount of infusion or decoction and, for extra safety, add a bit of milk.

In large amounts, tannins may cause stomach distress, nausea, and vomiting. Blackberry root bark contains the most tannins, followed by the leaves and, in distant third, the fruits. People with chronic gastrointestinal conditions, such as colitis, probably should not use the roots.

Wise-Use Guidelines

Anyone who is not allergic to blackberries may feel free to eat them. For adults who are not pregnant, nursing, or allergic, blackberry leaf is safe in the amounts typically recommended.

You should use medicinal amounts of blackberry leaf only in consultation with your doctor. If it causes minor discomfort, such as nausea or vomiting, reduce the dosage or stop using it altogether. Let your doctor know if you experience any unpleasant effects or if the symptoms for which you are using the herb do not improve significantly within 2 weeks.

Growing Information

Blackberry bushes grow wild around most of North America. They have long, tangled, thorny stems; lush foliage; and a profusion of berries that turn red as they ripen and become a juicy, purplish blue-black by midsummer.

Blackberry bushes are so vigorous and invasive that they quickly become a thick, thorny, impenetrable mass. Rooting them out is almost impossible, as any gardener who has tried can attest. Even when the bushes are removed, stray root fragments continue to send up new shoots. To minimize problems, plant this shrub in containers or surround its roots with sheet metal.

Blackberries grow easily from ½-inch root cuttings taken in autumn and stored through the winter in cool sand (around 50°F). Plant cuttings vertically 1 to 3 feet apart in 3 to 4 inches of soil.

Blackberries adapt to many conditions but grow best in loose, moist, rich soil amended with manure or finished compost. The plants flower in spring and bear fruit throughout the summer.

Harvest the leaves and roots anytime. For ease of harvesting the berries, train the branches along supports and prune them mercilessly.

Black Cohosh

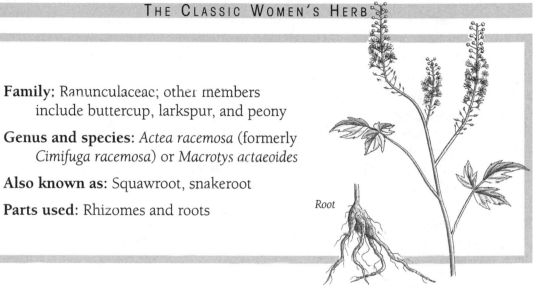

Family: Ranunculaceae; other members include buttercup, larkspur, and peony

Genus and species: *Actea racemosa* (formerly *Cimifuga racemosa*) or *Macrotys actaeoides*

Also known as: Squawroot, snakeroot

Parts used: Rhizomes and roots

Root

One of the 19th century's most popular patent medicines was Lydia E. Pinkham's Vegetable Compound, introduced in 1876 to treat "female weakness"—that is, premenstrual syndrome, menstrual cramps, and menopausal complaints. Pinkham's compound—developed by its namesake, a Lynn, Massachusetts, homemaker and practitioner of folk herbalism—contained several medicinal herbs. Chief among them was black cohosh, an age-old Algonquin treatment for gynecological complaints.

Pinkham's product also contained an enormous amount of alcohol. During the 19th century, respectable ladies did not drink liquor. Critics charged that the main weakness treated by the Vegetable Compound was a thirst for alcohol. Based on modern research findings, however, it seems clear that the black cohosh in Pinkham's product helped treat menstrual and menopausal symptoms.

After World War II, Pinkham's Vegetable Compound was reformulated to contain very little alcohol. Ironically, the revamped version also contained no black cohosh, the ingredient that supported the product's advertising as a remedy for female complaints.

Healing History

The *black* in black cohosh refers to the plant's dark medicinal roots. The word *cohosh* is Algonquin for "rough," another reference to the roots.

Native Americans boiled black cohosh's gnarled roots in water and drank the decoction for fatigue, sore throat, arthritis, and rattlesnake bite—hence another of the plant's popular names, snakeroot. But black cohosh was used primarily by Native American women for gynecological problems and for recovery after childbirth.

Wild black cohosh grew most profusely in the Ohio River valley, which seems fitting. After all, the herb was championed by 19th-century American Eclectic physicians, forerunners of today's naturopaths, whose medical school was located in Cincinnati on the banks of the Ohio. The Eclectics called the herb by a different name, macrotys, and recommended it for fever, rashes, insomnia, malaria, yellow fever, and all "hysterical" (gynecological) ailments. The Eclectic medical text *King's American Dispensatory* (1898) stated, "In dysmenorrhea [menstrual cramps], it is of greatest utility, being surpassed by no other drug."

Non-Eclectic ("regular") physicians remained unimpressed by black cohosh. But Lydia Pinkham sided with the Eclectics and included the herb in her compound.

Black cohosh does not grow in China, but Chinese physicians use several related plants to treat headache, measles, diarrhea, bleeding gums, and some gynecological problems. Homeopaths recommend microdoses of black cohosh for menstrual problems and childbirth.

Contemporary herbalists recommend the herb primarily for premenstrual syndrome (PMS), menstrual cramps, and menopausal symptoms. Since the mid-1990s, its popularity for women's health concerns has been growing, with many herb companies now marketing black cohosh products.

Therapeutic Uses

Black cohosh owes its medicinal properties to several compounds in its root: acetein, formononetin, and triterpenes. In the 1940s, German scientists discovered that these compounds are estrogenic, meaning that they mimic the effects of the female sex hormone estrogen. By the 1950s, a commercial extract of black cohosh, called Remifemin, was in wide use in Germany as a treatment for PMS, menstrual cramps, and menopausal hot flashes. (Herbal medicine is much more mainstream in Germany than in the United States.)

Most contemporary herbalists consider black cohosh estrogenic. Technically, the herb suppresses the secretion of luteinizing hormone (LH), which is produced by the pituitary gland. But this produces an estrogenic effect.

Premenstrual syndrome (PMS). Germany's Commission E, the expert panel that evaluates herbal medicines for the German counterpart of the FDA, endorses black cohosh as a treatment for PMS. The panel's position is based on more than 40 years of testimonials and clinical experience in Germany.

Menstrual cramps. For the same reasons, Commission E also endorses black cohosh as a treatment for menstrual cramps.

Menopausal complaints. Most studies of black cohosh have examined the herb as a treatment for hot flashes and other menopausal discomforts. From 1982 through 1991, eight clinical trials involving a total of 1,170 women were conducted by German researchers. The studies differed somewhat in design, but all of them investigated the effectiveness of the black cohosh extract Remifemin (40 drops twice a day or two 40-milligram tablets daily for 6 to 12 weeks).

All of the trials produced the same results with regard to relief of menopausal symptoms: fewer, briefer hot flashes; less vaginal dryness; improved mood; and relief from fatigue. In the largest of the studies, involving 629 women, 80 percent of the participants reported significant improvement in their discomfort within a month. Many experienced complete relief within 6 to 8 weeks. The herb caused no significant side effects. Commission E endorses black cohosh as a treatment for menopausal discomforts.

Hormone replacement alternative. The ovaries manufacture most of the estrogen in women's bodies. During menopause, production of the hormone slowly declines. Among women of any age who have their ovaries removed, estrogen production also declines, but more suddenly.

To make up for the loss of estrogen, mainstream physicians prescribe hormone replacement therapy. German researchers compared pharmaceutical hormone replacement with black cohosh (two tablets of Remifemin twice a day) in 60 women who had their ovaries removed before age 40. After 6 months, both groups reported similar satisfaction with their treatment, but the black cohosh caused no significant side effects.

High blood pressure. A study published in *Nature* revealed that black cohosh reduces blood pressure by opening blood vessels in the limbs (peripheral vasodilation). The herb may help manage high blood pressure, but consult your physician before using it for this purpose.

Intriguing Possibilities

One study found that black cohosh relieves pain and has anti-inflammatory activity, possibly explaining its traditional use as a treatment for arthritis. Another report suggests that it helps preserve bone, promoting its potential use in osteoporosis prevention. Other research involving the herb showed cholesterol and blood pressure reduction, anti-ulcer effects, and blood

sugar regulation, pointing toward the herb's possible value in controlling diabetes.

More research needs to be done to determine whether black cohosh will prove useful in treating any of those conditions. Other preliminary findings of animal studies hint that the herb may have antibiotic, sedative, and stomach-soothing properties.

Rx Recommendations

For a decoction, use ½ teaspoon of powdered root per cup of water and boil for 30 minutes, then strain if you wish. Let cool before drinking. Black cohosh has an unpleasant aroma and a sharp, bitter taste; you can add lemon and honey and/or mix the herb with a beverage herb. Take 2 tablespoons every few hours, up to 1 cup a day.

As a homemade tincture, take 2 to 4 teaspoons twice a day.

When using commercial preparations, follow the package directions

For children over age 2 and adults over age 65, start with low-strength preparations and increase the strength if necessary.

The Safety Factor

If you want to use black cohosh, double-check the label to be sure that you have black cohosh, not blue cohosh. The latter should not be used by most women. (For more information about blue cohosh, see page 94.)

Nineteenth-century researchers gave laboratory animals doses of black cohosh 90 times the recommended human equivalent. They reported that the herb may cause dizziness, diarrhea, vomiting, tremors, depressed heart rate, miscarriage, and other worrisome effects. These studies continue to be cited today. A 1986 FDA report, for example, warned of black cohosh causing potentially hazardous side effects.

On the other hand, in the eight studies that examined black cohosh as a treatment for menopausal discomforts, no significant side effects turned up. In fact, the only side effect was stomach upset, which was reported by 7 percent of the participants in the largest study. The consensus of the modern scientific research is that black cohosh is safe when used in the recommended doses for periods of up to 6 months. No studies of longer-term use have been completed to date.

Wise-Use Guidelines

Estrogen, and presumably estrogenic herbs, can stimulate the growth of breast cancer. But black cohosh, which is an LH suppressant, does not appear to have this effect, according to research presented at a 1999 conference on plant estrogens at the University of Ghent in Belgium. Nonetheless, if you have breast cancer, are a breast cancer survivor, or have a family history of the disease, you should consult your doctor before taking black cohosh.

In addition, women who are pregnant or nursing or whose physicians have advised them not to take birth control pills should probably not use black cohosh.

If you are taking postmenopausal hormone replacement therapy, consult your physician before taking black cohosh.

Let your doctor know if you experience any unpleasant effects or if the symptoms for which you are using the herb do not improve significantly within 4 weeks.

Growing Information

Black cohosh is a leafy perennial that reaches 9 feet. It has knotty black roots and a smooth stem with large, toothed, compound leaves and small, multiple white flowers that develop in midsummer on long projections called racemes.

Black cohosh grows from seeds sown in spring or root divisions taken in spring or fall. Harvest the roots in fall after the fruits have ripened and cut them lengthwise to dry.

Black Haw

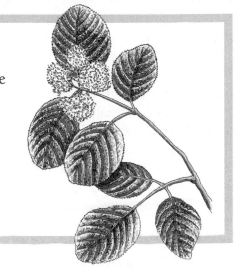

Family: Caprifoliaceae; other members include honeysuckle and elder

Genus and species: *Viburnum prunifolium*

Also known as: Viburnum

Part used: Bark

Indiana poet James Whitcomb Riley wrote, "What is sweeter, after all / Than black haws in early fall?" He was referring to the shrub's blue-black fruits, which are the size of small olives.

It's the reddish brown bark of this native American shrub, however, that has a long folk history as a remedy for gynecological complaints—a history that has been confirmed by modern science.

Native American women drank a decoction of black haw bark for menstrual cramps, childbirth recovery, and menopausal discomforts, but especially to prevent miscarriage. Later, Southern white women and their black slaves adopted these uses as well.

Healing History

Before the Civil War, many slave owners forced slave women to take black haw to prevent them from ending their pregnancies with abortion-inducing herbs. Slaves were a valuable asset, and slaveholders wanted the women to bear as many children as possible. The women were often raped by plantation owners or foremen, and many attempted to terminate the resulting pregnancies as a quiet protest against slavery.

A popular abortion-inducing herb was cotton root, which was readily available to slaves on Southern plantations. As explained in *King's American Dispensatory* (1898), the textbook of the 19th-century American Eclectic physicians who were forerunners of today's naturopaths, "It was customary for planters to compel female slaves to drink an infusion of black haw daily whilst pregnant to prevent abortion from taking the cotton root."

An Eclectic physician from Mississippi introduced black haw to the North, where it quickly became an herbal mainstay for gynecological complaints. The Eclectics valued it highly: "As a uterine tonic, it is unquestionably of great utility . . . for menstrual pains . . . and a good remedy for menopause. . . . But the condition for which black haw is most valued is threatened abortion. By its quieting effect upon the irritable womb, women who have been previously unable to go to term have been aided to pass through pregnancy without mishaps."

Modern herbalists continue to recommend black haw for menstrual cramps and threatened abortion. Some herbals encourage women to drink black haw tea throughout pregnancy, but this turns out not to be a good idea.

Therapeutic Uses

Here is another case where modern science supports folk wisdom, or at least some of it. Scientists have confirmed that black haw may be a good treatment for certain gynecological complaints.

Menstrual cramps. A study published in the British journal *Nature* found that black haw contains a uterine relaxant called scopoletin, thus supporting the herb's value in treating menstrual cramps. In Germany, where herbal medicine is more mainstream than in the United States, black haw preparations are widely recommended for menstrual cramps. These products are not available in the United States, but the herb itself is fairly easy to obtain.

Miscarriage. Black haw has been used for centuries to prevent miscarriage. As a uterine relaxant, it may indeed do the job. Unfortunately, it also contains salicin, a close chemical relative of aspirin. Because aspirin has been linked to birth defects, pregnant women should not take

black haw, except possibly under a physician's supervision to prevent premature delivery.

Fever and pain (including headache and arthritis). The aspirin-like chemical in black haw may reduce fever and relieve pain.

Rx Recommendations

For relief of menstrual cramps, fever, headache, and general aches and pains, prepare a decoction using 2 teaspoons of dried black haw bark per cup of water. Boil for 10 minutes, then strain and cool. Drink up to 3 cups a day. The herb has an extremely bitter taste, so you may want to add lemon and honey or mix it with a beverage tea.

As a homemade tincture, take up to 2 teaspoons three times a day.

When using commercial preparations, follow the package directions.

Do not give black haw to children under age 2 or to children under age 16 who have colds, flu, or chickenpox. For other children and adults over age 65, start with low-strength preparations and increase the strength if necessary.

The Safety Factor

Like aspirin, the salicin in black haw is a pain reliever (analgesic), which may contribute to the herb's ability to relieve menstrual cramping. But aspirin has been implicated as a cause of birth defects in the children of women who take it while pregnant. Aspirin is most hazardous to the unborn early in pregnancy. Recognizing this, the classic British herbal *Potter's New Cyclopaedia of Botanical Drugs and Preparations* says that black haw should be used only during the final 5 weeks of pregnancy as a means of preventing potential premature delivery.

Any woman facing a possible premature birth should discuss her situation with her obstetrician. Drugs (including herbs) are a last resort and should be used only with the consent of a doctor.

Do not give black haw to children under age 16 who have fevers related to colds, flu, or chickenpox. The salicin may raise the risk of Reye's syndrome, a rare but potentially fatal childhood disease.

Large doses of black haw may cause upset stomach, nausea, vomiting, and/or ringing in the ears (tinnitus), especially in people who are sensitive to aspirin.

Wise Use Guidelines

For adults who are not pregnant or nursing, black haw is considered safe in the amounts typically recommended.

You should use medicinal amounts of black haw only in consultation with your doctor. If it causes minor discomfort, such as stomach upset or ringing in the ears, reduce the dosage or stop using it altogether. Let your doctor know if you experience any unpleasant effects or if menstrual cramps do not improve significantly within 2 menstrual cycles.

Growing Information

In the North, black haw is a deciduous spreading shrub with reddish brown bark. In the South, it becomes a small tree. The leaves are pointed, serrated ovals resembling plum leaves. They turn red in the fall.

Depending on location, black haw blooms from early spring to summer. The flowers are large, clustered, white, and showy.

Black haw grows best in rich, moist, well-drained soil under full sun. It tolerates poorer soil and partial shade as long as it gets adequate moisture.

The branch bark may be collected in summer; the trunk bark should be collected in fall. Dry it in the shade.

Blue Cohosh

Family: Berberidaceae; other members include may apple, mandrake, and barberry

Genus and species: *Caulophyllum thalictroides*

Also known as: Papoose root and blue berry

Parts used: Roots

Native Americans referred to blue cohosh as papoose root, believing that it triggered labor and hastened childbirth. They were right. Science has proven that the herb contains a compound that can induce labor. This substance is so powerful, in fact, that blue cohosh should be used only under medical supervision.

Blue cohosh is not related to black cohosh. They belong to different botanical families, but the Native Americans used both as gynecological herbs and called them both cohosh. The word *cohosh* is Algonquin for "rough," a reference to the plant's gnarled roots. *Blue* reflects the herb's bluish stem and dark blue berries.

Healing History

Besides using blue cohosh to induce labor, menstruation, and abortion, Native Americans relied on it to treat sore throat, hiccups, infant colic, epilepsy, and arthritis. Some of the women even drank a strong decoction as a contraceptive.

Nineteenth-century American Eclectic physician John King popularized blue cohosh as a labor inducer and menstruation promoter in the first edition of his *King's American Dispensatory* in the 1850s. The Eclectics, forerunners of today's naturopaths, also prescribed the herb for menstrual cramps, breast pain, bladder and kidney infections, insomnia, bronchitis, and nausea.

Non-Eclectic ("regular") physicians never adopted blue cohosh, but it was listed in the *U.S. Pharmacopoeia*, a standard drug reference, from 1882 to 1905 as a labor inducer.

Modern herbals recommend blue cohosh as a labor inducer and menstruation promoter. Some herbalists also suggest it for asthma, anxiety, coughs, arthritis, and high blood pressure.

Therapeutic Uses

Blue cohosh's traditional uses in gynecology appear to stand up to scientific scrutiny.

Labor inducement. Researchers have discovered that a chemical in blue cohosh, caulosaponin, provokes strong uterine contractions. This finding supports the herb's traditional use among Native Americans.

Caulosaponin also narrows the arteries that supply blood to the heart, and blue cohosh has produced heart damage in laboratory animals. Heart damage in humans seems quite possible from overdose.

On the other hand, the herb does not appear to be significantly more hazardous than oxytocin (Pitocin), the standard drug used to induce labor. The drug may also cause heart damage and other serious side effects, including death of the mother and baby.

The use of oxytocin requires constant professional monitoring. Blue cohosh should also be used under strict medical supervision. If you'd like to use it at term, discuss your desire with your obstetrician and/or midwife and take it *only* with your doctor's consent and supervision.

Menstruation promotion. As a powerful uterine stimulant, blue cohosh could certainly trigger menstruation, but women should not use it for this purpose. It's too powerful, and its potential side effects are too serious.

Intriguing Possibilities

Researchers in India have discovered tantalizing evidence that Native Americans may have been on the right track in using blue cohosh as a contraceptive. The herb appears to inhibit ovulation in animals, according to a report published in the *Journal of Reproduction and Fertility*.

European researchers have identified some antibiotic and immune-stimulating properties in blue cohosh, possibly explaining the herb's use by Eclectic physicians as a treatment for bladder and kidney infections.

Blue cohosh also has anti-inflammatory activity, lending credence to its traditional use as a treatment for arthritis.

Medicinal Myth

Despite its traditional reputation as a treatment for high blood pressure, studies show that blue cohosh is more likely to cause this serious condition than to control it.

Rx Recommendations

Blue cohosh is a powerful herb that should be taken only under the supervision of a qualified herbal practitioner or a physician experienced in herbal medicine. As a decoction, it tastes somewhat sweet at first, then bitter and unpleasant.

The Safety Factor

No one with high blood pressure, heart disease, diabetes, glaucoma, or a history of stroke should use blue cohosh, nor should women who are pregnant or trying to conceive take it. In addition to the side effects already mentioned, animal studies have found that blue cohosh causes severe birth defects when taken early in pregnancy. It should be used only at term to induce labor, and then only under medical supervision.

As a powder, blue cohosh root irritates mucous membranes. Handle it with care, and be careful not to inhale the powder or introduce it into your eyes.

Growing Information

Blue cohosh is not a garden herb, but it's easy to recognize in early spring in forests from the Appalachians to the Mississippi. Before other forest-floor plants have shown signs of new life, blue cohosh's blue-purple stem and single large leaf have risen 2 to 3 feet. As spring turns to summer, blue cohosh produces three branches with three compound leaves each.

In summer, the plant produces small yellowish flowers and dark blue berries, which are poisonous and potentially fatal to children. Make sure that they do not eat the berries.

Boneset

Family: Compositae; other members include daisy, dandelion, and marigold

Genus and species: *Eupatorium perfoliaturn*

Also known as: Feverwort, agueweed, and sweat plant

Parts used: Leaves and flowers

Let's clear up one matter right away: Boneset has nothing to do with mending broken bones. The herb may help treat minor viral and bacterial illnesses by revving up the immune system's response to infection.

Boneset's name comes from its traditional use as a treatment for breakbone fever, an old term for dengue (pronounced *DENG-ee*) fever. Dengue is a mosquito-borne viral disease that causes muscle pain so intense that people imagine that their bones are breaking, hence the condition's traditional name.

Today, dengue is rare in the United States, except in southern Florida and Texas and among overseas travelers, who sometimes return from the tropics with it. Ironically, boneset has never been shown to provide significant relief from dengue fever.

Healing History

Native Americans introduced boneset to early colonists as a sweat inducer, an old treatment for fever. They used the herb for all fever-producing illnesses, including influenza, cholera, dengue, malaria, and typhoid. This is how boneset earned its other popular names: feverwort, sweat plant, and agueweed (*ague* is an archaic term for fever).

Native Americans also used boneset to relieve arthritis and to treat colds, indigestion, constipation, and loss of appetite.

White settlers adopted boneset so enthusiastically that it became one of early America's most popular healing herbs. During the Civil War, soldiers used it not only to treat fever but also as a tonic to keep them healthy. (Modern science shows this is not a good idea; see "The Safety Factor" on page 99.)

In his classic book *American Medicinal Plants*, Dr. C. F. Millspaugh had this to say about boneset: "There is probably no plant more extensively or frequently used than this. The attic or woodshed of almost every farm house has bunches hanging from the rafters, ready for immediate use should some family member or neighbor be taken with a cold."

Dr. Millspaugh also considered boneset excellent against malaria, a major health problem in 19th-century America. He wrote that he'd seen the herb cure cases of malaria that didn't respond to Peruvian cinchona bark, the source of the antimalarial drug quinine.

Boneset was listed as a treatment for fever in the *U.S. Pharmacopoeia*, a standard drug reference, from 1820 through 1916 and in the *National Formulary*, the pharmacists' reference, from 1926 through 1950. But the herb fell from favor over time, replaced by another fever fighter, aspirin.

Contemporary herbalists continue to recommend boneset for fever. In his *Holistic Herbal*, medical herbalist David Hoffmann describes it as "perhaps the best remedy for influenza."

Therapeutic Uses

Modern critics of herbs tend to ridicule boneset as passionately as physicians praised it a century ago. One expert says, "It simply doesn't work." Another claims, "Boneset lacks therapeutic merit." A third writes, "In view of [boneset's] singular lack of effectiveness, it seems incredible that the plant held official status from 1820 to 1950."

The critics have a point: Boneset has never been shown to suppress fever as well as aspirin. But several studies seem to suggest that the herb has some therapeutic value after all.

Colds and flu. European studies show that boneset helps treat minor viral and bacterial infections by stimulating white blood cells to more effectively destroy disease-causing microorganisms. In Germany, where herbal medicine is more mainstream than in the United States, physicians currently use boneset to treat viral infections such as colds and flu.

Arthritis. One study suggests that boneset is mildly anti-inflammatory, lending some support to its traditional use in treating arthritis.

Intriguing Possibility

Studies conducted worldwide suggest that possible immune-stimulating compounds in boneset have anticancer effects. More research is needed, however, before the herb can be used to treat tumors.

Medicinal Myth

Its traditional use notwithstanding, boneset has never been shown to be effective against dengue fever or malaria.

Rx Recommendations

To treat colds, flu, and arthritis and relieve minor inflammation, use an infusion or tincture of boneset. To prepare an infusion, use 1 to 2 teaspoons of dried leaves per cup of boiling water and steep for 10 to 20 minutes. Drink up to 3 cups a day. You'll find the taste very bitter and astringent, so you can add sugar or honey and lemon or mix it with an herbal beverage tea.

As a homemade tincture, take $\frac{1}{2}$ to 1 teaspoon up to three times a day.

When using commercial preparations, follow the package directions.

Do not give boneset to children under age 2. For older children and adults over age 65, start with low-strength preparations and increase the strength if necessary.

The Safety Factor

In large amounts, boneset may cause nausea, vomiting, and violent diarrhea. In addition, the herb contains pyrrolizidine alkaloids (PAs), chemicals that produce liver damage and liver tumors in laboratory animals when administered in large amounts. Boneset's effect on human cancer, if any, is unclear, because the plant also contains anticancer substances.

The PAs in some healing herbs, such as comfrey (see page 152), have caused liver damage in a few cases in which people have taken more than the recommended dose for long periods of time. It's not a good idea to take boneset frequently as a tonic.

Also, do not eat fresh boneset. It contains tremerol, a toxic chemical that causes nausea, vomiting, weakness, muscle tremors, increased respiration, and possibly—at high doses—even coma and death. Drying the herb eliminates the tremerol and the possibility of poisoning.

Wise-Use Guidelines

The FDA lists boneset as an herb of undefined safety. For adults who are not pregnant or nursing and do not have a history of alcoholism, cancer, or liver disease, boneset is considered safe in the amounts typically recommended.

You should use medicinal amounts of boneset only in consultation with your doctor. If it causes minor discomfort, such as stomach upset or a laxative effect, reduce the dosage or stop using it altogether. Let your doctor know if you experience any unpleasant effects or if the symptoms for which you are using the herb do not improve significantly within 2 weeks.

Do not take boneset for more than 2 weeks at a time, and do not exceed the recommended amounts.

Growing Information

Boneset is easy to identify because its long, narrow, pointed leaf pairs are not distinct; rather, they are connected and pierced by the stem. The herb has round, erect, hairy, hollow stems that grow to 5 feet, then split into three branches, each of which produces tiny, densely clustered white to bluish florets from midsummer through fall.

A hardy perennial, boneset grows easily from seeds planted in spring or root divisions planted in spring or fall. It prefers rich, moist, well-drained soil under full sun but tolerates poorer soil and partial shade.

Harvest it as it flowers by cutting the entire plant a few inches above the ground.

Buchu

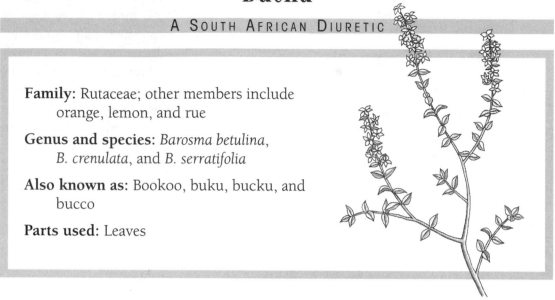

Family: Rutaceae; other members include orange, lemon, and rue

Genus and species: *Barosma betulina*, *B. crenulata*, and *B. serratifolia*

Also known as: Bookoo, buku, bucku, and bucco

Parts used: Leaves

Buchu is southern Africa's contribution to American herbal healing. The leaves of this 5-foot shrub contain an oil that increases urine production.

Healing History

The native people of what is now Namibia and South Africa used buchu for urinary problems long before they had any contact with Europeans. In the 17th century, when Dutch (Afrikaner) colonists settled the region, they adopted buchu as a treatment for urinary tract infections, kidney stones, arthritis, cholera, and muscle aches.

Later, English settlers adopted buchu and relied on it to treat so many illnesses that medical botanists now claim that it has been used for "almost every disease that afflicts mankind."

In 1847, New York patent medicine entrepreneur Henry T. Helmbold introduced Helmbold's Compound Extract of Buchu as a remedy for urinary problems, kidney stones, and "diseases arising from imprudence [venereal diseases]." The American public responded as enthusiastically as the African colonists had. Helmbold grew rich and called himself Helmbold, the Buchu King.

Therapeutic Uses

The Buchu King has long been forgotten, but herbalists have considered buchu an effective diuretic ever since.

Premenstrual syndrome (PMS). Many women complain of bloating from water retention before their periods. Buchu is an ingredient in several teas marketed in health food stores to relieve the bloating of PMS.

Urinary tract infections. Most modern

herbals continue to recommend buchu as a treatment for urinary tract infections. One study of the herb's effects on the bacteria that cause the infections showed no benefit. Still, herbal experts stand behind buchu as an infection fighter.

High blood pressure and congestive heart failure. Physicians prescribe diuretics to treat high blood pressure and congestive heart failure. These are serious conditions requiring professional care, so consult your physician about including buchu in your treatment plan.

Medicinal Myth

For years, buchu was an ingredient in herbal weight-loss products. Diuretics can cause temporary loss of excess water weight, but no science-based weight-loss program endorses the use of diuretics for permanent weight control.

Rx Recommendations

For relief of premenstrual bloating, try an infusion or tincture of buchu. You might also try these preparations for relief of chronic urinary tract infections.

To prepare an infusion, use 1 to 2 teaspoons of dried, crumbled leaves per cup of boiling water and steep for 10 to 20 minutes. Drink up to 3 cups a day. Buchu has a minty aroma and a pleasant, minty taste.

As a homemade tincture, take ½ to 1 teaspoon up to three times a day.

When using commercial preparations, follow the package directions.

Do not give buchu to children under age 2.

For older children and adults over age 65, start with low-strength preparations and increase the strength if necessary.

The Safety Factor

Diuretics deplete the body's stores of potassium, an important nutrient. If you take buchu, you should increase your consumption of foods rich in potassium, such as bananas and fresh vegetables.

Women who are pregnant or nursing should not take diuretics without a physician's approval.

Wise-Use Guidelines

The FDA views buchu as safe. No harmful effects have been reported in association with the herb's use. For adults who are not pregnant or nursing and are not taking other diuretics, it is considered safe in the amounts typically recommended.

You should use medicinal amounts of buchu only in consultation with your doctor. If it causes minor discomfort, such as stomach upset or diarrhea, decrease the dosage or stop using it altogether. Let your doctor know if you experience any unpleasant effects or if the symptoms for which you are using the herb do not improve significantly within 2 weeks.

Growing Information

This 5-foot shrub with finely toothed opposite or alternate leaves is not grown in the United States.

Buckthorn

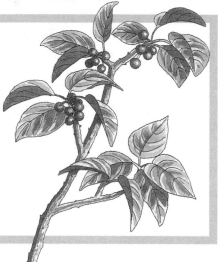

Family: Rhamnaceae; other members include cascara sagrada

Genus and species: *Rhamnus cathartica* and *R. frangula*

Also known as: Purging buckthorn, frangula, and alder buckthorn

Parts used: Berries and bark

The species name for buckthorn, *cathartica*, is no joke. The herb is a potent laxative—so powerful, in fact, that authorities recommend using it only as a last resort, when other, gentler laxatives have failed.

Healing History

Buckthorn became popular in herbal healing in Europe around the 13th century. At the time, physicians believed that the key to curing disease lay in purging "foul humors." Not surprisingly, powerful laxatives were widely prescribed.

Buckthorn was a favorite because it produced quick, reliable results. Of course, it didn't cure any diseases. All it did was produce dramatic purgative results and leave people with intestinal cramps.

Down through the ages, herbalists have recommended buckthorn for treating jaundice, he-morrhoids, gout, arthritis, and promoting menstruation. The herb also has a long history as a cancer treatment. In America, it was an ingredient in the popular but highly controversial Hoxsey Cancer Formula (see page 32).

Therapeutic Uses

Buckthorn doesn't treat jaundice or arthritis, and it's more likely to aggravate hemorrhoids than to help them. But its laxative action is so powerful that it's considered a purgative.

Constipation. No one disputes the laxative effect of buckthorn. It has been an ingredient in pharmaceutical laxatives and herbal laxatives. Commission E, the expert panel that evaluates herbal medicines for the German counterpart of the FDA, approves the herb as a laxative.

Buckthorn contains chemicals called an-thraquinones. They're dramatic purgatives—too dramatic for most people. That's why buckthorn should be considered a last-resort treatment for constipation.

Intriguing Possibility

Harry Hoxsey may have been on the right track. Buckthorn has an anti-tumor effect, according to research published in the *Journal of the National Cancer Institute.* Other studies must be conducted, however, before the herb can be used as a cancer treatment.

Rx Recommendations

In Germany, physicians prescribe an infusion containing ½ teaspoon each of dried buckthorn bark, fennel seeds, and chamomile flowers (which soothe the stomach). Steep the blend in 1 cup of boiling water for 10 minutes, then strain. Drink it before going to bed. You'll find the taste initially sweet, then bitter.

If you prefer a decoction, boil 1 teaspoon of dried buckthorn in 3 cups of water. Steep for 30 minutes, then strain. Drink it cool, 1 tablespoon at a time, before going to bed.

As a homemade tincture, take ½ teaspoon before going to bed.

When using commercial preparations, follow the package directions.

The Safety Factor

Because of buckthorn's powerful laxative action, people who have chronic gastrointestinal problems, including ulcers, colitis, Crohn's disease, diverticulitis, and hemorrhoids, should not use it. It's also not appropriate for women who are pregnant or nursing.

Don't take buckthorn for more than 2 weeks at a time. If you use it for too long, it causes lazy bowel syndrome, an inability to have bowel movements without chemical stimulation.

If you use bulk buckthorn, be sure that it has been dried thoroughly. Otherwise, it causes vomiting, severe abdominal pain, and violent diarrhea. Most herbalists recommend drying the berries or bark for at least a year (some say 2 years) before using them. Commercial preparations use aged bark.

You can artificially dry fresh buckthorn by baking it at 250°F for several hours. If you experience nausea and abdominal distress after taking the herb, seek professional medical attention immediately.

Wise-Use Guidelines

Adults who are not pregnant or nursing, do not have any of the gastrointestinal conditions mentioned above, and are not using other laxatives may take buckthorn very cautiously for short periods of time in the amounts typically recommended.

You should use medicinal amounts of buckthorn only in consultation with your doctor. If violent diarrhea or intestinal cramps occur, decrease the dosage or stop using it altogether. Let your doctor know if you experience any unpleasant effects or if constipation does not improve within a few days.

Growing Information

Buckthorn is a shrub or small tree that reaches about 20 feet. It has shiny, dark green leaves and produces black, pea-size berries. It is not a garden plant.

Burdock

Family: Compositae; other members include daisy, dandelion, and marigold

Genus and species: *Arctium lappa*

Also known as: Great burdock and burr

Parts used: Primarily roots; also leaves and seeds

Burdock (the name is a combination of *bur-*, for its tenacious burrs, and *-dock*, an Old English term for "plant") seems to reach out and grab anything that comes near it. The same could be said for its place in modern herbal healing. While many scientists have dismissed burdock as useless, it seems destined to hang on as a healing herb, particularly as a potential treatment for cancer.

Healing History

Burdock has had its ups and downs in the past. When it wasn't being reviled as a weed, it was being recommended as a healing treatment for a surprising variety of conditions.

Early Chinese physicians considered burdock a remedy for colds, flu, throat infections, and pneumonia. India's traditional Ayurvedic healers used it in similar ways.

The medieval German abbess/herbalist Hildegard of Bingen prescribed burdock to treat cancerous tumors. And during the 14th century in Europe, the herb's leaves were pounded into wine and used to treat leprosy.

England's overly imaginative 17th-century herbalist Nicholas Culpeper recommended burdock for uterine prolapse, a condition in which the ligaments supporting the uterus weaken and cause it to fall into the vagina. Culpeper's bizarre prescription: Place burdock on the crown of the head to draw the womb back up.

Later European herbalists prescribed burdock root for fever, cancer, eczema, psoriasis, acne, dandruff, gout, ringworm, skin infections, syphilis, gonorrhea, and problems associated with childbirth. And America's 19th-century Eclectic physicians, forerunners of today's naturopaths, considered the herb an excellent diuretic. They prescribed it for urinary tract infections, kidney problems, and painful urination in addition to skin infections and arthritis.

Centuries after Hildegard recommended burdock for cancer, the herb's reputation as a tumor treatment spread to Russia, China, India, and the Americas. From the 1930s to the 1950s, burdock was an ingredient in the alternative cancer treatment marketed by ex–coal miner Harry Hoxsey (see page 32).

Contemporary herbalists have abandoned burdock as a cancer treatment (perhaps prematurely). But they continue to recommend it for skin problems, wound healing, urinary tract infections, arthritis, sciatica, ulcers, and even anorexia nervosa.

Therapeutic Uses

Many modern herb experts give a thumbs-down to burdock as a healing herb. In *Natural Product Medicine*, Ara Der Marderosian, Ph.D., and Lawrence Liberti write, "There is little evidence to suggest burdock is useful in treatment of any human disease." And in *Tyler's Honest Herbal*, Varro E. Tyler, Ph.D., writes, "However, despite its long folkloric use, no solid evidence exists that burdock exhibits any useful therapeutic activity."

Most traditional claims for burdock have not withstood scientific scrutiny. The herb does not treat leprosy, arthritis, uterine prolapse, or congestive heart failure. Still, several studies suggest that it may prove to be therapeutic after all.

Infections. German researchers have discovered that fresh burdock root contains chemicals called polyacetylenes, which kill disease-causing bacteria and fungi. Although dried burdock has smaller amounts of these chemicals, their presence may help explain the herb's traditional use against the fungal infection ringworm as well as against several types of bacterial infections, including gonorrhea, skin infections, and urinary tract infections.

Still, burdock is no substitute for professional medical treatment of fungal and bacterial infections.

Intriguing Possibilities

Burdock has been used extensively around the world as a cancer treatment. Several studies have shown that certain substances in the herb do, in fact, have anti-tumor activity.

An article published in *Chemotherapy* identified arctigenin, a chemical in burdock, as an "inhibitor of experimental tumor growth." And a study reported in *Mutation Research* determined that burdock decreases mutations in cells exposed to mutation-causing chemicals. (Most substances that cause genetic mutations also cause cancer.)

Of course, cancer requires professional care. If you'd like to try burdock in conjunction with standard therapy, discuss it with your physician.

Finally, burdock has an as-yet-unexplained anti-poisoning effect. Experimental animals that were fed the herb were somehow protected against several chemicals known to be toxic.

In view of these tantalizing findings, let's hope that scientists cling to burdock research as tenaciously as the plant's burrs cling to just about anything.

Rx Recommendations

If your physician gives the okay, you can try burdock in conjunction with other cancer therapy. You can also incorporate the herb into treatment regimens for certain infections, such as gonorrhea and those that affect the urinary tract. Use it as a decoction or tincture.

To prepare a decoction, boil 1 teaspoon of root in 3 cups of water for 30 minutes, then let cool. Drink up to 3 cups a day. Burdock has a sweet taste similar to celery root.

As a homemade tincture, take ½ to 1 teaspoon up to three times a day.

When using commercial preparations, follow the package directions.

Do not give burdock to children under age 2. For older children and adults over age 65, start with low-strength preparations and increase the strength if necessary.

The Safety Factor

No one questioned the safety of burdock until the *Journal of the American Medical Association* linked the herb to one case of poisoning that could have proved fatal. A woman who drank a strong decoction experienced blurred vision, dry mouth, and hallucinations, all classic symptoms of atropine poisoning.

Burdock does not contain atropine, but belladonna, a plant that looks similar, does. Presumably, some belladonna accidentally adulterated the woman's burdock.

One case of adulteration is not cause for alarm. Still, if you decide to try burdock, be sure to buy it from a reliable source. And if you develop any of the symptoms of atropine poisoning mentioned above, seek emergency medical treatment immediately.

The *Toxicology of Botanical Medicines* identifies burdock as a uterine stimulant. For this reason, it should not be used by pregnant women.

Allergic reactions to burdock are possible.

Wise-Use Guidelines

The FDA lists burdock as an herb of undefined safety. Except for that one case of atropine poisoning, however, it apparently has never caused significant problems. For adults who are not pregnant or nursing, burdock is considered safe in the amounts typically recommended.

You should use medicinal amounts of burdock only in consultation with your doctor. If it causes minor discomfort, such as stomach upset or diarrhea, decrease the dosage or stop taking it altogether. Let your doctor know if you experience any unpleasant effects or if the symptoms for which you are using the herb do not improve significantly within 2 weeks.

Growing Instructions

Burdock's medicinal root has brown bark and a white, spongy, fibrous interior that becomes hard when dried. Its stem is multibranched, with long, egg-shaped leaves. Each branch is topped by a bristled "flower"—actually a clump of many purplish flowers—that produces its infamous burrs.

Burdock grows easily from seeds planted in spring. Thin seedlings to 6-inch spacing. Burdock prefers moist, rich, deeply cultivated soil and full sun, but it tolerates poorer soils. Many herbalists mix wood chips and sawdust into burdock beds to keep the soil loose so the roots are easier to harvest.

Burdock roots deeply, so it's not advisable to transplant established plants. Harvest the roots during the fall of the first year or the spring of the second.

Caraway

Family: Umbellifcrae; other members include carrot, celery, parsley, fennel, dill, and angelica

Genus and species: *Carum carvi*

Also known as: Carum

Parts used: Fruits (seeds)

Seeds

Caraway is best known as the seed that flavors rye bread. The reason that it's in rye bread, as well as many other foods, is that it has been used since ancient times to calm the digestive tract and expel gas.

Caraway seeds have been found in prehistoric food remains from 3500 B.C. The ancient Egyptians loved the aromatic seeds. They were recommended for digestive upsets in the *Ebers Papyrus*, one of the world's oldest surviving medical documents, dating to about 1500 B.C.

Healing History

Caraway is one of only a handful of herbs whose major medicinal uses have remained unchanged throughout history. The Greek physician Dioscorides mentioned the seeds to aid digestion, and herbals down through the ages have recommended them for indigestion, gas, and infant colic.

In Shakespeare's day, baked apples with caraway seeds were considered a stomach soothing dessert. In *Henry IV*, a meal ends with "a pippin and a dish of caraway."

Seventeenth-century English herbalist Nicholas Culpeper said that caraway "helpeth digestion . . . and easeth the pains of the wind colic." America's 19th-century Eclectic physicians, forerunners of today's naturopaths, believed that the seeds "gently excite the digestive powers . . . [and can be] used in flatulent colic, especially of children."

Throughout history, in Europe, the Middle East, and early America, caraway was a favorite addition to laxative herbs because it tempered their frequently violent effects.

Caraway's only other traditional uses relate to women's health—for relieving menstrual cramps, promoting menstruation, and aiding milk production in nursing mothers.

Therapeutic Uses

The Egyptians were right about caraway. It's amazing that a treatment used 3,500 years ago can still be effective today.

Digestive problems. Modern researchers have discovered that two chemicals in caraway seeds, carvol and carvene, soothe the smooth muscle tissue of the digestive tract and help expel gas.

In Germany, where herbal medicine is much more mainstream than in the United States, a popular over-the-counter digestive product called Enteroplant has two active ingredients: peppermint oil (90 milligrams) and caraway oil (50 milligrams). German researchers gave 45 people with chronic indigestion either a placebo or Enteroplant—one capsule three times a day with meals. After 4 weeks, those taking the placebo reported no change in abdominal distress. Of those taking Enteroplant, 94.5 percent reported significant improvement in their symptoms, with 63 percent declaring that they were free from pain.

In a separate German study, another herbal digestive aid—this one containing peppermint, caraway, fennel, and wormwood—produced similar relief from indigestion symptoms in only 2 weeks. No wonder Commission E, the expert panel that evaluates herbal medicines for the German counterpart of the FDA, endorses caraway as a treatment for indigestion and abdominal distress.

Women's health concerns. Antispasmodics, which appear to be present in caraway, soothe not only the digestive tract but also other smooth muscles, such as those of the uterus. Thus, caraway may relax the uterus, not stimulate it. Women might try the herb for relief of menstrual cramps.

Rx Recommendations

You can chew fresh caraway seeds a teaspoon at a time or mix them into food. Add them to any recipe that would benefit from their unique flavor. They're often used in breads, soups, salads, stews, cheeses, sauerkraut, pickling brines, and meat dishes.

Caraway oil is also used to flavor two digestive-aid liqueurs: Scandinavian Aquavit and German Kummel.

For a pleasant-tasting infusion that may aid digestion or relieve gas or menstrual cramping, use 2 to 3 teaspoons of crushed seeds per cup of boiling water. Steep for 10 to 20 minutes, then strain. Drink up to 3 cups a day.

If you prefer a homemade tincture, take 1/2 to 1 teaspoon up to three times a day.

When using commercial preparations, follow the package directions.

You may give low-strength caraway infusions to infants for colic and gas.

The Safety Factor

There have been no reports of harm from caraway.

Although the herb has antispasmodic properties, which means that it may relax the uterus, it has been used throughout history to promote menstruation. Pregnant women should exercise caution and not take the herb medicinally.

Wise-Use Guidelines

Caraway seed is on the FDA's list of herbs generally regarded as safe. Adults who are not pregnant or nursing can safely use caraway in the amounts typically recommended.

You should use medicinal amounts of caraway only in consultation with your doctor. If it causes minor discomfort, such as increased stomach upset, decrease the dosage or stop using it altogether. Let your doctor know if you experience unpleasant effects or if stomach distress does not improve significantly within 2 weeks.

Growing Information

Caraway is an attractive biennial that reaches 2 feet. It has feathery leaves and umbrella-like clusters of tiny white flowers, which bloom in early summer.

Caraway grows easily from seeds planted in spring ½ inch deep and 8 inches apart. The plants like rich, well-drained soil and full sun. Keep them moist but not wet.

The first year, caraway produces a small rosette of leaves and a long tap root. Don't transplant it once it has become established. During the second year, caraway sends up its stem, reveals its feathery leaves, and produces its seeds.

Seeds appear in midsummer. Harvest them as soon as they ripen. Leave some seeds behind, and the plants will self-sow.

Cascara Sagrada

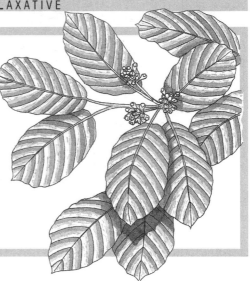

Family: Rhamnaceae; other members include buckthorn

Genus and species: *Rhamnus purshiana*

Also known as: Cascara, sacred bark, and chittem bark

Part used: Bark

The 16th-century Spanish explorers who first visited northern California had a problem: constipation. The Native Americans in the area had a solution, a tea made from a healing herb that they held sacred. The herb worked, and the Spanish named it *cascara sagrada*, or "sacred bark." It has been the answer to millions of prayers ever since.

Healing History

The Spanish recognized cascara sagrada as a relative of buckthorn, the powerful laxative herb used in Europe since ancient times. But cascara was much gentler. The explorers sent some back to Spain, where its comparatively mild action was hailed as a wonder of the New World.

But the Spanish explorers were more in-terested in finding gold than in spreading lax-atives around the newly discovered continent. For a long time, cascara remained a West Coast folk remedy, known as chittem bark, a polite variant of the Gold Rush '49ers' name, sh—tin' bark.

In 1877, an Eclectic physician in Detroit extolled cascara's mildness in a home medical guide, prompting Parke, Davis, the pharma-ceutical firm, to market a commercial prepara-tion. Cascara sagrada has been popular ever since. It entered the *U.S. Pharmacopoeia*, a standard drug reference, in 1890 and remains there today.

In Appalachian folk medicine, cascara sagrada has also been used to treat cancer. It was an ingredient in the popular but highly controversial Hoxsey Cancer Formula, an al-ternative therapy marketed from the 1930s to the 1950s by ex–coal miner Harry Hoxsey (see page 32).

Therapeutic Uses

Modern herbals recommend cascara sagrada for constipation and endorse the assertion of Eclectic physicians, who were forerunners of today's naturopaths, that it "restores bowel tone."

Constipation. Commission E, the expert panel that evaluates herbal medicines for the German counterpart of the FDA, endorses cascara sagrada as a safe, effective laxative. Many European laxative products contain the herb.

In the United States at one time, cascara was an ingredient in dozens of over-the-counter laxatives. Today, it is used less frequently, and senna (see page 368) has largely taken its place. Cascara sagrada is still an ingredient in two over-the-counter laxatives, Caroid and Nature's Remedy. It is also the active ingredient in one prescription laxative, Cascara Sagrada Aromatic Fluid Extract.

Cascara sagrada contains chemicals called anthraquinones that stimulate the intestinal contractions known as the urge. The Spanish were right in believing that the herb is milder than some other anthraquinone laxatives, notably aloe and buckthorn. Compared with these herbs, cascara is less likely to cause nausea, vomiting, and intestinal cramps, although these reactions are still possible.

Research has also supported the Eclectics' observation that cascara sagrada restores bowel tone. According to the natural-product text *Pharmacognosy*, "Cascara sagrada . . . not only acts as a laxative but also restores natural tone to the colon."

Intriguing Possibility

Harry Hoxsey may have been on the right track. Cascara sagrada contains aloe-emodin, which has demonstrated anti-leukemia action in laboratory animals, supporting the herb's use as a cancer treatment. Unfortunately, aloe-emodin is also quite toxic, and scientists say more research is needed before it can be used to treat leukemia.

Rx Recommendations

To benefit from the laxative action of cascara sagrada, take a commercial preparation, a decoction, or a homemade tincture.

When using a commercial preparation, follow the package directions.

To prepare a decoction, boil 1 teaspoon of well dried bark in 3 cups of water for 30 minutes, then strain and let cool to room temperature. Drink 1 to 2 cups a day. The taste is quite bitter. You may find that a tincture is more palatable; take ½ teaspoon at bedtime.

Do not give cascara sagrada to children under age 2. For older children and adults over age 65, start with low-strength preparations and increase the strength if necessary.

The Safety Factor

Anthraquinone laxatives are considered last resorts for constipation. First, increase your fiber intake, drink more fluids, and exercise more. If that doesn't work, try a bulk-forming laxative, such as psyllium (see page 325). And if that doesn't provide relief, try cascara sagrada.

Do not use cascara for more than 2 weeks. Over time, it causes lazy bowel syndrome, an inability to have bowel movements without chemical stimulation. If constipation persists, consult a physician.

Cascara bark must be stored for at least a year before use. The fresh herb contains chemicals that can cause violent diarrhea and severe intestinal cramps. Drying changes these chemicals and gives the herb milder action. Fresh bark may also be artificially dried by baking it at 250° F for several hours.

Cascara sagrada should not be used by anyone with ulcers, ulcerative colitis, Crohn's disease, irritable bowel syndrome, hemorrhoids, or other gastrointestinal conditions. Pregnant women should not take it either.

Wise-Use Guidelines

For adults who are not pregnant or nursing, are not taking other laxatives, and do not have digestive disorders, cascara sagrada is considered relatively safe when used cautiously in the amounts typically recommended.

You should use medicinal amounts of cascara only in consultation with your doctor. If it causes nausea, vomiting, diarrhea, or intestinal cramps, reduce the dosage or stop using it altogether. Let your doctor know if you experience any unpleasant effects or if constipation does not improve within a few days.

Growing Information

Cascara sagrada is an unassuming, 20-foot tree with reddish brown bark and thin, finely serrated leaves. It grows in the northwestern United States and is not a garden herb.

Catnip

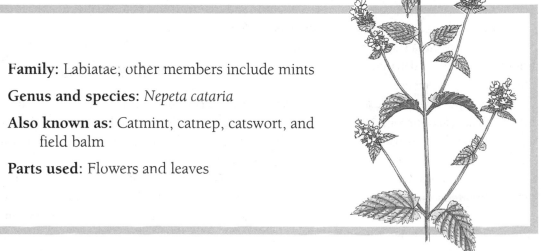

Family: Labiatae; other members include mints

Genus and species: *Nepeta cataria*

Also known as: Catmint, catnep, catswort, and field balm

Parts used: Flowers and leaves

You don't have to be an herbalist to appreciate catnip's effect on cats. But here's a case where one species' intoxicant is another's calmer.

In people, catnip helps soothe the nerves and digestive tract. It may also help relieve menstrual cramps and can provide handy first-aid for gardeners.

Healing History

From Europe to China, catnip has been used medicinally for at least 2,000 years. In teas, its pleasant, lemon-minty vapors were considered a cold and cough remedy, relieving chest congestion and loosening phlegm. Old herbals praised catnip's ability to promote sweating, a traditional treatment for fever.

Catnip has a long history of use as a tranquilizer, sedative, digestive aid, menstruation promoter, and treatment for menstrual cramps,

flatulence, and infant colic. Parents used to give weak catnip tea to colicky infants and even hang a small bag of the herb around their necks so they could inhale its soothing vapors.

A blend of equal parts of catnip and saffron was once recommended as a remedy for smallpox and scarlet fever. Catnip leaves were chewed to relieve toothache and, as crazy as this sounds today, smoked to treat bronchitis and asthma.

Catnip was a popular beverage tea in pre-Elizabethan England. During the Age of Exploration, it was replaced by the more stimulating Chinese herb that we call tea (*Camellia sinensis*). But not all English catnip lovers switched to Chinese tea without regrets. In her book *The Herb Garden*, a certain Miss Bardswell clucked, "Catmint Tea was . . . a good deal more wholesome."

Colonists introduced catnip into North America. The plant quickly went wild and now grows across the continent. Native Americans adopted it and used it as the settlers did, for indigestion and infant colic and as a beverage.

Early Americans believed that catnip roots made even the kindest person mean. Hangmen used to consume the roots before executions to get in the right mood for their work.

Catnip was listed as a stomach soother in the *U.S. Pharmacopoeia*, a standard drug reference, from 1842 to 1882 and in the *National Formulary*, the pharmacists' reference, from 1916 to 1950.

A report published in the *Journal of the American Medical Association* in 1969 claimed that catnip produces marijuana-like intoxication. The wire services picked up the story, newspapers ran screaming headlines, and bewildered pet shop owners reported a sudden run on cat toys.

The report was quickly discredited by correspondents who flooded the medical journal with letters pointing out that the catnip photos that were printed with the article actually showed marijuana. Catnip has no history as a human intoxicant, and authorities quickly dismissed the notion that smoking catnip causes anything—except a sore throat.

Unfortunately, the same cannot be said for the popular press. As Varro E. Tyler, Ph.D., writes in *Tyler's Honest Herbal*, "It is unfortunate that once an erroneous statement has appeared in print, it is almost impossible to eradicate. Catnip now is listed in practically all books devoted to drugs of abuse as a mild intoxicant." For the record: It isn't.

Cat intoxication is another matter. All cats are attracted to catnip, but only about two-thirds exhibit strong "feline catnip euphoria," according to a report published in *Economic Botany*. Kitty euphoria is an inherited trait, and not all cats have the necessary gene.

Contemporary herbalists continue to have great faith in catnip. One writes, "Surely a plant with such a powerful impact on our feline friends . . . could not be destitute of medicinal value in humans." Modern herbals recommend catnip as a tranquilizer, sedative, digestive aid, and treatment for colds, colic, diarrhea, flatulence, and fever.

Therapeutic Uses

Studies confirm that catnip is definitely not just for cats. While modern herbalists tend to overstate the herb's value, scientists have confirmed several of its traditional uses.

Digestive problems. Like other mints, catnip may soothe the smooth muscles of the digestive tract, an ability that classifies it as an antispasmodic. Have a cup of catnip tea after meals if you're prone to indigestion or heartburn.

Insomnia and anxiety. German researchers report that the chemicals in catnip responsible for cats' intoxication (nepetalactone isomers) are similar to the natural sedatives in valerian (valepotriates). This finding supports catnip's traditional use as a mild tranquilizer and sedative. Try a cup of tea when you feel tense or before bed and see if it works for you.

Infections. Catnip has some antibiotic properties, which lends credence to the herb's traditional use in some cases of diarrhea and fever. As an antibiotic, catnip is not particularly powerful, but it may help prevent infection after garden mishaps.

Women's health concerns. Antispasmodics calm not only the digestive tract but also other smooth muscles, such as the uterus. Catnip's antispasmodic effect supports its traditional role in relieving menstrual cramps.

Catnip was also used traditionally as a menstruation promoter. Current research suggests that it should not stimulate the uterus, but pregnant women should still exercise caution and not take medicinal amounts.

Rx Recommendations

Enjoy a pleasant, minty infusion of catnip as a digestive aid, as a mild tranquilizer, or to soothe menstrual cramps.

For an infusion, use 2 teaspoons of dried herb per cup of boiling water. Steep for 10 to 20 minutes, then strain. (Do not boil catnip; boiling dissipates its healing oil.) Drink up to 3 cups a day.

If you prefer a homemade tincture, take ½ to 1 teaspoon up to three times a day.

When using commercial preparations, follow the package directions.

You may give weak, cool catnip infusions cautiously to collcky infants. For older children and adults over age 65, start with low-strength preparations and increase the strength if necessary.

To treat minor garden mishaps, press some crushed catnip leaves on cuts and scrapes until you can wash and bandage them.

The Safety Factor

Catnip is considered nontoxic, but some people may experience upset stomach or allergic reactions.

Wise-Use Guidelines

The FDA lists catnip as an herb of undefined safety, but no significant toxic reactions have ever been reported. For adults who are not pregnant or nursing, catnip is considered safe in the amounts typically recommended.

You should use medicinal amounts of catnip only in consultation with your doctor. If it causes minor discomfort, such as stomach upset, decrease the dosage or stop using it altogether. Let your doctor know if you experience any unpleasant effects or if the symptoms for which you are using the herb do not improve significantly within 2 weeks.

Growing Information

Catnip is a gray-green aromatic perennial that grows to 3 feet and bears all the hallmarks of the mint family: a square stem, fuzzy leaves, and twin-lipped flowers.

The herb grows easily from seeds or root divisions planted in spring or fall. It thrives in almost any well-drained soil with full sun or partial shade. Some growers say that keeping the soil on the dry side produces more aromatic plants. Thin seedlings to 18-inch spacing.

Harvest the leaves and flowers in late summer when the plants are in bloom. Dry and store them in opaque, tightly sealed containers to preserve the volatile oil.

Gardeners' mythology holds that cats are not attracted to catnip in the ground. An old rhyme says, "If you set it / The cats will get it. / But if you sow it / The cats won't know it." Don't believe it. Cats often destroy sown plants.

The current consensus is that sowing, per se, does not keep cats away. The key is to prevent bruising of the leaves. Carefully cultivated, completely unbruised plants reportedly hold little attraction for cats. Any bruising, however, releases the plant's aromatic oil, and the cats come running.

Cat's Claw

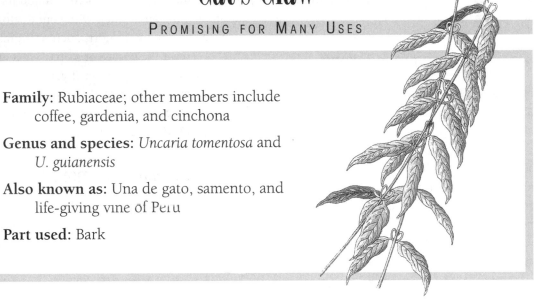

Family: Rubiaceae; other members include coffee, gardenia, and cinchona

Genus and species: *Uncaria tomentosa* and *U. guianensis*

Also known as: Una de gato, samento, and life-giving vine of Peru

Part used: Bark

Cat's claw, a vine from the highlands of the Peruvian Amazon, is a newcomer to American herbal medicine. It was introduced here in the early 1990s after studies in Europe and Asia showed that the herb reduces inflammation, stimulates the immune system, kills viruses, helps protect against heart disease, and may help prevent and treat certain cancers.

Healing History

The Ashanica Indians of the Peruvian Amazon believe that cat's claw is a life giver, hence one of its common names. They drink a cup or two of a decoction of the root or bark weekly in the belief that the herb prevents disease, reduces pain, and prolongs life. They also rely on cat's claw as a treatment for dysentery, ulcers, inflammatory conditions, infections, and tumors. Scientific research generally supports these uses.

The Ashanica have no written language, and ethnobotanists and anthropologists have been unable to determine from oral histories how long the Ashanica have used cat's claw medicinally. Scientists speculate, however, that the plant has been around for centuries.

In 1974, Austrian researchers isolated six medicinal compounds from cat's claw root and bark. Collectively, these compounds are known as oxindole alkaloids. The two that show the most promise, medicinally speaking, are rhynchophylline and isorynchophylline.

In 1989 and 1990, an Austrian company was awarded U.S. patents for a chemical process that extracts the oxindole alkaloids from cat's claw.

Therapeutic Uses

Research involving cat's claw is still in its infancy, but studies to date have validated—and expanded on—its traditional uses. It has anti-inflammatory, immune-stimulating, and anti-tumor action, and, in addition, it appears to reduce risk factors for cardiovascular disease.

Enhanced immunity. German, Austrian, and Canadian researchers report that cat's claw stimulates the immune system. South American scientists have found that cat's claw extract stimulates white blood cells to devour more pathogenic microorganisms. This tends to validate the herb's traditional use as a treatment for infections.

Viral infections. In laboratory studies, Italian researchers discovered that cat's claw reduced the ability of two viruses to cause infection. This finding also seems to confirm the herb's traditional use against infections.

Inflammatory diseases. In a cell-culture study, researchers at Louisiana State University Medical Center determined that cat's claw has significant anti-inflammatory effects. This seems to support its traditional use for inflammatory conditions.

Heart attack and stroke. Researchers at Shanghai College of Traditional Chinese Medicine have found that cat's claw reduces cholesterol and blood pressure, inhibits the formation of arterial plaque deposits, and helps prevent the blood clots that trigger heart attacks and most strokes.

Intriguing Possibilities

Scientists at the National Cancer Institute found "encouraging" evidence of cat's claw's anti-tumor effects. A 1993 study by Italian researchers showed that the herb contains no cancer-initiating (mutagenic) compounds but does contain cancer-preventive compounds.

As part of the study, the researchers gave a longtime smoker, whose urine contained mutagenic compounds, a daily dose of cat's claw. After 15 days, the number of mutagenic compounds in the urine had declined.

To date, there have been no rigorous clinical trials of cat's claw, so its effects in humans remain unclear. On the other hand, an increasing number of anecdotal reports in the herb literature suggest that the herb helps treat Crohn's disease, chronic prostatitis, canker sores, sinus infections, and flu.

Rx Recommendations

Most herbalists familiar with cat's claw recommend a dose of 2 to 3 grams three times a day, either in a decoction or as capsules. To make a decoction, simmer 1 to 2 teaspoons of herb in a cup of boiling water for 10 to 20 minutes. Drink up to 3 cups a day

The Safety Factor

Approximately a dozen Amazonian herbs are popularly known as cat's claw. The name also refers to a shrub (*Acacia greggii*) that grows along the Texas-Mexico border. This shrub is poisonous; it contains cyanide, so be very careful when you buy cat's claw. Look for botanical identification: *Uncaria tomentosa* or *U. guianensis*. If the product does not list the plant's Latin name, don't buy it.

Don't confuse cat's claw with another medicinal herb, devil's claw (*Harpagophytum procumbens*). This is an African plant with aspirin-like pain-relieving and anti-inflammatory effects.

There have been no reports of serious

adverse reactions to cat's claw. A toxicological analysis by Spanish researchers showed no known toxic compounds. However, cat's claw is a newcomer on the botanical medicine scene, so caution is advised. Pregnant or nursing women should not use it. And if you develop any odd symptoms while taking it, stop.

Wise-Use Guidelines

You should use medicinal amounts of cat's claw only in consultation with your doctor. If it causes minor discomfort, such as stomach upset or diarrhea, reduce the dosage or stop using it altogether. Let your doctor know if you experience unpleasant effects or if the symptoms for which you are using the herb do not improve significantly within 2 weeks.

Growing Information

Cat's claw is a climbing, woody vine that often reaches 100 feet as it grows up trees in the high Peruvian Amazon. It climbs with the help of hooks that resemble cat's claws; hence the plant's name. The hooks grow out of the stem at leaf junctions. If the stem is cut, drinkable water exudes from it.

The medicinal constituents of cat's claw are found in its roots and bark. In recent years, as the herb has gained prominence in herbal medicine, rampant overcollection has become a threat. In the mid-1990s, the Peruvian government banned the use of cat's claw root and required that the vine be harvested by cutting the stem above ground. This allows the plant to survive and regenerate.

Cat's claw is not grown in the United States.

Celery

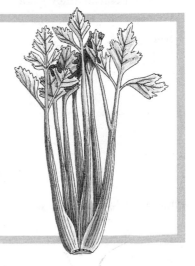

Family: Umbelliferae; other members include carrot and parsley

Genus and species: *Apium graveolens*

Also known as: Marsh parsley and wild celery

Parts used: Stalks and fruits (seeds)

Dieters often eat celery stalks, believing that chewing the stringy vegetable burns more calories than it contains. Most experts dismiss this as a myth.

Celery does more than add crunch to salads, however. Scientists have discovered a surprising number of healing benefits in its stalks and seeds. This herb may help relieve gout, insomnia, high blood pressure, and high cholesterol.

Healing History

The ancient Greeks gave celery wine to winning athletes, and celery elixirs have been used in healing throughout history. A contemporary echo of this, minus any medicinal claims, is the celery-flavored soft drink Dr. Brown's Cel-Ray Soda.

India's traditional Ayurvedic physicians have prescribed celery seed since ancient times as a diuretic to treat water retention. They also recommend it as a treatment for colds, flu, indigestion, arthritis, and diseases of the liver and spleen.

The medieval German abbess/herbalist Hildegard of Bingen wrote, "Whoever is plagued by [the arthritis of] gout . . . should powder celery seeds . . . because this is the best remedy." English herbalist John Gerard claimed celery "provoketh urine" as an aid to weight loss and expelled "phlegm out of the head." And 17th-century England's Nicholas Culpeper recommended celery seed as a diuretic for dropsy (congestive heart failure).

Later herbalists suggested celery to treat insomnia, obesity, nervousness, and several cancers, to promote menstruation, and to induce abortion. It has even been recommended as an aphrodisiac.

Oddly, America's 19th-century botanical

physicians, the Eclectics, forerunners of today's naturopaths, were not impressed with celery. They considered the herb a mere footnote to its close relative, parsley. If parsley was unavailable, the Eclectics grudgingly recommended celery as "a nerve tonic" and a remedy for arthritis and chest congestion.

Contemporary herbalists recommend celery as a diuretic, tranquilizer, sedative, and menstruation promoter and as a treatment for gout, arthritis, obesity, anxiety, and lack of appetite (gustatory, not sexual).

Therapeutic Uses

There hasn't been that much research on the medicinal benefits of celery, but the studies to date validate several of the herb's age-old uses in healing.

Gout. Some 800 years after Hildegard of Bingen endorsed celery as "best" for gout, science has validated her claim. Gout is caused by a buildup of uric acid that forms crystals in the joints, notably the big toe.

In the mid-1990s, James A. Duke, Ph.D., retired USDA herbal medicine authority and author of several highly regarded herbal medicine references—and a gout sufferer—came across a study suggesting that celery can reduce uric acid levels and has anti-inflammatory action. As he recalls, "My HMO doctor had urged me to take the gout-preventive drug allopurinol—one pill a day for the rest of my life. I did, for a while. Then I read a study showing that celery extract can eliminate uric acid. It seemed as though four daily 800-milligram tablets of celery seed extract would provide protection equivalent to the allopurinol I'd been taking.

"Now, I'm a believer. My uric acid level has stayed below the level that triggers gout. I haven't had any gout attacks since I began taking celery seed extract."

Of course, one testimonial does not prove that celery seed extract works. If you'd like to try it, talk with your doctor.

High blood pressure. In Chinese medicine, celery is recommended as a treatment for high blood pressure. Until the 1990s, this seemed ludicrous to mainstream physicians. As a vegetable, celery contains an unusually large amount of salt (sodium), which raises blood pressure in many people.

In 1992, Minh Le, the father of a University of Chicago medical student, was diagnosed with high blood pressure. His doctor prescribed standard antihypertensive medication. Le ignored his doctor's advice and began eating a ¼ pound of celery (about four stalks) a day. Before long, his blood pressure dropped from 158/96 to 118/82.

Le's son, Quang Le, and University of Chicago pharmacologist William Elliot, Ph.D., isolated a compound from celery (3-n-butyl phthalide) and injected rats with an amount equal to four stalks of celery. The animals' blood pressure dropped 13 percent, and their cholesterol declined 7 percent.

If you want to add celery to a treatment plan for high blood pressure, consult your doctor. It might help. But if you're especially salt-sensitive, it may do more harm than good.

High cholesterol. A high-fiber diet helps reduce cholesterol, and celery supplies an abundance of fiber. In addition, the 3-n-butyl phthalide it contains helped cut cholesterol in the animal study mentioned above.

Congestive heart failure. Diuretics are often prescribed to treat both high blood pressure and congestive heart failure, which involves serious fluid buildup in the body. Celery seed has been shown to have diuretic action, which supports its traditional role as a treatment for congestive heart failure. If you'd like to use celery seed for this purpose, discuss it with your doctor.

Diabetes. Several studies have indicated that celery seed reduces blood sugar (glucose) levels, an important part of managing diabetes. Diabetes requires professional treatment. If you'd like to use celery seed as part of your treatment plan, discuss it with your physician.

Anxiety and insomnia. Celery seed oil contains phthalides, chemicals that have sedative effects in animals. Of course, findings in animals don't always apply to humans, but if you're anxious, nervous, or wakeful, try the herb and see if it works for you.

Women's health concerns. Celery seed stimulates uterine contractions in animals, lending support to its traditional uses in promoting menstruation and inducing abortion. For this reason, pregnant women should exercise caution and not consume the seeds. The stalks, however, are not harmful.

Other women may want to try celery seed to bring on their periods. But don't use the herb to try to induce abortion.

Diuretics help relieve the bloated feeling caused by premenstrual fluid retention. Women who are bothered by premenstrual syndrome might try some celery seed during the uncomfortable days right before their periods.

Intriguing Possibilities

Celery contains psoralens, chemicals that have been used to treat psoriasis and, more recently,

a form of cancer called cutaneous T-cell lymphoma. Further research is needed to determine whether celery is indeed effective for these diseases.

Medicinal Myth

Celery seed's diuretic action lends some credence to its traditional use in treating obesity, because it would tend to eliminate water weight. Keep in mind, however, that lost water weight usually returns.

Celery may aid weight loss in the short term, but the key to permanent weight control is a low-fat, high-complex-carbohydrate diet and regular aerobic exercise.

Rx Recommendations

To treat gout, try adding four 800 milligram tablets of celery seed extract a day to your treatment program, in consultation with your physician.

To treat high blood pressure, high cholesterol, or congestive heart failure, add four stalks of celery a day to your treatment program, in consultation with your doctor.

For a pleasant-tasting, relaxing infusion that might help treat diabetes, use 1 to 2 teaspoons of freshly crushed seeds per cup of boiling water. Steep for 10 to 20 minutes, then strain. Drink up to 3 cups a day.

As a tincture, take 1/2 to 1 teaspoon up to three times a day.

Do not give celery seed preparations to children under age 2. For older children and adults over age 65, start with low-strength preparations and increase the strength if necessary.

The Safety Factor

All diuretics should be used in consultation with a physician. They can deplete the body's stores of potassium, an essential nutrient, so people who use them should also eat foods high in potassium, such as bananas and fresh vegetables, to replace lost electrolytes.

Women who are pregnant or nursing should not take diuretics, including celery seed, without a physician's approval.

High blood pressure, elevated cholesterol, congestive heart failure, and diabetes are serious conditions. Celery seed may help manage them, but it should be used in consultation with your physician as part of an overall treatment plan.

Wise-Use Guidelines

Celery seed and oil are considered nontoxic and are on the FDA list of herbs generally regarded as safe. For adults who are not pregnant or nursing, celery seed should be safe when used in the amounts typically recommended.

You should use medicinal amounts of celery seed only in consultation with your doctor. If it causes minor discomfort, such as stomach upset or diarrhea, reduce the dosage or stop using it altogether. Let your doctor know if you experience any unpleasant effects or if the symptoms for which you are using the herb do not improve significantly within 2 weeks.

Growing Information

Celery grows best in well-watered, richly organic soil. Less ideal conditions produce tougher, stringier, more bitter stalks.

In mild areas, celery grows virtually year-round. Elsewhere, start seeds indoors in January and plant seedlings in early spring after the danger of frost has passed. Soak the seeds before planting.

Germination typically takes about 10 days. Transplant at approximately 3 months, when the seedlings are about 3 inches high. Space the plants about 6 inches apart, and water copiously. The juiciness of the stalks depends on how much water the plants receive. Harvest seeds when they mature.

The psoralens in celery sometimes cause rashes in agricultural workers. Gardeners take note: Wearing sunscreen prevents this reaction.

Chamomile

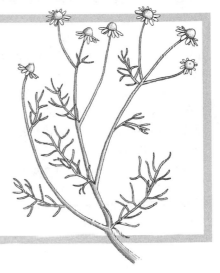

Family: Compositae; other members include daisy, dandelion, and marigold

Genus and species: *Matricaria chamomilla* (German or Hungarian) and *Anthemis nobilis* (Roman or English)

Also known as: Camomile, matricaria, anthemis, and ground apple

Parts used: Flowers

In *The Tale of Peter Rabbit*, the young bunny eats himself sick in Mr. McGregor's garden, then gets chased out at the wrong end of the angry man's hoe. When Peter gets home, his mother gives him chamomile tea.

Peter's mother was a wise herbalist. Chamomile helps treat indigestion and soothes jangled nerves. Perhaps Peter's mother feared that his ordeal might give him an ulcer. Chamomile helps prevent them. Or perhaps Mr. McGregor's hoe grazed Peter's tender skin. A chamomile compress can help heal superficial wounds.

Unfortunately, few people who sip tasty, apple-flavored chamomile tea realize what a healer they hold in their paws . . . sorry, hands.

Healing History

Chamomile is not one herb but two: German (or Hungarian) chamomile and Roman (or En-glish) chamomile. The two plants are botanically unrelated, but both produce the same light blue oil that's been healing people since ancient times.

Chamomile's daisylike flowers reminded the ancient Egyptians of the sun. They used the herb to treat fever, particularly the recurring fevers of malaria.

The Greek physician Dioscorides and the Roman naturalist Pliny recommended chamomile to treat headaches and kidney, liver, and bladder problems. India's ancient Ayurvedic physicians used the herb in similar ways.

Germans have used chamomile since the dawn of history to ease digestive upsets, promote menstruation, and relieve menstrual cramps.

The 17th-century English herbalist Nicholas Culpeper recommended chamomile for fevers, digestive problems, aches, pains, jaundice, kidney stones, dropsy (congestive heart failure), and "to bring down women's courses" (promote menstruation).

British and German immigrants introduced both chamomiles into North America. Most of the chamomile grown here today is the German variety.

America's 19th-century Eclectic physicians, forerunners of today's naturopaths, recommended chamomile poultices to speed wound healing and prevent gangrene. They prescribed infusions for digestive problems, malaria, typhus, menstrual cramps, and menstruation promotion as well as for all birth-related difficulties: to quiet fetal kicking, stop premature labor, relieve sore breasts and nipples, suppress milk production, and relieve infant colic.

Today, chamomile is one of the nation's best-selling herbs, but not as a medicinal. It's a favorite in beverage teas, by itself or in blends. Its apple aroma gives many herbal skin care products their fragrance, and it has been used in shampoos since the days of the Vikings because it adds luster to blond hair.

Medicinally, contemporary herbalists recommend chamomile as an external treatment for wounds and inflammation and as an internal treatment for fever, digestive upsets, anxiety, and insomnia.

Therapeutic Uses

In Germany, where herbal healing is more mainstream than in the United States, one pharmaceutical company markets a popular chamomile product called Kamillosan. The Germans use it externally for wounds and inflammations and internally for indigestion and ulcers. (The product is not available in the United States.)

Chamomile is so popular in Germany that many there call the herb *alles zutraut*, or "capable of anything." An exaggeration, to be sure, but chamomile has a lot going for it.

Digestive problems. Dozens of studies support chamomile's traditional use as a digestive aid. Several chemicals in chamomile oil—primarily bisabolol—have a relaxing effect on the smooth muscle lining the digestive tract, making the herb an antispasmodic. In fact, one study found that chamomile relaxes the digestive tract as well as the opium-based drug papaverine.

Commission E, the expert panel that evaluates herbal medicines for the German counterpart of the FDA, endorses chamomile for gastrointestinal conditions.

Ulcers. Chamomile may help prevent stomach ulcers and speed their healing. In one experiment, two groups of animals were fed a chemical known to cause ulcers. The animals that also received chamomile developed significantly fewer sores. When the animals that got ulcers were divided into two groups, those that were fed chamomile recovered more quickly.

Anxiety. Chamomile's long history as a tranquilizer has a scientific basis. Argentinian researchers discovered that a compound in chamomile oil, apigenin, binds to the same cell receptors as the family of tranquilizers and anti-anxiety drugs that includes diazepam (Valium). This suggests that chamomile would have similar effects.

Japanese researchers worked with chamomile oil vapors in a study of animals under stress. Among the animals exposed to the chamomile vapor, stress hormone levels fell significantly.

Infections. The Eclectic physicians were onto something when they suggested using chamomile compresses to keep wounds from becoming infected. Some studies show that chamomile oil applied to the skin reduces the time required for burns to heal. The herb also has anti-inflammatory action, thanks to the azulene compounds it contains. Commission E endorses chamomile as a wound treatment.

Other studies show that the herb kills *Candida albicans*, the yeast fungi that cause vaginal infections, as well as staphylococcus bacteria. Chamomile also impairs replication of the polio virus.

Enhanced immunity. No one knew why chamomile prevented infections until British researchers discovered that it stimulates the immune system's infection fighting white blood cells (macrophages and B-lymphocytes). Drink some chamomile tea when you have a cold or the flu. It does no harm, and it just might help.

Women's health concerns. Antispasmodics relax not only the digestive tract but also other smooth muscles, such as the uterus. Chamomile's antispasmodic properties support its age-old use to soothe menstrual cramps and reduce the risk of premature labor.

Oddly, however, chamomile was also used to stimulate menstruation. The apparent contradiction remains unresolved, but European researchers have isolated a substance in chamomile that stimulates uterine contractions.

Women should feel free to try chamomile both to soothe menstrual cramps and to promote the onset of menstruation, but women who are pregnant or trying to conceive should steer clear of medicinal amounts.

Arthritis. In animal studies, chamomile successfully relieves arthritis-related joint inflammation. Findings in animals don't necessarily apply to people, but chamomile has been used traditionally to treat arthritis. Try it and see if it works for you.

Rx Recommendations

Use an infusion or tincture to take advantage of chamomile's many proven healing benefits.

For a pleasant, refreshing, apple-flavored infusion, use 2 to 3 heaping teaspoons of flowers per cup of boiling water. Steep for 10 to 20 minutes, then strain. Drink up to 3 cups a day.

As a homemade tincture, take 1/2 to 1 teaspoon up to three times a day.

When using commercial preparations, follow the package directions.

You can give weak infusions of chamomile cautiously to children under age 2 for colic. For older children and adults over age 65, start with low-strength preparations and increase the strength if necessary.

Try a chamomile infusion when you feel anxious, or add chamomile flowers to a hot bath. Just tie a handful of chamomile flowers into a cloth and run the bath water over it. Don't forget to inhale the vapors.

For cuts, scrapes, and burns, brew a strong infusion, then soak a clean cloth in the liquid and apply it as a compress.

The Safety Factor

Controversy about chamomile erupted in 1973, when a report in the *Journal of Allergy and Clinical Immunology* claimed that chamomile tea might cause a potentially fatal allergic reaction, called anaphylaxis, in people who were allergic to its botanical relative, ragweed. Herb conservatives immediately urged the millions of people with ragweed allergy to shun chamomile. Outraged herb advocates insisted that chamomile had been vilified unfairly.

To settle the issue, researchers compiled all

of the reports of chamomile-induced allergic reactions from all of the world medical literature for the 95-year period from 1887 to 1982. The grand total: No deaths and 50 allergic reactions—45 involving Roman chamomile and just 5 involving German chamomile, the type typically used in the United States.

Chamomile poses no significant health hazard. The only people who should think twice about using the herb (and its close relative, yarrow) are those who have previously experienced anaphylaxis from ragweed.

This doesn't mean that adverse reactions are impossible. Large amounts of highly concentrated preparations have caused some nausea and vomiting.

Wise-Use Guidelines

Chamomile is on the FDA's list of herbs generally regarded as safe. For adults who are not pregnant or nursing, it is safe when used in the amounts typically recommended.

You should use medicinal amounts of chamomile only in consultation with your doctor. If it causes minor discomfort, such as nausea or vomiting, reduce the dosage or stop using it altogether. Let your doctor know if you experience any unpleasant effects or if the symptoms for which you are using the herb do not improve significantly within 2 weeks.

Growing Information

German chamomile is an annual that reaches 3 feet. The Roman herb is a perennial ground-cover that rarely exceeds 9 inches. Both have downy stems, feathery leaves, and daisylike flowers with yellow centers and white rays.

Most chamomile seed available in the United States is the annual German variety. It grows easily when sown in spring after the danger of frost has passed. Scatter the tiny seeds on well-prepared beds, then gently tamp them down. Seedlings up to 2 inches tall transplant well; taller plants do not.

German chamomile prefers sandy, well-drained soil in partially shaded gardens and tends to shrivel under full sun. It flowers at about 6 weeks, producing lush flowers even in the short summers of northern climes. The flowering lasts for several weeks, and if some flowers are left unharvested, the plant will sow itself. Don't leave too many, though, as this herb may become a pest.

Perennial Roman chamomile comes in two subtypes: single-flower and double-flower. Herbalists prefer the double-flower variety, which adapts to almost any soil but favors moist, well-manured loam. The tiny seeds may be sown, but most gardeners prefer to propagate the plant from offshoots. Plant them about 18 inches apart in early spring. Roman chamomile is quite hardy, but if your winters are particularly severe, protect the plants with mulch.

Oddly enough, Roman chamomile does best when it's stepped on. In Britain, it is often used as a groundcover on garden paths. Walking on it releases the herb's lovely apple fragrance and does not hurt the plant. After harvesting, dry the flowers and store them in sealed containers to preserve their volatile oil.

Chaparral

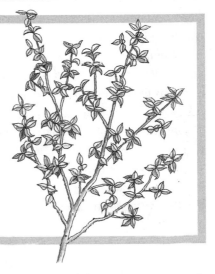

Family: Zygophyllaceae; other members include caltrop, star thistle, and bean caper

Genus and species: *Larrea divaricata* and *L. tridentata*

Also known as: Stinkweed, greasewood, and creosote bush

Parts used: Twigs and leaflets

Chaparral stinks. Literally. And it tastes downright unpleasant. Because of these characteristics, one of the herb's major benefits may come as something of a surprise: It's used as a mouthwash.

We're not talking minty fresh here. You wouldn't want to reach for it before puckering up for your morning kiss. But don't let that stop you. The unassuming chaparral shrub, native to the American Southwest, contains a chemical that may spell death to some of the germs that cause tooth decay. The same chemical, called NDGA (nordihydroguaiaretic acid), also kills other microorganisms that turn fats and oils rancid.

Healing History

If, as some people believe, effective medicine smells foul and tastes terrible, chaparral should be a wonderful healer. Its leaves exude a waxy resin that smells like creosote and is the source of its popular names: stinkweed, greasewood, and creosote bush (although the plant contains no actual creosote).

Native Americans in the Southwest rubbed chaparral resin on burns. They used chaparral tea to treat colds, bronchitis, chickenpox, snakebite, and arthritis. And they heated the tips of chapparal twigs and applied the hot resin to painful teeth.

White settlers adopted the plant, using it externally for bruises, rashes, dandruff, and wounds and internally for diarrhea, upset stomach, menstrual problems, venereal diseases, and cancers of the liver, kidney, and stomach.

Chaparral was listed as an expectorant (to clear mucus from the respiratory system) and bronchial antiseptic in the *U.S. Pharmacopoeia*, a standard drug reference, from 1842 to 1942. Today, few herbalists mention it. Those who do suggest using it externally to prevent wound infections and internally to treat intestinal parasites and bacterial and viral illnesses.

Therapeutic Uses

Chaparral is an intriguing and increasingly controversial herb.

Wounds. The NGDA in chaparral is a potent antiseptic with antibacterial and antifungal action, lending credence to the herb's traditional use as a wound treatment. It is approved by the USDA as a preservative in lard and animal shortenings, although since the 1960s, it has been supplanted by other commercial preservatives.

Tooth decay and gum disease. Because of chaparral's traditional use as a treatment for toothache, scientists tested the herb against the bacteria that cause tooth decay and gum disease. A study published in the *Journal of Dental Research* showed that chaparral mouthwash reduces cavity formation by 75 percent.

Oral microorganisms also cause gum disease, the leading cause of tooth loss in adults. Chaparral mouthwash is no substitute for regular brushing and flossing, but it may provide added protection.

General degenerative illness prevention. NGDA is a powerful antioxidant. It helps prevent the cell damage that's at the root of many degenerative diseases, including heart disease, cataracts, and, especially, many cancers.

Cancer. Investigations of chaparral's effects on cancer have been very mixed. Laboratory studies by the National Cancer Institute (NCI) show that the herb has definite anti-tumor effects, but NCI animal studies have shown no cancer-treating benefit.

Meanwhile, the medical literature contains several case studies of tumor shrinkage in people who have used chaparral. One such study, published in *Cancer Chemotherapy Reports*, tells of a man diagnosed with malignant melanoma, the most serious skin cancer. His doctors urged surgery, but the man refused, saying that he would treat himself with chaparral tea. Eight months later, the man showed "marked regression" of his cancer.

Melanoma is a life-threatening disease that requires professional medical care. Do not rely solely on chaparral as a treatment. Cancer patients might decide—in consultation with their physicians—to use the herb in conjunction with other therapies.

Arthritis. Some animal studies confirm that chaparral has anti-inflammatory action, lending support to its traditional use in treating arthritis.

Intriguing Possibility

Life-extension advocates say that antioxidants like NGDA help slow the aging process and may even extend the human life span. One French study found that NGDA significantly lengthens the average life span of laboratory animals. Other scientists claim that the chemical almost doubles the average life span of laboratory insects.

While science has not yet found a way to extend the human life span, these results are certainly intriguing.

Rx Recommendations

To prepare a mouthwash or an infusion, use 1 tablespoon of dried leaves and stems per quart of boiling water. Steep for 1 hour, then strain. Gargle or drink up to 3 cups a day. Because of its unpleasant taste, you may want to add honey and lemon to the infusion or mix it with a beverage tea.

Do not give chaparral to children under age 2. Older children and adults over age 65 may use a full-strength gargle, but for internal use, they should start with low-strength preparations and increase the strength if necessary.

The Safety Factor

Chaparral is safe for use as a mouthwash, assuming that you spit it out.

Although NGDA is a food preservative approved by the USDA, the FDA removed it from the list of substances generally regarded as safe in 1968. The decision resulted from research showing that experimental animals fed large amounts of NGDA for long periods developed kidney and lymphatic problems.

Neither of those problems has ever been documented in humans who have used chaparral, but to be prudent, people with kidney and lymph conditions should not take the herb. Likewise, stop using chaparral if you develop signs of kidney or lymphatic problems, such as urinary difficulties or swollen glands.

Since 1990, there have been 18 reports of liver damage in people taking chaparral. All but a few were using tablets or capsules, not the tea traditionally preferred in herbal medicine. One person developed liver damage after only 3 weeks, but most took chaparral for at least 3 months. Several were using other liver-damaging substances, such as alcohol and a variety of over-the-counter and prescription drugs, at the same time. In all cases, the liver abnormalities cleared up after treatment with chaparral was discontinued.

In 1992, after a half-dozen cases of liver damage had been reported, the American Herbal Products Association (AHPA) asked member herb marketers to voluntarily suspend chaparral sales pending the outcome of an investigation. Scientists at the University of Texas Health Sciences Center reviewed case reports supplied by the FDA. They found no pattern clear enough to warrant action against chaparral. So, in 1995, the AHPA rescinded its voluntary suspension of chaparral sales. The FDA has taken no action against sale of the herb.

Still, in light of the possibility of liver damage, no one with liver disease or a history of it should ingest chaparral. Nor should it be used by anyone who is alcoholic or taking any medication—including over-the-counter drugs—regularly.

Others who wish to try chaparral should use an infusion, not tablets or capsules, and should not take it for longer than a few months. Stop using chaparral if you develop any signs of liver trouble, such as nausea, fatigue, fever, or jaundice (dark-colored urine or yellowing of the eyes).

Pregnant or nursing women should not take chaparral.

Wise-Use Guidelines

You should use chaparral cautiously, for a short period of time, and only in consultation with your doctor. If it causes minor discomfort, such as stomach upset or diarrhea, reduce the dosage or stop using it altogether. Let your doctor know if you experience any unpleasant effects or if the symptoms for which you are using the herb do not improve significantly within 2 weeks.

Growing Information

Chaparral is not a garden herb. It's a woody, olive green or yellow shrub that dominates the Southwest's arid landscape. It grows to about 10 feet and resembles a dwarf oak. Its roots radiate far beyond its above-ground parts and contain chemicals that kill other plants.

Chaste Tree

Family Verbenaceae; other members include verbenas and many tropical trees and shrubs

Genus and species: *Vitex agnus-castus*

Also known as: Vitex, monk's pepper, and wild pepper

Parts used: Fruits (berries)

Since ancient times, Europeans believed that the small, dark, peppercorn-like fruits of the chaste tree suppressed a woman's libido. Those who took religious vows of chastity used the fruits to suppress their sexual urges, hence the name chaste tree.

This herb has no documented effect on libido, but it does change the balance of female sex hormones in ways that make it helpful in treating several women's health conditions.

Healing History

As a native Mediterranean plant, chaste tree was well-known to leading ancient Greek physicians. Hippocrates, known as the father of medicine, recommended it as a treatment for injuries and inflammations.

Dioscorides, author of the West's first guide to herbal medicine, *De Materia Medica* (*On Med-*

icines), recognized chaste tree's effect on the female reproductive system, especially its ability to increase milk production in nursing mothers. He recommended chaste tree to treat lactation problems and to expel the placenta and control bleeding after delivery. "If blood flows from the womb," Dioscorides wrote, "let the woman drink dark red wine in which the leaves of the chaste tree have been steeped."

During the 1st century A.D., the Roman naturalist Pliny cited chaste tree as an aphrodisiac, although most ancient writers believed that it put a damper on sexuality. In Homer's *Iliad*, the herb is mentioned as a symbol of virginity. In ancient Rome, the vestal virgins carried chaste tree twigs as symbols of their chastity. (The plant's species name, *agnus-castus*, means "chaste lamb.")

During the Middle Ages, chaste tree flowers were strewn on the ground before the feet of novitiates as they entered convents and monasteries, symbolically preparing them for their vows of chastity. Monks ate the fruits to suppress sexual urges, hence one of the plant's common names—monk's pepper.

During times of war or social upheaval, when Asian black pepper was difficult to obtain, Europeans used peppery chaste tree fruits as a substitute. This gave rise to another of the plant's common names, wild pepper.

Nineteenth-century American Eclectic physicians, forerunners of today's naturopaths, prescribed chaste tree berries to increase milk production in nursing women.

Therapeutic Uses

Modern research has shown that chaste tree affects the pituitary gland, increasing the production of luteinizing hormone and decreasing the secretion of follicle-stimulating hormone. These changes influence the balance of female sex hormones, reducing levels of estrogen and increasing levels of progesterone.

Premenstrual syndrome (PMS). Shifting the estrogen-progesterone balance can help relieve the irritability, breast tenderness, fluid retention, and other symptoms of PMS. In Germany, where herbal medicine is more mainstream than in the United States, an over-the-counter tincture of chaste tree (called Agnolyt) has been marketed since the 1950s as a treatment for PMS discomforts. German women consider the herb particularly effective for relieving PMS-related bloating and breast tenderness.

Several studies support the use of chaste tree for PMS symptoms. In one German trial, 1,542 women took 50 drops of tincture of chaste tree every day for 6 months. Ninety percent reported significant or complete relief of their PMS symptoms.

In another German trial, this one lasting 3 months, 175 women with PMS took either chaste tree or 200 milligrams of vitamin B_6, a treatment with demonstrated effectiveness for premenstrual complaints. Among the women taking B_6, 61 percent found the treatment helpful. Among those using chaste tree, that figure rose to 77 percent.

British researchers conducted their own 3-month study, in which 600 women took either medically inactive placebos or chaste tree. Once again, the herb showed significant benefit for relieving premenstrual discomfort.

Menstrual problems. Chaste tree's hormonal effects also help regulate the menstrual cycle. In one German study, 126 women with a variety of menstrual problems—scanty flow, heavy flow, and midcycle spotting—took 40 drops of chaste tree tincture every day for several months. The women experienced statistically significant normalization of their menstrual cycles.

Women with erratic cycles, scanty or unusually heavy menstrual flow, midcycle spotting, nonovulatory periods, or menstrual cramps might try chaste tree in consultation with a physician.

Lactation problems. The ancients were right: Chaste tree fruits help increase milk production in nursing women. A German study demonstrated this benefit when the participants took the herb for at least several weeks. The researcher who led the study described chaste tree as safe for breastfed infants.

Libido reduction. In men, chaste tree reduces levels of androgens, the male sex hormones. Most men produce much more testosterone and other androgens than is necessary to fuel normal libido, so suppressing androgens probably has little effect. But in men with low levels of androgens, the herb might reduce libido, suggesting that some of the monks who took it to inhibit sexual urges may have indeed benefited from it.

Rx Recommendations

Most studies with chaste tree have used tinctures in which 100 milliliters of the solution has been standardized to contain the equivalent of 9 grams of berries. The standard dose is 40 drops daily for at least 12 weeks.

Chaste tree is a slow-acting herb. It usually takes several months to show benefit, except in the case of lactation, which often improves within a few weeks.

Capsules of chaste tree are also now available. The recommended dose is one 175-milligram capsule daily. Follow the package directions.

The Safety Factor

Chaste tree has never been linked to any significant side effects, but minor problems are possible. In the 6-month German study of PMS, 17 women dropped out because of stomach upset. A few cases of itching and rash have also been reported.

Do not give chaste tree to girls who have not reached puberty.

Wise-Use Guidelines

For adult women who are not pregnant and do not have hormonal abnormalities, chaste tree may be used in the recommended doses in consultation with a physician. Let your doctor know if you experience any unpleasant side effects, if PMS symptoms do not improve after three menstrual cycles, or if milk production does not improve after taking the herb for 2 to 3 weeks.

Growing Information

Chaste *tree* is something of a misnomer. The plant is more of a shrub, generally growing to about 10 feet, although in favorable conditions, it may reach 20. It's most commonly found along moist riverbanks in southern Europe and around the Mediterranean.

Chaste tree has finger-shaped leaves, slender violet flowers that bloom in summer, and dark brown or black berrylike fruits the size of peppercorns that appear in fall. The berries are edible and have a peppery fragrance and flavor.

European colonists introduced chaste tree to the United States. Today, it grows along the Eastern Seaboard from Maryland to Florida and throughout the South as far west as Arkansas, Oklahoma, and Texas.

Cinnamon

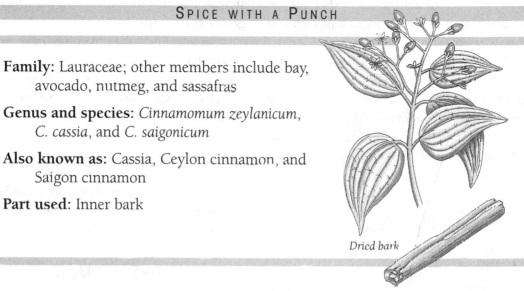

Family: Lauraceae; other members include bay, avocado, nutmeg, and sassafras

Genus and species: *Cinnamomum zeylanicum*, *C. cassia*, and *C. saigonicum*

Also known as: Cassia, Ceylon cinnamon, and Saigon cinnamon

Part used: Inner bark

Dried bark

We sprinkle it on toast, add it to cookie dough, stir it into hot apple cider, and find it in candies. But cinnamon is more than a sweet treat. It's one of the world's oldest healers—and modern science has confirmed its value for preventing infection and indigestion.

Healing History

Cinnamon originally grew in southern Asia. Ancient Chinese herbals from as early as 2700 B.C. mention the aromatic herb as a treatment for fever, diarrhea, and menstrual problems. India's ancient Ayurvedic healers used it in similar ways.

When ancient travelers introduced the herb to the Egyptians, they added it enthusiastically to their embalming mixtures. The Egyptian demand for cinnamon (and other Asian spices) played a major role in ancient trade.

The biblical Hebrews, Greeks, and Romans adopted cinnamon as a spice, perfume, and treatment for indigestion. After the fall of Rome, trade with Asia came to a virtual halt, but somehow, cinnamon still found its way to Europe. The 12th-century German abbess/herbalist Hildegard of Bingen recommended it as "the universal spice for sinuses" and as a treatment for colds, flu, cancer, and "inner decay and slime."

By the 17th century, Europeans considered cinnamon primarily a kitchen spice. In healing, they used it only to mask the bitterness of other herbs.

As time passed, however, cinnamon slowly regained its former reputation as a healer. America's 19th-century Eclectic physicians, forerunners of today's naturopaths, prescribed it for stomach cramps, flatulence, nausea, vomiting, diarrhea, and infant colic. The Eclectic medical text *King's American Dispensatory* (1898) also endorsed it for uterine problems: "[Cinnamon's] most direct action is on the uterine muscle fibers, causing contraction and arresting bleeding. For postpartum and other uterine hemorrhages, it is one of the most prompt and efficient remedies."

Modern herbalists recommend cinnamon to relieve nausea, vomiting, diarrhea, and indigestion and as a flavoring agent for bitter-tasting healing herb preparations. They can't quite agree about how it affects the uterus. Some say it stimulates uterine contractions, while others say it calms the uterus.

Therapeutic Uses

Of course, cinnamon delights the tastebuds, but it benefits other parts of the body as well.

Infections. Cinammon is included in toothpaste and dental floss for more than just flavor. Like all of the other culinary spices, it's a powerful antiseptic. It kills many decay- and disease-causing bacteria, fungi, and viruses. Try sprinkling some on minor cuts and scrapes after they've been thoroughly washed.

Perhaps toilet paper should be permeated with cinnamon. One German study showed that it "suppresses completely" the bacteria that cause most urinary tract infections (*Escherichia coli*) and the fungus responsible for vaginal yeast infections (*Candida albicans*).

Pain. There's another reason to dust a bit of cinnamon on cuts and scrapes. It contains eugenol, a natural anesthetic oil that may help relieve the pain of household mishaps.

Digestive problems. Along with lending flavor to foods, cinnamon assists the body in digesting cakes, cookies, ice cream, and other high-fat treats. According to a study published in the British journal *Nature*, cinnamon helps break down fats in the digestive system, possibly by boosting the activity of a particular digestive enzyme (trypsin).

Commission E, the expert panel that evaluates herbal medicines for the German counterpart of the FDA, endorses cinnamon for indigestion, abdominal distress, bloating, and flatulence.

Intriguing Possibility

Japanese researchers report that cinnamon helps reduce blood pressure. If yours is high, it won't hurt to use more of this spice.

Medicinal Myth

Despite some modern herbalists' contention that cinnamon helps calm the uterus, the weight of historical evidence suggests the opposite. For this reason, pregnant women should limit their use of cinnamon to culinary amounts.

Rx Recommendations

For a warm, sweet, spicy infusion, use ½ to ¾ teaspoon of powdered herb per cup of boiling water, steep for 10 to 20 minutes, and strain if you wish. Drink up to 3 cups a day.

Do not give cinnamon infusions to children under age 2. For older children and adults over age 65, start with low-strength preparations and increase the strength if necessary.

To treat minor cuts and scrapes, wash the affected area thoroughly, then sprinkle on a little powdered cinnamon.

The Safety Factor

Culinary amounts of powdered cinnamon are nontoxic, although allergic reactions are possible.

Cinnamon oil is a different story. On the skin, it may cause redness and burning. Used internally, it can cause nausea, vomiting, and possibly even kidney damage. Do not ingest the oil.

Wise-Use Guidelines

Cinnamon is on the FDA list of herbs generally regarded as safe. For adults who are not pregnant or nursing, it is considered safe in the amounts typically recommended.

You should use medicinal amounts of cinnamon only in consultation with your doctor. If it causes minor discomfort, such as stomach upset or diarrhea, decrease the dosage or stop using it altogether. Let your doctor know if you experience any unpleasant effects or if the symptoms for which you are using the herb do not improve significantly within 2 weeks.

Growing Information

Cinnamon is not grown in the United States. Most of our supply comes from Asia and the West Indies. The trees reach a height of 30 feet. Collectors strip the aromatic bark from young branches no more than 3 years old.

Clove

Family: Myrtaceae; other members include myrtle, tea tree, and eucalyptus

Genus and species: *Eugenia caryophyllata* or *Syzygiurn aromaticurn*

Also known as: Clavos and caryophyllus

Parts used: Flower buds

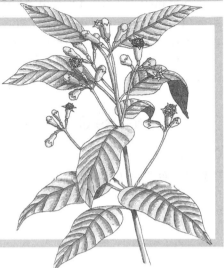

Step into any spice shop, take a deep breath, and enjoy the rich, warm aroma that fills the air. Chances are the dominant fragrance is clove, one of the world's most aromatic healing herbs.

Step into your dentist's supply room and, although things smell quite different, chances are that clove oil is one of the items on the shelf. It's a dental anesthetic—and more.

Healing History

Clove is the bud of a highly aromatic Asian tropical evergreen tree. During the Han dynasty (207 B.C. to A.D. 220), those who addressed the Chinese emperor were required to hold cloves in their mouths to mask bad breath.

Traditional Chinese physicians have long used clove to treat indigestion, diarrhea, hernia, and ringworm, along with athlete's foot and other fungal infections. Likewise, India's tradi-tional Ayurvedic healers have prescribed clove since ancient times to treat respiratory and digestive ailments.

Clove first arrived in Europe around the 4th century A.D. as a highly coveted luxury. The medieval German abbess/herbalist Hildegard of Bingen recommended the rare herb in her anti-gout mixture.

Demand for clove and other Asian herbs helped launch the Age of Exploration. Magellan's flotilla carried some clove back to Spain in 1512, when the explorers completed their first voyage around the world.

Once the herb became readily available in Europe, it was prized as a treatment for indigestion, flatulence, nausea, vomiting, and diarrhea. It was also used to treat cough, infertility, warts, worms, wounds, and toothache.

America's 19th-century Eclectic physicians, forerunners of today's naturopaths, recommended clove to treat digestive complaints and added it to bitter herbal medicine preparations to make them more palatable. The Eclectics were also the first to extract clove oil from the herbal buds. They used it on the gums to relieve toothache, a practice adopted by modern dentists.

Contemporary herbalists recommend clove for digestive complaints and its oil for toothache.

Therapeutic Uses

Clove oil is 60 to 90 percent eugenol, which is the source of its anesthetic and antiseptic properties.

Toothache and oral hygiene. Dentists use clove oil as an oral anesthetic and to disinfect root canals. It is an ingredient in the toothache remedies Dentapaine and Orajel; in Numzit, an anesthetic for teething pain; and in the lip balms Blistex and Orabase. In addition, several products for oral discomfort contain eugenol, including Dent-Zel-Ite Toothache Relief, Dentemp Temporary Filling Mix, and Red Cross Toothache Medication.

Commission E, the expert panel that evaluates herbal medicines for the German counterpart of the FDA, endorses clove oil as an oral anesthetic. Keep in mind, though, that toothaches require professional care. Clove oil and products that contain either it or eugenol may provide temporary relief, but you need to see a dentist promptly.

Digestive problems. Like all culinary spices, clove helps relax the smooth muscle lining the digestive tract, supporting the herb's age-old use as a digestive aid.

Parasites and infections. Clove kills intestinal parasites and "exhibits broad antimicrobial properties against fungi and bacteria," according to one of many reports supporting the herb's traditional use as a treatment for diarrhea, intestinal worms, other digestive ailments, and ringworm.

Hay fever. Research shows that clove has some antihistamine action. If you have hay fever, clove probably won't replace pharmaceutical antihistamines, but it may provide additional relief.

Rx Recommendations

For temporary relief of toothache prior to professional care, dip a cotton swab in clove oil and apply it to the affected tooth and surrounding gum. When using commercial clove oil or eugenol preparations, follow the package directions.

To make a warm, pleasant-tasting infusion, use 1 teaspoon of powdered herb per cup of boiling water and steep for 10 to 20 minutes, then strain if you wish. Drink up to 3 cups a day.

Do not give medicinal amounts of clove to children under age 2. For older children and adults over age 65, start with low-strength preparations and increase the strength if necessary.

The Safety Factor

Small amounts of clove oil are used in foods, beverages, and toothpaste. The oil should never be ingested, however. As little as 1 teaspoon can cause serious toxicity. Externally, clove oil may cause skin irritation.

Some smokers switch to clove cigarettes, thinking that they're safer than tobacco. They aren't. Most clove cigarettes are 50 to 60 percent tobacco, and when clove burns, it releases many carcinogens. The *Journal of the American Medical Association* has reported many toxic reactions to clove cigarettes.

Wise-Use Guidelines

For adults who are not pregnant or nursing, powdered clove is considered nontoxic. Still, you should use medicinal amounts of clove and clove oil only in consultation with your doctor. If either form of the herb causes minor discomfort, such as stomach upset or diarrhea, reduce the dosage or stop using it altogether. Let your doctor know if you experience any unpleasant effects or if the symptoms for which you are using the herb do not improve significantly within 2 weeks.

Growing Information

Clove does not grow in the United States. The aromatic clove evergreen, which has leathery leaves and reaches 60 feet in height, is native to the Philippines.

Today, Tanzania produces about 80 percent of the world's clove supply. The plant also grows in Indonesia, Sri Lanka, Brazil, and the West Indies.

Cocoa (Chocolate)

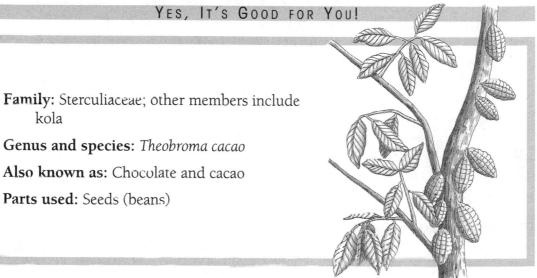

Family: Sterculiaceae; other members include kola

Genus and species: *Theobroma cacao*

Also known as: Chocolate and cacao

Parts used: Seeds (beans)

Chocoholics of the world, rejoice! Your favorite vice may be just what the doctor ordered for a long, sweet life.

Cocoa and its derivative, chocolate, are rich in antioxidants that may contribute to longevity. They also contain compounds that support good digestion, boost blood flow to the heart, and help clear up chest congestion. So unwrap a chocolate kiss and read on.

Healing History

Imagine a world without chocolate. It would be desolate indeed. But that's how it was until 1519, when Spanish conquistador Hernando Cortez saw Mexico's Aztec ruler, Montezuma, sip a bitter drink called *xocoatl* from a golden goblet. Cortez was more interested in the goblet's gold than in its contents—until the Aztecs informed him that the drink was made from beans so valuable that 100 could buy a healthy human slave. After conquering Mexico, Cortez shipped some *xocoatl*, which he called chocolatl, back to Spain as a gift for the king.

Before the arrival of the Spanish, the Aztecs and Mayans drank enormous amounts of *xocoatl* (the name means "bitter water"). The common folk could afford it only for special occasions, such as to seal marriage vows. Priests used it in prayer offerings. But royalty couldn't get enough. Surviving records suggest that a century before the arrival of Cortez, the Aztec royal court consumed an astonishing 32,000 cocoa beans a day.

Cortez's gift to his king became an instant sensation with the Spanish court. Chocolate proved so popular that the Spanish tried to keep it secret from the rest of Europe, and they succeeded for more than 100 years. During the late 16th century, Mexico was exporting some

200 tons of cocoa beans to Spain each year. Some ships carrying the beans were captured, and eventually, the secret got out.

By the mid-17th century, chocolate had spread throughout Western Europe. It became especially popular in Switzerland, England, Belgium, and Holland, where the bitter drink was enriched and sweetened with milk and sugar.

Oddly, until the 19th century, chocolate was solely a beverage—sometimes bitter, sometimes sweet, but always a liquid. It was only about 150 years ago that it was fashioned into the blocks and candies that we so love today.

For centuries, Central Americans have used cocoa to treat fever, coughs, and problems associated with pregnancy and childbirth. They have also applied cocoa butter to soothe burns, chapped lips, balding heads, and the sore nipples of nursing mothers.

America's 19th-century Eclectic physicians, forerunners of today's naturopaths, recommended cocoa butter externally as a wound dressing and salve. They prescribed hot cocoa internally as a treatment for asthma, as a substitute for coffee, and as "a very useful nutritive for invalids and persons convalescing from acute illness."

Few contemporary herbalists view cocoa or chocolate as a healing herb. It's their loss.

Therapeutic Uses

Cocoa's genus name, *Theobroma*, means "food of the gods," a high tribute to a humble bean. But its derivative, chocolate, is much more than a revered sweet treat. It possesses remarkable healing powers, thanks largely to the antioxidants, caffeine, and theobromine that it contains.

General degenerative illness prevention. Antioxidants—among them vitamins C and E and the mineral selenium—help prevent the cell damage that sets the stage for degenerative conditions such as heart disease, stroke, and many cancers. These nutrients also help keep fats from spoiling.

Although chocolate is high in fat (more on this later), it doesn't spoil when left unrefrigerated. This observation led researchers at the University of California at Davis and the National Institutes of Public Health and Environment in the Netherlands to analyze cocoa for antioxidants. They discovered that it (and chocolate) contains large amounts of flavonoids and catechins, both categories of antioxidant nutrients.

Two tablespoons of cocoa contain 146 milligrams of antioxidants, while a 1½-ounce piece of milk chocolate boasts 205 milligrams. Dark chocolate has even more antioxidants because it's not diluted by milk and sugar as milk chocolate is. In comparison, a standard 5-ounce serving of red wine contains 210 milligrams of antioxidants.

Studies have shown that a glass of red wine a day can reduce the risk of heart attack. A piece of chocolate a day appears to confer the same benefit, according to a team of Harvard researchers who tracked the diet and health status of 7,814 male Harvard graduates.

The study compared men who ate no candy bars with those who ate one to three bars a month. The researchers found that those who ate the chocolate had a 36 percent lower death rate from all causes. As the consumption of sweets increased beyond three candy bars a month, the health benefits decreased, but even the most ardent chocolate lovers had a 16 percent lower death rate than men who completely abstained from chocolate.

Fatigue and lethargy. Cocoa has 10 to 20 percent of the amount of caffeine in coffee—about 13 milligrams a cup compared with instant coffee's 65 milligrams and drip coffee's 100 to 150 milligrams. As a result, cocoa and chocolate may relieve drowsiness and provide mild stimulation without causing as much jitteriness, insomnia, and irritability as coffee. Try some when you feel lethargic (purely as herbal medicine, of course).

Digestive problems. The theobromine in cocoa relaxes the smooth muscle lining the digestive tract, which may be why many people have room for chocolate after a heavy meal. Try some to soothe your stomach after eating.

Bronchial congestion. Theobromine and caffeine are close chemical relatives of theophylline, which, until recently, was a standard asthma medication. Theophylline opens the bronchial passages; theobromine and caffeine have similar effects.

If you're really congested, or if you have asthma, the large dose of decongestant caffeine in coffee may be more beneficial. But even the low dose in cocoa or chocolate may provide some relief from the chest congestion of colds and flu.

Enhanced mood. Several years ago, a burst of publicity surrounded a report suggesting that chocolate contains a compound that plays a key role in the biochemistry of the feeling of being in love. The compound, phenylethylamine (PEA), is an antidepressant chemically similar to amphetamine. It's what makes lovers feel as if they're walking on clouds. When the love affair ends, PEA levels drop precipitously.

This finding may explain why lovers often offer gifts of chocolate on Valentine's Day—to boost their paramours' PEA levels and heighten their loving feelings. It may also explain why those with broken hearts sometimes binge on chocolate—to replace their lost PEA and recoup some of its mood-elevating effects.

Rx Recommendations

Kiss guilt goodbye. Now you have some genuine, good-for-you reasons to brew yourself a heavenly cup of cocoa. Try the herb as a gentle pick-me-up or digestive aid. And if you have respiratory congestion from a cold, flu, or asthma, there's no harm in sipping steamy hot cocoa, as long as you also seek appropriate professional medical care.

To make cocoa, use 1 to 2 heaping teaspoons of herb per cup of hot water or low-fat or fat-free milk.

Some children and adults are extra-sensitive to the stimulant compounds in cocoa and chocolate. If insomnia, irritability, or hyperactivity becomes a problem, reduce consumption.

The Safety Factor

Chocolate cake is sometimes called devil's food, and it's no wonder. Chocolate has long been vilified as a cause of obesity, heart disease, tooth decay, acne, kidney stones, infant colic, headaches, and heartburn. Much of this reputation is undeserved.

Chocolate's fat content may contribute to obesity and heart disease. But the chocolate in confections is rarely as much of a problem as the high-fat, high-cholesterol butter and cream used in them.

Cocoa and chocolate contain no cholesterol (except milk chocolate, whose dairy ingredients have a small amount). They are high in fat, however. Here's how various kinds of chocolate stack up.

Type	Calories (per oz)	Calories from Fat (%)
Cocoa	75	65
Bittersweet chocolate	135	75
Baker's chocolate	143	93
Milk chocolate	147	56

Even worse, much of the fat in cocoa and chocolate is saturated fat, the type that's most closely associated with elevated cholesterol, heart disease, and several cancers. But wait: A good deal of that saturated fat is in the form of stearic acid, which does *not* raise cholesterol.

Scientists have now come up with a mathematical formula that provides a realistic assessment of the fat-related health hazard from chocolate. In this ranking system, heart-healthy canola oil rates a 1, while butter, which is very high in saturated fat, gets an 11. Here's a comparison of one serving of each of the various types of chocolate.

Type	Rating
Dark chocolate	4
Fudge syrup	4
Semisweet baking chocolate	4.5
Semisweet chocolate chips	4.5
Milk chocolate	5.5
Chocolate chip cookies	6
Cake	7
Fudge	7.5
Truffle	7.5
Brownie	9
Pudding	9
Ice cream	10.5

As for chocolate's contribution to tooth decay, it has been blown out of proportion. Some research even suggests that the antioxidants in cocoa help inhibit the growth of bacteria that cause tooth decay. Again, the problem with chocolate candy is not its cocoa content but rather its sugary, gooey ingredients.

There is no evidence that chocolate causes acne, kidney stones, or infant colic. It does contain chemicals called tyramines that can trigger headaches in some people, particularly those prone to migraines.

Many people find that a cup of hot chocolate soothes their stomachs after meals. The only glitch here is that cocoa and chocolate may cause heartburn. The herb relaxes the valve at the end of the esophagus, the tube that carries food into the stomach. When this valve (the lower esophageal sphincter) does not shut tightly, it allows stomach acid to splash up into the esophagus, causing heartburn. If cocoa or chocolate gives you heartburn, reduce your consumption or give it up altogether.

The real safety issue with cocoa and chocolate has to do with their caffeine content. Caffeine is a powerfully stimulating, classically addictive drug. It has been linked to insomnia, irritability, and anxiety attacks; elevated blood pressure, cholesterol, and blood sugar (glucose) levels; and increased risk of birth defects. (For a complete discussion of caffeine's many effects, see Coffee on page 144.)

Although cocoa and chocolate contain only 10 to 20 percent as much caffeine as coffee, consuming large amounts of them may trigger caffeine's classic effects. People with insomnia, anxiety problems, high cholesterol, high blood pressure, diabetes, or heart disease should limit their caffeine intake.

Wise-Use Guidelines

Cocoa and chocolate are on the FDA list of herbs generally regarded as safe. For adults who are not pregnant or nursing and have no history of insomnia, anxiety problems, high cholesterol, high blood pressure, diabetes, or heart disease, cocoa and chocolate are safe in the amounts typically consumed.

You should use medicinal amounts of cocoa only in consultation with your doctor. If you experience heartburn, headache, or caffeine effects, reduce your intake or stop using it altogether. Let your doctor know if you notice any unpleasant effects or if the symptoms for which you're using the herb do not improve significantly within 2 weeks.

Growing Information

Cocoa (or cacao) should not be confused with coconut or with coca, the source of cocaine. Cocoa trees are small, oval-leafed evergreens that grow in tropical lowlands. They do not grow in the United States.

Wild cocoa trees grow to 30 feet, but cultivated trees are pruned to about 15 feet to allow easier harvesting of the seeds (beans). Central and South America still grow and export cocoa beans, but an estimated 80 percent of the world crop now comes from Africa.

Once harvested, cocoa beans are roasted and ground into a liquid known as cocoa liquor. The liquor then undergoes Dutching, the addition of a minute amount of lye to enhance its flavor (the amount is so small that it poses no health hazard). Then the liquor is further processed to remove its fat, known as cocoa butter. The final product, chocolate, is a combination of the defatted cocoa powder with some cocoa butter added back.

The powder that we know as cocoa is simply dried cocoa liquor, perhaps with a little sugar added. Baker's chocolate is processed cocoa liquor with no sugar added. Bittersweet chocolate has some sugar added, semisweet contains more sugar, and milk chocolate has the most, plus milk to make it creamy.

Coffee

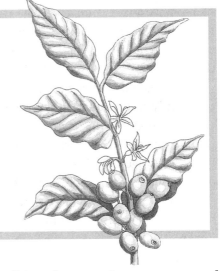

Family: Rubiaceae; other members include gardenia, cat's claw, and cinchona

Genus and species: *Coffea arabica, C. liberica,* and *C. robusta*

Also known as: Arabica, mocha, java, espresso, cappuccino, and latté

Parts used: Seeds (beans)

The next time one of your skeptical friends starts giving you a hard time about using medicinal herbs, here's the perfect comeback: "Do you drink coffee?"

The fact is, coffee is America's most widely used herbal infusion. The average American drinks 28 gallons a year, using 10 pounds of coffee beans.

Coffee does more than wake us up in the morning. It helps treat colds, flu, allergies, and asthma. It improves athletic performance. It helps prevent kidney stones and jet lag. It relieves pain and combats depression, possibly even reducing the risk of suicide. It may also promote weight loss in some people who are seriously obese.

On the other hand, coffee can produce significant side effects. Its active constituent, caffeine, is an addictive drug. Over time, regular users develop a tolerance, and if they suddenly give up caffeine, they experience symptoms of withdrawal.

Caffeine has also been accused, often mistakenly, of causing or contributing to many other health problems. Ironically, its main downsides—impaired fertility in women and increased risk of osteoporosis—have not been well-publicized.

Caffeine is definitely not risk-free. No drug is. Authorities generally agree, however, that for most people, drinking a cup or two a day is safe.

Healing History

Our word *coffee* comes from Caffa, the name of the region in Ethiopia where the fabled beans were first discovered. Archeological evidence suggests that prehistoric East Africans loved coffee's remarkable stimulant properties. They ate the red, unroasted beans ("cherries") before tribal wars, extended hunts, and other activities that required alertness, strength, and stamina.

The beverage that we know as coffee emerged around A.D. 1000, when Arabs began roasting and grinding coffee beans and drinking the hot beverage as we do today. Around the same time, the noted Arab physician Avicenna penned the first medical description of coffee's stimulant effects.

Although coffee is enormously popular today, it was quite slow in developing its global reputation. For 500 years, it remained in the Middle East. Then, in 1517, Sultan Selim I introduced the beverage into Constantinople (now Istanbul). At around the same time, spice traders introduced it into Italy. Over the next 100 years, it spread throughout Europe.

The first coffeehouse opened at Oxford University in England in 1650. It was remarkably similar to Starbucks and other contemporary coffeehouses—a place to enjoy coffee, conversation, reading, and writing. Coffeehouses quickly spread to London, where they became hotbeds of political discussion and dissent. In 1675, King Charles II ordered all of London's coffeehouses closed, claiming that they were contributing to sedition.

Coffee arrived in New York City in 1696, 30 years before it reached Brazil, which is now one of the world's major coffee-exporting nations.

Until the 17th century, Arabia supplied all of the world's coffee through the port of Mocha (hence one popular name for coffee). Then the Dutch introduced the plant into Java, and the island quickly became synonymous with coffee.

In 1732, Bach composed the "Coffee Cantata" in celebration of the beverage, despite some feeling that it threatened Germany's traditional brew, beer. As coffee became more pop-

ular in Germany, the backlash in favor of beer intensified. In 1777, Frederick the Great of Prussia issued a manifesto denouncing coffee in favor of beer.

Fernando Illy of Italy invented the espresso machine in 1904. Merck, the pharmaceutical manufacturer, introduced decaffeinated coffee in 1910. And in 1938, Nestlé introduced Nescafé instant coffee. It is still the leading brand.

Coffee has always been more popular as a beverage than as a healing herb, but European herbalists believed that its stimulant effect could help treat opium and alcohol sedation.

In their medical text *King's American Dispensatory* (1898), America's 19th-century Eclectic physicians, forerunners of today's naturopaths, prescribed coffee as "an agreeable stimulant . . . that frequently overcomes the soporific [sedative] effects of opium, morphine, and alcohol." They also recommended it to treat asthma, constipation, menstrual cramps, and dropsy (congestive heart failure).

The Eclectics also recognized coffee's down side, however. As noted in *King's*, "If taken too freely, [coffee causes] irritability, trembling, confusion, ringing in the ears, and disorders of the bowel. On the other hand, if one is accustomed to moderate amounts, headache will result if the coffee be withdrawn."

Folk healers have used coffee for centuries to treat asthma, fever, headache, colds, and flu. But few modern herbalists include it among the healing herbs. This is odd, considering that coffee is America's most popular medicinal herb.

Therapeutic Uses

Caffeine, the stimulant in coffee (as well as in tea, cocoa, chocolate, cola, maté, and guarana), is also an ingredient in many cold, flu, anti-drowsiness, and menstrual remedies. These uses are direct outgrowths of coffee's role in traditional herbal healing.

The caffeine content of coffee depends on how it's prepared. A cup of instant contains about 65 milligrams, a cup of drip or percolated has 100 to 150 milligrams, and a cup of espresso delivers about 350 milligrams.

Caffeine is such an integral part of our culture that we seldom realize how much of a drug it is. The fact is, caffeine is classically addictive. Regular users develop a tolerance and require increasing amounts to obtain the expected stimulant effect. Deprived of caffeine, these people usually develop withdrawal symptoms, primarily headache and constipation.

The media regularly report health problems linked to caffeine and coffee, many of which have been debunked, but they never discuss coffee's many potential therapeutic benefits.

Fatigue and lethargy. No doubt about it: Coffee is a powerful central nervous system stimulant. For those who drive long distances, it helps prevent dozing at the wheel. It also counteracts the sedative effects of antihistamines, which is one reason for its inclusion in many cold remedies. It does not, however, help people sober up after overindulging in alcohol.

Enhanced athletic performance. Attention, athletes: Coffee improves physical stamina and athletic performance. This was proven in a British study in which researchers had 18 runners race about a mile on nine different days after giving them 1 to 2 cups of either regular or decaffeinated coffee. With the help of caffeine, the runners ran 4.2 seconds faster.

In a similar study, researchers had distance runners run and cycle until they were clinically exhausted. A few days later, the athletes were retested an hour after drinking 5 cups of coffee. With caffeine in their systems, their stamina improved by 44 percent in the running test and by 51 percent in the cycling test.

The International Olympic Committee regulates caffeine use by Olympic athletes, allowing no more than 12 micrograms of caffeine per milligram of urine. To reach that level, an athlete would have to drink at least 5 cups of coffee within 3 hours before Olympic events.

To experience caffeine's performance-enhancing benefit, you must consume more than you already tolerate. A person who uses no caffeine might improve performance by drinking just a cup or two of coffee, but a 1-cup-a-day athlete might have to drink 2 to 3 cups before noticing any effect.

Colds, flu, and allergies. Caffeine is a decongestant. As such, it can be used to treat ailments that cause chest congestion, such as colds, flu, and allergies.

Asthma. Some years ago, North Carolina pharmacists Joe and Terry Graedon, authors of *The People's Pharmacy* books and syndicated column, received a letter from a woman who had just returned from her honeymoon. While in Hawaii, the woman, who had asthma, began wheezing. She reached for the inhaler she always carried with her, but it was nowhere to be found. Wheezing more and feeling panicky, she ransacked her luggage. Nothing. In all of the wedding and honeymoon commotion, she'd forgotten to pack her inhaler.

She imagined her honeymoon ruined by a trip to the emergency room. Then she recalled something that she'd read in *The People's Pharmacy*—that caffeine is chemically similar to some asthma medications. In a pinch, the Graedons had written, it can be used to stop an asthma attack. It is a bronchodilator, which means that it opens narrowed bronchial tubes and eases breathing.

The wheezing newlywed rushed to the hotel snack bar and quickly downed 3 cups of coffee. Within minutes, she was breathing more easily. She told the Graedons, "You saved my honeymoon."

This woman's experience is not unique. A survey of 70,000 Italian households found that as the consumption of coffee increased, the incidence of asthma attacks declined.

Pain. Compared with plain aspirin or ibuprofen, the combination of either painkiller and a small amount of caffeine—60 milligrams, about the amount in 1 cup of instant coffee, ½ cup of brewed coffee, 1 cup of strong tea, or a 12-ounce cola—relieves pain faster and more effectively. Caffeine has no intrinsic pain-relieving effect, but it is a mild antidepressant.

Pain and mood are connected. You hurt less when you feel happier and more when you feel depressed. Researchers believe that coffee's ability to boost mood is the reason that it enhances the pain-relieving effects of aspirin and ibuprofen.

The next time you have a headache or an injury that makes you reach for aspirin or ibuprofen, wash down the pill with a caffeinated beverage. Or take Excedrin, which is a combination of aspirin and caffeine.

Suicide prevention. Caffeine's mood-elevating effects appear to explain why regular coffee drinkers have a lower than expected risk of suicide. For more than 20 years, Harvard researchers have tracked the diet, lifestyle, and health status of a group of about 85,000 female nurses in the ongoing Nurses' Health Study.

Based on the information gathered to date, the women who drink no coffee have a somewhat higher suicide rate than those who drink 2 to 3 cups a day.

Kidney stones. Kidney stones cause excruciating pain in the lower back and groin. The traditional preventive measure involves drinking plenty of water to dilute the urine, which minimizes the risk of stones. The Nurses' Health Study, however, has shown that compared with taking no preventive measures, drinking a daily glass of water cuts kidney stone risk by 2 percent, while a having a cup or two of coffee daily reduces risk by 10 percent. (Tea, which also contains caffeine, lowers risk by 8 percent.)

Gallstones. Gallstones affect 20 million Americans and send 800,000 to hospitals each year. Harvard researchers tracked 46,008 male health professionals who were initially free of gallstones. Over the following 8 years, 1,081 of the men developed stones. Compared with the study participants who drank no coffee, those who consumed 2 to 3 cups a day were 40 percent less likely to have gallstones. Drinking smaller amounts of coffee also provided some protection.

Menstrual problems. Coffee appears to protect against heavy menstrual flow, which not only is inconvenient but also may contribute to iron-deficiency anemia. Researchers surveyed 403 healthy premenopausal women enrolled in California's Kaiser Permanente health maintenance organization about their diet, lifestyle, and health status. Compared with those who drank no coffee, the women who drank more than 2 cups a day (300 milligrams of caffeine) had a significantly lower risk of menstrual periods lasting at least 8 days.

Caffeine is a vasoconstrictor, the researchers

explain. It constricts blood vessels, including those in the uterus. In this way, it can help reduce menstrual flow.

Jet lag. Jet lag is the disorientation, insomnia, and fatigue that develop after flying across time zones. Coffee may help shift the body's natural time cycle (its circadian rhythm) after abrupt time-zone changes. Some jet-lag experts recommend drinking coffee in the morning when traveling west and in the late afternoon when traveling east.

Overweight. The caffeine in coffee raises metabolic rate, the speed at which the body burns calories. As metabolic rate increases, fat accumulation decreases, and the body may shed unwanted pounds.

In medically supervised weight-loss programs, severely obese individuals who supplement a low-calorie diet and regular exercise with caffeine and other stimulants lose a little more weight—not much, but enough to keep caffeine in the programs.

Unfortunately, caffeine's side effects can be a problem (more on this later). And caffeine helps only those who are severely obese—that is, at least 20 percent more than their recommended weight. It does not help those with more modest weight-loss goals, in the range of 5 to 10 pounds.

Rx Recommendations

Coffee has a wonderful, rich, pleasantly bitter taste. The growing sales of decaffeinated products demonstrate that taste alone is sufficient incentive for millions of people to drink coffee regularly. But you might enjoy having a regular caffeinated brew as a stimulating pick-me-up, stamina booster, decongestant, antidepressant,

or kidney stone and jet lag preventive, or as part of a medically supervised weight-loss program.

To make an infusion—that is, a standard cup of java—use 1 heaping tablespoon of ground beans per cup of water, then proceed with your favorite brewing method. Or buy instant and follow the directions on the label. Drink up to 3 cups a day.

Coffee-flavored food items such as yogurt and ice cream also contain some caffeine. If you eat them, be aware that they count toward your caffeine intake and may increase your tolerance.

Do not give coffee to children under age 2. For older children and adults over age 65, start with low-strength brews and increase the strength if necessary.

The Safety Factor

Coffee is classically addictive and causes so many side effects that one report observed, "If caffeine were a newly synthesized drug, its manufacturer would almost certainly have great difficulty getting it licensed under current [FDA] regulations. If it were licensed, it would almost certainly be available only by prescription."

If you're a coffee drinker, you know that when you consume more than you're used to, you get jittery and irritable, and you have trouble falling asleep. If you're concerned about caffeine giving you a short temper, consider reducing your coffee intake or switching to decaf. The same is true if you don't sleep as soundly as you'd like. Or try drinking caffeinated coffee only in the morning. That way, the caffeine's stimulant effect will wear off by bedtime.

Individual reactions to caffeine vary, but over time, large amounts—on the order of 8 or more cups a day—may cause caffeinism, a condition with the same symptoms as anxiety neurosis. They include nervousness and irritability, chronic muscle tension, insomnia, heart palpitations, diarrhea, heartburn, and stomach upset. In fact, many people are misdiagnosed with anxiety neurosis when the problem is actually caffeinism, according to a report in the *American Journal of Psychiatry*.

What's more, regular use of caffeine produces a tolerance, meaning that over time, you need even more coffee to achieve the desired stimulation. Once you're addicted to caffeine, suddenly eliminating coffee produces a withdrawal syndrome: a headache that may last for several days, often accompanied by sluggishness and constipation.

If you want to wean yourself from coffee or switch to decaf, do it gradually to minimize or prevent the discomforts of withdrawal. When switching from caffeinated coffee, mix increasing amounts of decaf with decreasing amounts of regular over the course of several weeks until you're drinking 100 percent decaf.

Coffee also increases the secretion of stomach acid. People with ulcers or other chronic digestive disorders should drink coffee sparingly, if at all.

Three cups of brewed coffee can boost blood pressure by as much as 15 percent. If you have high blood pressure, which is a risk factor for heart disease and stroke, discuss your coffee consumption with your physician.

Can Coffee Make You Sick?

Coffee has been accused of increasing the risk of several serious health problems, including heart disease, cancer, birth defects, and hyperactivity in children. The latest news on this front is largely reassuring.

High blood pressure? As previously mentioned, caffeine is a vasoconstrictor. As the blood vessels narrow, blood pressure rises. While caffeine produces a sharp spike in blood pressure in people using it for the first time, several studies show that in people with normal blood pressure, the rise is temporary, and blood pressure soon returns to normal.

If your blood pressure is normal, you won't get high blood pressure from modest caffeine consumption. If you take medication for high blood pressure, however, you should discuss your caffeine intake with your doctor.

High cholesterol? Some years ago, a Scandinavian study that followed 38,500 men and women for 3 years found that as coffee consumption increased, so did cholesterol levels and heart attack risk. Compared with people who abstained from coffee, those who drank 9 cups a day had about three times the risk of heart attack. Although very few people drink 9 cups of coffee a day, the association was troubling because the risk increased with every cup.

It's considerably less troubling today. The same researchers have continued their study for 12 years, during which the association between coffee consumption and elevated cholesterol and heart attack risk has plummeted. Now, the 9-cup-a-day coffee drinkers are only 1.3 times more likely to have heart attacks than their non-coffee-drinking counterparts. Statistically, this difference is hardly significant, and those who drink only a cup or two a day show barely any increase in risk.

What has changed? The Scandinavians' preferred coffee-brewing method. They used to boil their coffee, a process that extracts compounds from the beans that raise cholesterol and increase heart attack risk. In recent years, though, they have switched to drip coffee, made with a process that filters out the harmful compounds. Instant coffee doesn't contain these compounds either.

The vast majority of Americans drink drip or instant coffee. A recent analysis of long-term data from the Nurses' Health Study found no increase in heart disease risk based on coffee consumption.

Most recently, Swedish researchers discovered that coffee raises blood levels of homocysteine, another risk factor for heart disease. The increase was small, and the researchers concluded that a cup or two a day does not pose a hazard. Public health authorities are no longer concerned that typical coffee consumption increases heart attack risk.

Cancers? In various studies over the years, coffee has been linked to cancers of the breast, bladder, ovaries, pancreas, and prostate gland. All of these reports have been disputed. Most have been thoroughly debunked. In fact, the researchers who accused caffeine of promoting bladder cancer later repudiated their own findings.

At this point, there is no solid evidence that a cup or two a day significantly increases cancer risk, but the possibility remains because roasting coffee introduces carcinogens into the beans.

Birth defects? Studies performed in the early 1980s found that animals that were fed extraordinarily high doses of caffeine bore young with an increased risk of birth defects. No human study has shown that a daily cup or two of coffee produces the same results. Still, the FDA advises pregnant women to limit their intake of caffeine or give it up altogether. Nature seems to have the same opinion, since many women lose their taste for coffee while pregnant.

Hyperactivity in children? Caffeine is clearly a stimulant, but no evidence exists that it contributes to hyperactivity. In fact, stimulants such as the drug methylphenidate (Ritalin) are often used to treat the condition. It's not clear why stimulants calm hyperactive children, but they often help.

Researchers at the University of Chicago analyzed 12 studies of caffeine and behavior in children. None found any increase in hyperactivity, and a few even concluded that caffeine has calming benefits.

For Women, Cause for Concern

For all the publicity surrounding coffee's purported side effects, the media have generally underreported the proven risks associated with caffeine consumption by women.

Impaired fertility. In a 10-year study, researchers at Johns Hopkins University School of Medicine tracked 1,430 mothers, analyzing their diet and lifestyle habits, including coffee consumption. During that time, there were 2,501 pregnancies among the women. The more coffee they drank, the longer it took them to become pregnant. A 3-cup-a-day coffee habit reduced fertility by about 26 percent.

If you're trying to conceive, limit your caffeine consumption or go caffeine-free. On the other hand, don't count on coffee as a contraceptive. Even in large amounts, its fertility-reducing effect is highly unreliable.

Increased bone loss. Caffeine pulls calcium out of bone. Several studies have shown that the more coffee women drink, the more calcium they excrete in their urine. Women can minimize loss of the mineral somewhat by adding milk to their coffee or by choosing coffee-and-milk beverages such as cappuccino. Women who drink coffee regularly should make a point of consuming lots of calcium as well.

Higher risk of fibrocystic breasts. A few studies have linked caffeine to painful, non-cancerous breast lumps called fibrocysts, a common but annoying condition. Women who have fibrocystic breasts might try cutting out all caffeine—in coffee, tea, cocoa, chocolate, soft drinks, and over-the-counter drugs— to see if it makes a difference.

Increased likelihood of premenstrual syndrome (PMS). One study found that compared with women who abstained from brewed coffee, those who drank 2 to 4 cups a day were five times more likely to experience PMS. If premenstrual symptoms are a problem for you, consider reducing your coffee consumption or switching to decaf.

Elevated risk of stress incontinence. Coffee contributes to stress incontinence, the urine leakage associated with coughing, laughing, or sneezing. For reasons that remain unclear, coffee is associated with weakening of the muscles that hold the urine tube (the urethra) closed, a condition known as detrusor instability.

Brown University researchers surveyed 259 women with various types of urinary incontinence. Compared with those who drank little or no coffee, those who consumed 5 cups a day were 2.4 times more likely to have stress incontinence.

Because coffee is America's most popular herbal medicine, the debate over its safety is sure to continue, with headlines trumpeting any research findings of adverse effects. But public health experts generally agree that for people who have no medical reason to abstain, it's safe to drink one to two cups of coffee a day. Beyond that, the risk of side effects increases.

Wise-Use Guidelines

For adults who are not pregnant or nursing; do not have gastrointestinal problems, high blood pressure, anxiety, fertility problems, or osteoporosis; and are not taking medications containing caffeine, coffee is considered safe in amounts of up to 2 brewed cups a day.

You should use medicinal amounts of coffee only in consultation with your doctor. If it causes insomnia, stomach distress, anxiety, or any of the other problems discussed above, reduce or eliminate it. Let your doctor know if you experience any unpleasant effects or if the symptoms for which you're drinking coffee do not improve significantly within 2 weeks.

Growing Information

Coffee grows in tropical areas around the world. The plant is an evergreen shrub or small tree with two-seeded, bright crimson fruits. The green seeds are extracted and roasted to produce the dark brown, oily beans recognized the world over.

Most of the world's coffee supply consists of the Arabian *arabica* species. *Liberica*, from Liberia, and *robusta*, from the Congo, are also cultivated worldwide.

You can grow a coffee plant purely as an ornamental if you live in a sunny, humid area where the temperature does not dip below 60°F. The plant requires full sun, moist air, moist soil, good drainage, and regular feeding.

Coffee plants are also available as houseplants. Again, they require full sun and high humidity. They grow well in greenhouses but not in homes with forced-air heat, which tend to be too dry. Consult your local nursery or plant store.

Comfrey

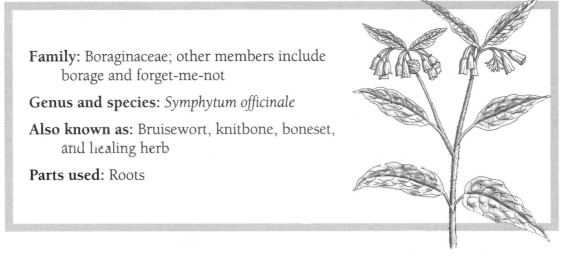

Family: Boraginaceae; other members include borage and forget-me-not

Genus and species: *Symphytum officinale*

Also known as: Bruisewort, knitbone, boneset, and healing herb

Parts used: Roots

Well into the 1980s, many herbalists touted comfrey as "an absolute must," "ideal for the amateur herbalist," and "perfectly safe and harmless." Then the herb was found to contain liver-damaging chemicals. Today, responsible herbalists recommend comfrey for external use only.

Healing History

The early Greeks used juicy comfrey root externally to treat wounds, believing that it encouraged torn flesh to grow back together. The Roman naturalist Pliny "verified" this practice with the observation that boiling comfrey in water produces a sticky paste that's capable of binding chunks of meat together. Comfrey paste hardens like plaster, and on ancient battlefields, cloths soaked in it were often wrapped around broken bones. When the paste dried, the result was a primitive but effective cast. This treatment earned comfrey the popular names knitbone and boneset (although comfrey shouldn't be confused with the herb boneset.)

During the 1st century A.D., the Greek physician Dioscorides began prescribing comfrey tea internally for respiratory and gastrointestinal problems.

By the 1500s, herbalists were recommending comfrey tea, not paste, to mend broken bones. One early English herbal suggested that it "helpeth [people who have] broken the bone of the legge."

The 17th-century English herbalist Nicholas Culpeper recommended comfrey roots, "full of glutinous and clammy juice," for "all inward hurts, and for outward wounds and sores in [all] fleshy or sinewy parts of the body. . . . [It] is especially good for ruptures and broken bones." Culpeper also prescribed the herb for fever, gout, hemorrhoids, gangrene, and respiratory and menstrual problems.

As plaster replaced comfrey paste for casting broken bones, names like knitbone were discarded. Comfrey came to be used internally to soothe inflamed mucous membranes. America's 19th-century Eclectic physicians, forerunners of today's naturopaths, prescribed it for diarrhea, dysentery, cough, bronchitis, and "female debility" (menstrual discomfort).

Mexican midwives still apply comfrey to torn vaginal tissue. In the Philippines, the herb is used to treat arthritis, diabetes, anemia, lung infections, and even leukemia.

By the mid-1990s, responsible herbalists had stopped recommending comfrey for internal use because of its potential to cause liver damage. Today, it's primarily used to heal wounds.

Therapeutic Uses

The ancient Greeks and Romans were right about comfrey aiding wound healing. But the herb's stickiness has nothing to do with its therapeutic powers.

Wounds. Comfrey contains allantoin, a chemical that helps protect the skin and promotes the growth of new skin cells. These properties validate the herb's more than 2,500 years of external use on everything from minor cuts and burns to major battle wounds. Studies show that comfrey also helps relieve inflammation, adding to its wound-treating effects.

The FDA considers allantoin safe in concentrations of up to 2 percent. It is an ingredient in many over-the-counter products for dry skin, diaper rash, and herpes, including Cutemol Emollient Skin Cream, Diabetic Pure Skin

Therapy, Derma-Heal, DiabetiDerm, Eucerin Light Moisture-Restorative, Herpalieve, Jergens Ultra Healing Lotion, Sofenol 5, and Stevens Skin Softener.

Such widespread commercial use suggests that comfrey root preparations may provide similar benefits. Commission E, the expert panel that evaluates herbal medicines for the German counterpart of the FDA, approves comfrey root powder for the treatment of minor wounds.

Comfrey is not absorbed through the skin, so external use poses no danger to the liver. Still, be sure to wash wounds thoroughly with soap and water before applying the herb.

Rx Recommendations

To use comfrey externally, sprinkle some dried, powdered root on clean cuts and scrapes, or make a paste from some powdered root and a few drops of water. Apply the paste to the wound and cover with a clean bandage. Change the bandage and reapply the comfrey daily.

The Safety Factor

Comfrey contains chemicals called pyrrolizidine alkaloids (PAs), which, in large amounts, cause serious liver damage. Animals fed plants containing PAs showed symptoms of poisoning, and some died. In humans, several cases of poisoning have also been reported after long-term ingestion of comfrey.

Tests by FDA researchers have shown that the PA content of comfrey varies greatly, with the root—the part most widely used in herbal medicine—containing the highest levels. Some herbalists have claimed that PAs are not water-soluble and that, as a result, comfrey tea should be free of PAs. But the FDA scientists have found PAs in comfrey tea as well.

The American Herbal Products Association, the herb industry trade organization, recommends that all comfrey products be labeled for external use only.

Wise-Use Guidelines

You should never ingest comfrey, and you should use it externally only in consultation with your doctor. If any wound does not stop bleeding quickly with firm, direct pressure, call your doctor or emergency medical service immediately. If a wound treated with comfrey does not begin to heal within a week, or if it shows signs of infection (warmth, tenderness, redness, swelling, or a yellow or greenish discharge), consult a physician promptly.

Growing Information

Comfrey is a hardy 5-foot perennial with large, hairy, lance-shaped leaves; thick, spreading roots; a hollow, bristly stem; and bell-like flowers, which may be white, blue, or purple.

Comfrey can be started from seeds, but it grows best from root cuttings taken in spring or fall. An inch-long piece of root planted in 3 inches of soil almost always produces a plant. Set cuttings 3 feet apart. The herb grows in any well-drained soil and tolerates full sun or partial shade. It spreads vigorously, so contain it in a pot or border it with sheet metal to a depth of 12 inches.

Gather the roots in autumn, after the first frost, or in spring before the first leaves appear. Wash harvested roots thoroughly and cut them into slices to dry. Grind them to a powder in a blender or coffee grinder and store in a sealed container.

Cranberry

Family: Ericaceae; other members include azalea, blueberry, and uva-ursi

Genus and species: *Vaccinium macrocarpon* or *Oxycoccus quadripetalus*

Also known as: No other common names

Parts used: Berries

Cranberry, or, more specifically, cranberry juice, is *the* herbal choice for preventing urinary tract infections (UTIs). The berries are also rich in antioxidant nutrients, which help prevent degenerative diseases, particularly those that affect the eyes.

Healing History

Cranberries were eaten for their tangy, refreshing taste long before anyone thought of them as healing herbs. The Pilgrims supposedly dined on cranberry dishes at the first Thanksgiving in 1621, but cranberry sauce did not become a national tradition until after the Civil War. General Ulysses S. Grant considered cranberry sauce an essential part of Thanksgiving, and he ordered it served to Union troops during the siege of Petersburg in 1864. Soldiers who were unfamiliar with the tart berries liked them, and the custom stuck.

Although the colonists were unaware of their high vitamin C content, the bright red berries became a favorite among New England sailors because those who ate them did not develop scurvy.

America's 19th-century Eclectic physicians, forerunners of today's naturopaths, did not consider the cranberry particularly beneficial. Their medical reference *King's American Dispensatory* (1898) contained this curious prescription, however: "A split cranberry, held in position by a daub of starch paste, will quickly relieve the pain and inflammation attending boils on the tip of the nose."

Today, we Americans eat cranberries not only at Thanksgiving but year-round. Our annual consumption is somewhere around 400 million pounds, an amount that's valued at more than $1 billion.

Therapeutic Uses

Cranberry's claim to fame as a UTI preventive comes not from herbal tradition but rather from 19th-century German chemists.

Urinary tract infections. During the 1840s, German researchers discovered that people who eat cranberries pass a bacteria-fighting chemical called hippuric acid in their urine. Sixty years later, American researchers speculated that urine acidified by a steady diet of cranberries might prevent UTIs—a common, recurrent, and often chronic health problem among women.

Women began drinking cranberry juice with gusto, and several studies endorsed the practice. But by the late 1960s, nay-sayers claimed that the tart berries did not significantly acidify urine and therefore could not prevent UTIs.

Now, more recent research shows that cranberry juice is indeed an effective preventive. A 1984 study, reported in the *Journal of Urology*, showed that 73 percent of women with recurrent UTIs experienced significant protection from infection after drinking a pint of commercial cranberry juice cocktail every day for 3 weeks. The researchers theorized that urinary acidity has nothing to do with the herb's effectiveness. Instead, they wrote, the juice prevents the germs that cause UTIs from adhering to the lining of the urinary tract, thus reducing the likelihood of infection.

Subsequent studies in the *New England Journal of Medicine* (1991), the *Journal of the American Medical Association* (1994 and 1998), and the *Journal of Family Practice* (1997) reached the same conclusion. Apparently, cranberries contain antioxidant compounds called proanthocyanidins that inhibit bacterial adherence in the bladder. Proanthocyanidins are members of the chemical family known as anthocyanosides.

General disease prevention. Like the better-known antioxidants—vitamins C and E, the mineral selenium, and carotenoids (including beta-carotene)—anthocyanosides help prevent degenerative diseases, notably heart disease, most strokes, and many cancers.

Researchers at the Jean Mayer USDA Human Nutrition Research Center on Aging at Tufts University in Boston analyzed and ranked dozens of common plant foods according to their total antioxidant contents. The best antioxidant sources turned out to be the dark-colored fruits and berries, such as cranberries, that contain generous amounts of anthocyanosides.

Cataracts. Cataracts are a major cause of vision impairment and blindness among older adults in the United States. The condition occurs when the normally clear lens of the eye develops cloudy spots as a result of oxidative damage.

For reasons that remain unclear, anthocyanosides have unusually powerful effects on the eyes. In one Italian study, 50 people with early-stage cataracts were given an extract of bilberry (another berry that's rich in anthocyanosides) three times a day, along with antioxidant vitamin E. The treatment stopped cataract progression in 97 percent of the study participants. Because cranberries contain generous amounts of anthocyanosides, they may also help prevent cataracts.

Macular degeneration. The nerve-rich retina in the back of the eye plays a key role in vision. One area of the retina, called the macula, is responsible for central vision (seeing what's directly in front of you) and fine detail. Macular degeneration is characterized by deterioration of the macula.

In a European study, 31 people with various types of retinal eye problems, including macular degeneration, were given an extract of bilberry. Those with macular degeneration experienced significant improvement in their vision. Since cranberries have many of the same eye-friendly nutrients as bilberries, they may also help this condition.

Diabetic retinopathy. Diabetes damages all the blood vessels in the body, including the tiny capillaries that nourish the retina. When injured, these capillaries can leak blood into the eye, causing the blurred vision of diabetic retinopathy.

Anthocyanosides strengthen retinal blood vessels, thus reducing leakage. In the European study of retinal eye problems mentioned above, people with diabetic retinopathy showed significant improvement when taking the bilberry extract. Cranberries may also help.

Incontinence. Cranberry juice helps deodorize urine. A report in the *Journal of Psychiatric Nursing* suggests that people with urinary incontinence incorporate cranberry juice into their diets to reduce embarrassing odor.

Rx Recommendations

Most of the studies showing that cranberry helps prevent UTIs have used cranberry juice cocktail, which is available in most supermarkets. Pure cranberry juice is highly acidic and too sour to drink, which is why water and sugar are added to the commercial juice, turning it into "cocktail." If you're prone to UTIs, try drinking a couple of glasses of cranberry juice cocktail daily to see if it helps prevent recurrence.

In the study of UTIs reported in the *Journal of Family Practice*, participants did not drink juice. Instead, they took one capsule of concentrated cranberry extract, containing 400 milligrams of cranberry solids, twice a day for at least a month. The solids were as effective as the juice. If you'd like to try an extract, they are available in many health food stores. Cranactin is a popular brand.

Many health food stores and supermarkets also sell dried cranberries as a snack food, similar to raisins.

The Safety Factor

For adults who are not taking other medications that affect the kidneys or urinary tract, cranberry juice and solids are considered safe in the amounts typically recommended. Cranberry juice is also considered safe for pregnant and nursing women. No problems have been reported from drinking cranberry juice, although some people may be allergic or sensitive to it.

You should use medicinal amounts of cranberry only in consultation with your doctor. If you develop UTI symptoms, let your doctor know. Treatment with antibiotics is usually necessary.

Growing Information

Cranberry is a small evergreen shrub that grows in mountain forests and damp bogs from Alaska to Tennessee. Its pink or purple flowers bloom from late spring to late summer and produce bright red fruits in fall.

Few gardeners have the conditions necessary to grow this herb. It requires wet, boggy, acidic soil amended with peat moss or leaf mold. Check with your local nursery to see if cranberry is viable in your area.

Dandelion

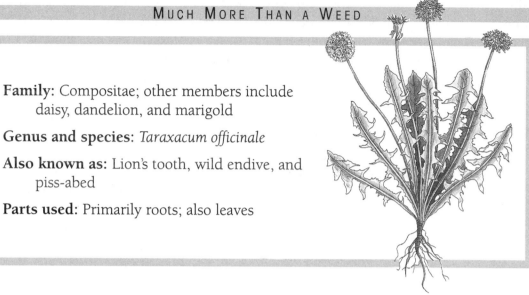

Family: Compositae; other members include daisy, dandelion, and marigold

Genus and species: *Taraxacum officinale*

Also known as: Lion's tooth, wild endive, and piss-abed

Parts used: Primarily roots; also leaves

Dandelion is so widely despised as a weed that many people have a hard time seeing it for what it really is: a nutritious healing herb with a medicinal reputation dating back more than 1,000 years.

Dandelion stimulates the flow of bile, and as a diuretic, it may help treat premenstrual syndrome, high blood pressure, and congestive heart failure. It may also help prevent gallstones and have other medically intriguing benefits as well.

Healing History

Chinese physicians have prescribed dandelion since ancient times to treat colds, bronchitis, pneumonia, hepatitis, boils, ulcers, obesity, dental problems, itching, and internal injuries. They also made poultices of chopped dandelion to treat breast cancer.

India's traditional Ayurvedic physicians

used the herb for similar therapeutic purposes. Tenth-century Arab physicians were the first to recognize that dandelion increases urine production.

During the Middle Ages, Europeans believed in the Doctrine of Signatures—the idea that plants' physical characteristics reveal their healing values. Under this doctrine, anything yellow was linked to the liver's yellow bile and considered a liver remedy. That's why dandelion gained a reputation as a treatment for jaundice and gallstones.

The Doctrine of Signatures also validated dandelion's use as a diuretic to treat water retention. The plant has a juicy root, stem, and leaves. Anything juicy was linked to urine production.

By the 17th century, dandelion was so well known as a diuretic that the English referred to it as piss-abed, from the French *pissenlit*. Meanwhile, the French thought the herb's leaves were shaped like lion's teeth and so dubbed it *dent de lion*, which became anglicized as *dandelion*.

Thanks to herbal exaggerators like 17th-century English herbalist Nicholas Culpeper, dandelion's medicinal reputation spread as widely as the plant itself across an untended lawn. Culpeper recommended the herb for every "evil disposition of the body."

In fact, dandelion was used for so many ailments that it became known as "the official remedy for disorders." This designation lives on today in dandelion's genus name, *Taraxacum*, from the Greek *taraxos*, meaning "disorder," and *akos*, for "remedy."

Early American colonists introduced dandelion to North America, and Native Americans quickly adopted the herb as a tonic. Dandelion root was an ingredient in Lydia E. Pinkham's Vegetable Compound, a popular 19th-century patent medicine for menstrual discomforts. Because it's a diuretic, dandelion no doubt helped relieve the bloating that many women experience before they menstruate.

Even though dandelion was included in the *U.S. Pharmacopoeia*, a standard drug reference, from 1831 to 1926, many 19th-century herbalists despised it for the weed it had become. According to *King's American Dispensatory* (1898), the text used by the American Eclectic physicians, who were forerunners of today's naturopaths, dandelion was "overrated. . . . Dandelion root possesses little medicinal virtue [except] slightly diuretic action."

Contemporary herbalists recommend dandelion almost exclusively as a diuretic for premenstrual syndrome, menstrual discomforts, swollen feet, high blood pressure, congestive heart failure, and weight loss.

Therapeutic Uses

The FDA continues to treat dandelion as a weed. The agency's official position is that "there is no convincing reason for believing it possesses any therapeutic virtues."

The folks at the FDA forgot to read their Ralph Waldo Emerson. "What is a weed?" Emerson wrote. "A plant whose virtues have not yet been discovered." As far as dandelion is concerned, truer words were never penned, although its virtues have been well-documented.

Gallstones. The Doctrine of Signatures was right on at least one count. Two German studies suggest that dandelion stimulates the flow of bile, which helps digest fats.

In Germany, where herbal medicine is more mainstream than in the United States, physicians routinely recommend dandelion to help improve the flow of bile and prevent gallstones. A German preparation called Chol-Grandelat—a combination of dandelion, milk thistle, and rhubarb—is prescribed for gallbladder disease. (This product is not available in the United States.)

Commission E, the expert panel that evaluates herbal medicines for the German counterpart of the FDA, endorses dandelion root and leaves as bile flow stimulants.

Premenstrual syndrome (PMS). Animal studies suggest that dandelion does indeed have diuretic action. Findings in animals don't always apply to people, but this one seems to.

Commission E recognizes dandelion as an effective diuretic. Since diuretics may help relieve the bloated feeling of PMS, women may want to try some before their periods to see if it works for them.

High blood pressure. As the fluid volume of blood decreases, so does blood pressure. That's why physicians often prescribe diuretics to treat high blood pressure. Dandelion may help.

Of course, high blood pressure is a serious condition that requires professional treatment. Use dandelion only in consultation with your physician.

Congestive heart failure. Congestive heart failure is characterized by chronic fatigue of the heart muscle. The condition is often treated with diuretics because they reduce blood volume, so the weakened heart has less fluid to pump around the body. As a natural diuretic, dandelion may be appropriate when taken in conjunction with other medications and therapies prescribed by a physician.

Like high blood pressure, congestive heart failure is a serious condition that cannot be self-treated. If you'd like to try dandelion, discuss it with your physician and use it in addition to standard medication.

Cancer. Dandelion leaves contain noteworthy amounts of beta-carotene and vitamin C. Both nutrients are antioxidants that help prevent the cell damage that sets the stage for cancer, not to mention other degenerative diseases.

Yeast infections. One study found that dandelion inhibits the growth of *Candida albicans*, the fungus responsible for vaginal yeast infections.

Overweight. In one study, animals fed dandelion lost a significant amount of weight. As a diuretic, the herb could help eliminate water weight.

In general, experts do not recommend diuretics for permanent weight control. Most advocate a low-fat, high-fiber diet and regular aerobic exercise. Lost water weight eventually returns as the body, which is mostly water, adjusts to ongoing treatment with diuretics and decreases its urine output.

Intriguing Possibilities

Dandelion may help reduce the amount of sugar in the blood, which means that it may help manage diabetes. Because diabetes is a serious condition that requires professional treatment, however, you should try dandelion only in consultation with your physician.

Some studies have shown that dandelion root has anti-inflammatory properties, suggesting the herb's possible value in treating arthritis. And a Japanese study hinted at dandelion's anti-tumor activity, although it's much too early to consider the herb as a cancer treatment.

Rx Recommendations

Eat fresh leaves in a salad or as a vegetable. If you're using dandelion as a diuretic (for premenstrual syndrome, high blood pressure, or congestive heart failure) or as a digestive aid, take it as a leaf infusion, root decoction, or tincture. The taste is reasonably pleasant, with a slightly bitter sharpness.

To make a leaf infusion, use ½ ounce of dried leaves per cup of boiling water. Steep for 10 minutes, then strain. Drink up to 3 cups a day.

For a root decoction, gently boil 2 to 3 teaspoons of powdered root per cup of water for 15 minutes, let cool, and strain if you wish. Drink up to 3 cups a day.

As a homemade tincture, take 1 to 2 teaspoons up to three times a day.

When using commercial preparations, follow the package directions.

As a potential preventive for vaginal yeast infections, add a couple of handfuls of dried leaves and flowers to bath water.

Do not give dandelion to children under

age 2. For older children and adults over age 65, start with a low-strength preparation and increase the strength if necessary.

The Safety Factor

Long-term use of diuretics such as dandelion can be hazardous. Diuretics deplete the body of potassium, an essential nutrient, so people who are using them should be sure to eat foods rich in potassium, such as bananas and fresh vegetables.

Fortunately, dandelion causes less potassium loss than other diuretics because the herb itself is high in potassium. Nevertheless, if you use dandelion for long periods, be sure to eat potassium-rich foods. Women who are pregnant or nursing should not take diuretics in any form without a doctor's approval.

Dandelion may cause a skin rash in people who are sensitive to it.

Wise-Use Guidelines

Dandelion is included in the FDA list of herbs generally regarded as safe. For adults who are not pregnant, nursing, or taking other diuretics, dandelion is considered safe in the amounts typically recommended.

You should take medicinal amounts of dandelion only in consultation with your doctor. If it causes minor discomfort, such as stomach upset or diarrhea, reduce the dosage or stop using it altogether. Let your doctor know if you experience any unpleasant effects or if the symptoms for which you're using the herb don't improve significantly within 2 weeks.

Growing Information

If you cultivate dandelions, be careful whom you tell. You may end up with some unhappy neighbors.

As every gardener knows, dandelions grow like weeds. This low-growing perennial has a deep taproot, a rosette of jaggedly toothed leaves that radiate from its base, and a smooth, hollow, 6- to 12-inch stem capped by a single yellow flower that gives rise to hundreds of tufted single-seed fruits. The root, leaves, and stem contain a milky fluid.

Harvest young leaves as they develop; as they mature, they become unpleasantly bitter. Herbalists generally recommend harvesting the root at the end of the second growing season. To prevent spreading, clip the flowers before seed tufts form.

Dandelion seeds may not be readily available, but check seed catalogs. Better yet, check nearby lawns or vacant lots. It's unlikely that anyone will mind if you take a few. Plant the seeds in early spring. They grow in almost any soil but prefer moist, well-drained loam.

Dill

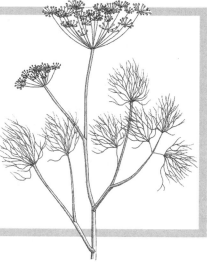

Family: Umbelliferae; other members include carrot, parsley, celery, fennel, and angelica

Genus and species: *Anethum graveolens*

Also known as: No other common names

Parts used: Fruits (seeds); leaves are used in cooking

Dill does more for pickles than provide flavor. It's also a natural preservative. In fact, preserving food was the original purpose of pickling.

Dill has been used in herbal healing since the dawn of Egyptian civilization, and for good reason. In addition to its preservative action, the herb is an infection fighter and a soothing digestive aid.

Healing History

Records found in 3,000-year-old Egyptian tombs show that ancient physicians used fragrant dill as a digestive aid and a remedy for intestinal gas. The 1st-century Greek physician Dioscorides prescribed dill so frequently that it was known for centuries as "the herb of Dioscorides." The Romans chewed dill seeds to promote digestion, and they hung dill garlands in their dining halls, believing that the herb would prevent stomach upset.

Traditional Chinese physicians have used dill as a digestive aid for more than 1,000 years. They recommend it especially for children because its action is milder than that of other digestive herbs such as caraway, anise, and fennel.

The Vikings were well-aware of dill's digestive benefits. The word *dill* comes from the Old Norse *dilla*, meaning to lull or soothe.

The 17th-century English herbalist Nicholas Culpeper claimed dill "stayeth the belly . . . and is a gallant expeller of wind." Culpeper also recommended the herb for hiccups and swelling and to "strengthen the brain."

Colonists brought dill to North America. Its seed infusion, known as dillwater, became a favorite among American folk healers for childhood ailments such as colic, cough, indigestion, gas, stomachache, and insomnia. In adults, the herb was used to treat hemorrhoids, jaundice, scurvy, and "dropsy" (congestive heart failure).

Contemporary herbalists view dill as the herb of choice for infant colic. They recommend chewing the seeds for bad breath and drinking dill tea both as a digestive aid and to stimulate milk production in nursing mothers.

Therapeutic Uses

If you use dill only in pickling spices or on salmon, you're missing out on a marvelous healer. While it won't cure hemorrhoids or increase milk production, some of its other traditional applications are supported by science.

Digestive problems. Research has validated dill's 3,000 years of use as a digestive aid. The herb helps relax the smooth muscles of the digestive tract. One study found dill to be an antifoaming agent, meaning that it helps prevent the formation of intestinal gas bubbles. Dill seed oil also inhibits the growth of several types of bacteria that attack the intestinal tract, suggesting that it may help prevent infectious diarrhea caused by these microorganisms.

Commission E, the expert panel that evaluates herbal medicines for Germany's counterpart of the FDA, endorses dill for indigestion.

Urinary tract infections. *Escherichia coli*, the bacteria that usually cause urinary tract infections, is one type of bacteria that is inhibited by dill.

Intriguing Possibilities

When injected into laboratory animals, dill extract stimulates respiration, slows heart rate, and opens blood vessels, all of which reduce blood pressure. Of course, people don't inject dill preparations, but these effects suggest that there's more to learn about dill's healing potential.

Rx Recommendations

To benefit from dill's breath-freshening effects, chew $\frac{1}{2}$ to 1 teaspoon of seeds.

If you're using the herb as a digestive aid, take it as an infusion or tincture. To make a pleasant-tasting infusion, use 2 teaspoons of crushed seeds per cup of boiling water, steep for 10 minutes, and strain. Drink up to 3 cups a day.

As a homemade tincture, take $\frac{1}{2}$ to 1 teaspoon up to three times a day.

When using commercial preparations, follow the package directions.

You may give small amounts of a weak infusion to children under age 2 for colic or gas. For older children and adults over age 65, start with low-strength preparations and increase the strength if necessary.

To prevent urinary tract infections, tie some dill seeds in a cheesecloth bag and add it to your bath. You can also use up to a teaspoon of dill seed oil in the bath.

The Safety Factor

Never ingest dill seed oil; as little as a teaspoon may be toxic.

In people who are sensitive to it, dill may cause skin rash. The leaves and seeds are generally considered nontoxic.

Wise-Use Guidelines

Dill appears in the FDA list of herbs generally regarded as safe. For adults, dill is safe when used in the amounts typically recommended.

You should use medicinal amounts of dill only in consultation with your doctor. If it causes minor discomfort, such as stomach upset or diarrhea, reduce the dosage or stop using it altogether. Let your doctor know if you experience unpleasant effects or if the symptoms for which you're using the herb do not improve significantly within 2 weeks.

Growing Information

Dill is an annual with a long taproot like its close relative, carrot. It has a delicate, fast-growing, spindly stem with lacy leaves. Yellow flowers appear in summer and produce great quantities of tiny ridged fruits (seeds).

Dill grows vigorously from seeds sown ¼ inch deep in early spring. Germination takes about 2 weeks. Thin seedlings to 12-inch spacing. The plants grow to 3 feet in rich, moist, slightly acidic soil under full sun, or in partial shade in the South. Shelter plants from the wind.

You may harvest the leaves once the plants have established themselves. Fresh dill leaves are much more aromatic than dried. To guarantee a supply of fresh leaves from late spring to late fall, plant seeds periodically throughout your growing season.

The seeds mature in about 2 months. Harvest them when they begin to turn brown.

Dill self-sows, so if you leave a few plants unharvested, you'll have this tasty healing herb every year.

Echinacea

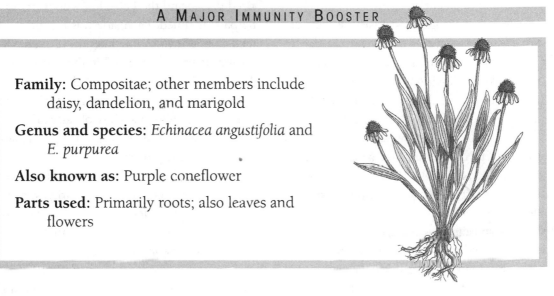

Family: Compositae; other members include daisy, dandelion, and marigold

Genus and species: *Echinacea angustifolia* and *E. purpurea*

Also known as: Purple coneflower

Parts used: Primarily roots; also leaves and flowers

Echinacea (pronounced *eh-kin-AY-sha*) has certainly had its ups and downs on its way to becoming one of the nation's best-selling herbal medicines. Since the 1870s, it has been reviled, then lionized, then forgotten, and finally resurrected.

Today, echinacea is widely accepted as *the* herbal remedy for colds and flu. Many studies published in mainstream medical journals agree that it is a safe, effective immune stimulant that helps the body combat all manner of infections.

Healing History

Echinacea is a tall, daisylike flower native to the American Great Plains. It was the primary medicine of the Native Americans in the region. They applied root poultices to wounds, insect bites and stings, and snakebites. They used echinacea mouthwash for painful teeth and

gums and drank echinacea tea to treat colds, smallpox, measles, mumps, and arthritis.

Plains settlers adopted the herb, but it remained a folk remedy until 1870, when a patent-medicine purveyor, Dr. H. C. F. Meyer of Pawnee City, Nebraska, used it in his Meyer's Blood Purifier. He promoted the remedy as "an absolute cure" for rattlesnake bite, blood poisoning, and a host of other ills. Claims like Dr. Meyer's are what earned patent medicines the derisive name snake oil.

Dr. Meyer truly believed that echinacea could cure rattlesnake bite, however, and he set out to prove it. In 1885, he sent a sample to John Uri Lloyd, professor at the Eclectic Medical Institute in Cincinnati. Lloyd was also one of the first presidents of the American Pharmaceutical Association and a cofounder (with his brothers) of Lloyd Brothers Pharmacists, a prominent 19th-century drug company. Lloyd identified the plant as echinacea, but after one look at Dr. Meyer's label with its claim of "absolute cure" for rattlesnake bite, he dismissed Dr. Meyer as a crackpot.

Dr. Meyer wrote back, insisting that echinacea was indeed a cure for rattlesnake bite. He was so confident that he offered to take a live rattlesnake to Cincinnati and let it bite him in Lloyd's presence to demonstrate his Blood Purifier's effectiveness. Lloyd declined the offer.

Undaunted, Dr. Meyer shipped some echinacea to Lloyd's Eclectic colleague, John King, who had mentioned the plant's Native American uses in the first edition of his Eclectic text, *King's American Dispensatory*, in the 1850s. King tested the herb, and after successfully using it to treat bee stings, chronic nasal congestion, leg ulcers, and a variety of infections, he extolled the plant and included it in subsequent editions of his book.

Eventually, Lloyd also accepted echinacea, declaring it useful for treating wounds, venomous bites and stings, blood poisoning (septicemia), diphtheria, meningitis, measles, chickenpox, malaria, scarlet fever, influenza, syphilis, and gangrene.

Lloyd's enthusiasm was not simply academic. His family business, Lloyd Brothers Pharmacists, developed several echinacea products, which enjoyed tremendous national popularity as infection treatments from the 1890s well into the 1920s. During the early 20th century, it was a rare home medicine cabinet that didn't contain tincture of echinacea. (The Lloyd brothers also owned the New York Giants baseball team and founded the Lloyd Library in Cincinnati, which today houses one of the world's largest collections of botanical literature and publishes the *Journal of Natural Products*, formerly *Lloydia*.)

Unfortunately, echinacea became a casualty of the war between orthodox physicians (known prior to World War I as "regulars"), who favored the emerging laboratory-synthesized drugs, and the Eclectics, who were more herbally inclined. Each side was hostile to the medicines touted by the other. In 1909, the following statement appeared in the *Journal of the American Medical Association*: "Echinacea . . . has failed to sustain the reputation given it by its enthusiasts . . . [who] make use of early unverified reports to endow their nostrums with remarkable therapeutic properties."

By World War II, as modern antibiotics became available, echinacea's popularity waned. It was listed in the *National Formulary*, the pharmacists' reference, from 1916 until 1950. But from the 1940s on, it was largely forgotten—that is, until the herbal revival of the 1970s.

Contemporary herbalists are as enthusiastic about echinacea as the Eclectics were. They tout it as a botanical antibiotic and immune-system stimulant for boils, colds and flu, bladder infections, tonsillitis, and other infectious diseases. Many recommend taking the herb daily as a tonic and immune-system enhancer.

Therapeutic Uses

Old Dr. Meyer would be tickled to learn how potent his favorite herb actually is. Echinacea has never been shown to cure rattlesnake bite, but from the 1950s through the 1980s, many studies (almost all of them German) concluded that echinacea has remarkable immune-stimulating and infection-fighting properties. By the 1990s, American researchers were studying the herb and coming to the same conclusion.

Enhanced immunity. Echinacea helps treat infection by revving up the immune system.

When disease-causing microorganisms attack, cells secrete chemicals that attract infection-fighting white blood cells (macrophages) to the area. The macrophages (literally, "big eaters") engulf and digest the invaders. Echinacea boosts their ability to destroy germs.

The herb also energizes other important white blood cells, the natural killer cells and T lymphocytes. And it increases secretion of interleukin-1, another component of the immune system.

Athletes who engage in ultra-strenuous activities, such as triathlons, often experience immune suppression. German researchers gave 42 triathletes one of three daily treatments: medically inactive placebos, mineral supplements, or echinacea. A month later, shortly after a triathlon, those who had taken the echinacea showed the least immune suppression.

Infections. In addition to its ability to stimulate the immune system, echinacea helps combat a broad range of disease-causing viruses, bacteria, fungi, and protozoa. This attribute lends support to the herb's traditional use for healing wounds and treating many infectious diseases.

Echinacea fights infection in several ways. First, the herb contains echinacoside, a natural antibiotic with broad-spectrum antimicrobial activity.

Second, it strengthens tissues against assault by invading microorganisms. Tissues contain hyaluronic acid (HA), a chemical that in part acts as a shield against germ attacks. Many germs produce the enzyme hyaluronidase to dissolve the HA chemical shield so they can penetrate tissues and cause infection. But echinacea contains another substance, echinacein, that counteracts the germs' tissue-dissolving enzyme and keeps them out of the body's tissues.

Third, echinacea mimics interferon, the body's own virus-fighting compound. Before a virus-infected cell dies, it releases a tiny amount of interferon, which boosts the ability of surrounding cells to resist infection. Echinacea appears to do the same thing. Researchers bathed cells in echinacea extract, then exposed them to two potent viruses (influenza and herpes). Compared with untreated cells, only a small number of the treated cells became infected.

German researchers report success in using echinacea to treat tonsillitis, bronchitis, tuberculosis, meningitis, wounds, abscesses, whooping cough (pertussis), ear infections, and especially colds and flu.

Colds and flu. By the late 1990s, more than a dozen studies had investigated echinacea as a cold treatment. While most showed significant benefit in the form of shorter, milder colds, there were enough that showed no benefit to keep critics carping that echinacea offered more hype than substance.

Then, in a 1999 report published in the *Journal of Family Practice*, two mainstream M.D.'s from the University of Wisconsin at Madison and a naturopathic physician from Bastyr University, the naturopathic medical school near Seattle, teamed up to analyze every published study of using echinacea to prevent and treat upper-respiratory infections.

On the treatment side, the researchers looked at eight studies involving more than 1,000 people. All of the studies were double-blind, meaning that neither the participants nor the researchers knew who was taking echinacea and who was taking placebo. Those who received the herb used various preparations—tablets, capsules, juices, and tinctures. All of the preparations contained the immune-boosting parts of the plant: the roots, leaves, and flowers.

Among the eight studies, this one was typical. In a large Swedish furniture factory, researchers identified 60 workers who were experiencing the initial stages of colds. Half of the workers were given placebos, and the rest were given tincture of echinacea (20 drops in water every 2 hours for the first day, then the same amount three times a day for up to 10 days). Among those taking placebos, the average recovery time was 8 days. That figure was reduced by half, to 4 days, among those taking the echinacea.

All eight studies showed similar results. Six were statistically significant. Two were not, but they showed a clear trend in the direction of benefit. The reviewers' verdict: Echinacea is a solid winner as a treatment for colds and flu. In all eight studies, compared with placebos, the herb produced an average 50 percent reduction in the severity of symptoms and a similar reduction in the number of days that people actually felt ill.

Commission E, the expert panel that evaluates herbal medicines for the German counterpart of the FDA, also endorses echinacea as a treatment for colds and flu.

On the prevention side, the researchers analyzed four studies with a total of 1,152 participants. Again, the studies were double-blind and used various preparations of all parts of the herb. None of these studies showed echinacea to have statistically significant preventive value. The reviewers concluded that the herb isn't useful in preventing colds and flu. (It should be noted that traditional herbalists have recommended echinacea only as a treatment for infectious illnesses, never as a preventive.)

The researchers concluded that treatment with echinacea should begin as soon as you feel the first twinges of a cold or flu coming on. Take it several times a day, then taper off as you begin to feel better.

Wounds. Science has confirmed echinacea's traditional use for wound healing. Echinacein—the same chemical that prevents germs from penetrating tissues—also helps broken skin knit faster by spurring the cells that form new tissue (fibroblasts) to work more efficiently.

Echinacea preparations can be applied to cuts, burns, psoriasis, eczema, genital herpes sores, and cold sores. Commission E supports the use of echinacea for wound treatment.

Yeast infections. In a German study, 203 women with recurrent vaginal yeast infections were treated with either a standard pharmaceutical anti-yeast cream or the cream plus oral doses of echinacea. Within 6 months, 60 percent of the women who used just the antifungal cream experienced recurrences. Among those who also took echinacea, that figure was only 16 percent—a highly significant difference.

Cancer chemotherapy and radiation therapy. Cancer patients undergoing chemotherapy typically experience reductions in their white blood cell counts, which increases their risk of infection. German researchers gave 15 people with advanced esophageal and colorectal cancers chemotherapy treatment plus echinacea and an extract of the thymus gland, a component of the immune system. Instead of falling, as would be expected, their white blood cell counts increased.

Radiation treatments can also depress white blood cell counts, suggesting that echinacea may help. If you're receiving cancer chemotherapy or radiation therapy, ask your medical and radiation oncologists about incorporating echinacea into your treatment plan.

Intriguing Possibility

In animals, echinacea has demonstrated promising anticancer activity against leukemia and a few tumors. It would be premature to describe the herb as a cancer treatment, but that day may come.

Rx Recommendations

You can use either a decoction or a tincture to take advantage of echinacea's infection-fighting potential.

To make a decoction, use 2 teaspoons of root material per cup of water. Bring it to a boil, then simmer for 15 minutes. Drink up to 3 cups a day. You'll find the taste initially sweet, then bitter.

As a homemade tincture, take 1 teaspoon up to three times a day.

When using commercial preparations, follow the package directions.

Do not give echinacea to children under age 2. For older children and adults over age 65, start with low-strength preparations and increase the strength if necessary.

The Safety Factor

Echinacea often causes a normal, harmless tingling sensation on the tongue.

Wise-Use Guidelines

The FDA lists echinacea as an herb of undefined safety. The evidence suggests that it's safe, although allergic reactions are possible.

The only people who should not use echinacea are those with autoimmune conditions, such as lupus, since it's possible that stimulating the immune system may aggravate such conditions. People who are HIV-positive should also exercise caution with echinacea. The AIDS virus attacks the cells of the immune system, so stimulating them may also stimulate the virus.

For adults who are not pregnant or nursing and do not have autoimmune conditions or HIV infection, echinacea is considered safe in the amounts typically recommended.

You should use medicinal amounts of echinacea only in consultation with your doctor. If it causes minor discomfort, such as stomach upset or diarrhea, reduce the dosage or stop using it altogether. Let your doctor know if you experience any unpleasant effects or if the symptoms for which you are using the herb do not improve significantly within 2 weeks.

Growing Information

Echinacea is a 2- to 5-foot perennial whose flowers resemble black-eyed Susans, with purple rays radiating from a cone-shaped center (hence its common name, purple coneflower). The herb has black roots, a single stem covered with bristly hairs, and narrow leaves.

Echinacea grows from seeds or root cuttings taken in spring or fall. Don't cover the seeds. When the temperature is in the seventies, simply tamp them into moist, sandy soil.

Echinacea grows in poor, rocky, slightly acidic soil under full sun. It also thrives in richer soils.

It takes 3 to 4 years for the roots to grow large enough to harvest. Pull them in autumn after the plant has gone to seed. Roots larger than $1/2$ inch in diameter should be split before drying.

Elecampane

Family: Compositae; other members include daisy, dandelion, and marigold

Genus and species: *Inula helenium*

Also known as: Wild sunflower, velvet dock, scabwort, and horseheal

Parts used: Roots

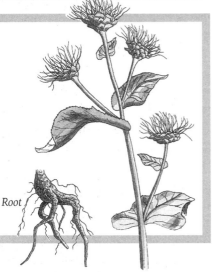

Root

Legend has it that Helen of Troy carried a handful of elecampane on the fateful day that the Trojan prince Paris abducted her from Sparta, igniting the Trojan War. Perhaps the woman whose face launched 1,000 ships had amoebic dysentery, pinworms, hookworms, or giardiasis.

We'll probably never know. We do know that elecampane, whose Latin name (*Inula helenium*) memorializes the Greek beauty, may help expel parasites from the intestine.

Healing History

According to Hippocrates, elecampane stimulates the brain, kidneys, stomach, and uterus. The ancient Romans used the herb to treat indigestion. The Roman naturalist Pliny wrote, "Let no day pass without eating some roots of elecampane to help digestion, expel melancholy,

and cause mirth." And the Roman physician Galen recommended the herb as "good for passion of the hucklebone [sciatica]."

Traditional Chinese and Indian Ayurvedic physicians recommended elecampane as a treatment for respiratory problems, particularly bronchitis and asthma.

During the Middle Ages, European herbalists prescribed elecampane to treat coughs, bronchitis, and asthma, but the herb was more popular as a veterinary medicine. It was reputed to cure scab disease in sheep, hence one of its popular names, scabwort. It was also considered a panacea for horses, and for that reason, it was known as horseheal.

As time passed, elecampane regained its reputation as a human digestive aid. It was the main ingredient in a medieval elixir known as *potio Paulina*.

The 17th-century London herbalist Nicholas

Culpeper touted elecampane "to relieve cough, shortness of breath, and wheezing in the lungs." Echoing Galen, he also endorsed the herb for sciatica and claimed that it restored vision and cured gout, sores, and "worms in the stomach."

In those days, elecampane root was candied and eaten as a confection. Lozenges combining elecampane and honey were a popular treatment for whooping cough (pertussis).

Early American colonists naturalized elecampane and used it as an expectorant, digestive aid, menstruation promoter, and diuretic for treating the water retention associated with dropsy (congestive heart failure). Native American tribes in the Northeast adopted the plant for respiratory problems.

America's 19th-century Eclectic physicians, forerunners of today's naturopaths, also used elecampane as a diuretic and menstruation promoter. Primarily, however, they prescribed the herb for "asthma, bronchial and chronic pulmonary [lung] affections, weakness of the digestive organs, itching, dyspepsia [indigestion], night sweats, and severe colds."

Present day herbalists generally recommend elecampane only for respiratory ailments, cough, asthma, bronchitis, and emphysema. Some recommend it as a digestive aid, as a treatment for menstrual and skin problems, and to banish intestinal parasites.

Therapeutic Uses

The FDA says that elecampane "was employed by the ancients for diseases in which it was probably of no service." The herb has not been well-researched, but the few scientific studies that have been done suggest that for once, Nicholas Culpeper wasn't completely off the deep end.

Intestinal parasites. European scientists have discovered that elecampane contains a chemical called alantolactone that really does help expel intestinal parasites, as Culpeper claimed. The herb also kills some bacteria and fungi, adding to its potential therapeutic action in the intestine.

Infestation with intestinal parasites, especially pinworms and the protozoan *Giardia lamblia* (which causes giardiasis), is a growing problem in the United States. Families with children in day care are particularly susceptible. Intestinal parasites are quite common in the tropics. If you travel overseas, do what Helen of Troy did: Take some elecampane with you.

Women's health concerns. Elecampane has not been shown to stimulate uterine contractions, but because of its long tradition as a menstruation promoter, women may want to try it to help bring on their periods.

Intriguing Possibilities

In animal tests conducted in Europe, elecampane was found to lower blood pressure. People with high blood pressure might try it, in consultation with their physicians.

Elecampane has also been shown to have a sedative effect in experimental animals. People with insomnia might try taking some before bed.

Rx Recommendations

Elecampane's main use is to help prevent and treat intestinal parasites. To try it for this purpose or—in consultation with your physician—to keep your blood pressure down, take it as either a decoction or a tincture.

To prepare a decoction, gently boil 1 to 2

teaspoons of dried, powdered root in 3 cups of water for 30 minutes, then strain if you wish. The taste is bitter. Take 1 to 2 tablespoons at a time with honey, up to 2 cups a day.

As a homemade tincture, use ¼ to ½ teaspoon up to three times a day.

When using commercial preparations, follow the package directions.

Do not give elecampane to children under age 2. For older children and adults over age 65, start with low-strength preparations and increase the strength if necessary.

The Safety Factor

Although elecampane has never been proven to stimulate the uterus, it has been used traditionally to promote menstruation. For this reason, pregnant women should not take it.

Animal studies have shown that small doses of elecampane lower blood sugar levels, while higher doses raise them. These studies have not been replicated in humans, but people with diabetes should steer clear of the herb.

People who are sensitive to elecampane may develop a rash from skin contact with the herb or its oil. Otherwise, no harmful effects have been reported.

Wise-Use Guidelines

Elecampane is included in the FDA list of herbs generally regarded as safe. For adults who are not pregnant or nursing and do not have dia-betes, elecampane is safe when used in the amounts typically recommended.

You should take medicinal amounts of elecampane only in consultation with your doctor. If the herb causes minor discomfort, such as stomach upset or diarrhea, reduce the dosage or stop using it altogether. Let your doctor know if you experience any unpleasant effects or if the symptoms for which you're using the herb do not improve significantly within 2 weeks.

Growing Information

Elecampane is a striking perennial that reaches 5 feet and produces a large flower (hence its common name, wild sunflower). The entire plant is covered with woolly hairs. The medicinal roots are large, branching, and fleshy.

Elecampane may be started from seeds sown indoors in late winter, then transplanted. Once plants have been established, however, the herb is best propagated from 2-inch root cuttings taken in fall from the buds (eyes) of 2-year-old roots. Cover the cuttings with moist, sandy soil and store them for the winter in a cool indoor room. Plant the cuttings 3 feet apart after the danger of frost has passed. Deeply cultivated soil produces the biggest roots.

Elecampane likes rich, moist, well-drained, slightly acid loam and full sun or partial shade. Harvest the roots during the fall of their second year. Older roots become too woody. To speed drying, slice roots into pieces.

Ephedra

Family: Ephedraceae; other members include broom and horsetail

Genus and species: *Ephedra sinica, E. vulgaris, E. nevadensis, E. antisyphilitica,* and other species

Also known as: Ma huang, Mormon tea, and whorehouse tea

Parts used: Stems and branches

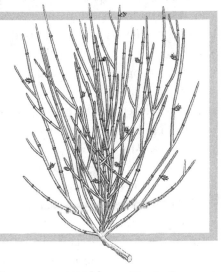

Ephedra—or, in Chinese, ma huang—is a powerful bronchial decongestant and stimulant. Many herbalists view ephedra as the world's oldest medicine. It is certainly one of the oldest.

Sadly, few people who take over-the-counter cold remedies containing the herb's laboratory equivalent (pseudoephedrine) have any idea that they are part of an herbal healing tradition that's estimated to date back some 5,000 years. Even more sadly, a small but widely publicized group who've used irresponsibly large amounts of ephedra have experienced serious consequences, including death.

Healing History

The origins of Chinese medicine are lost in legend. Authorities generally agree, however, that Chinese physicians began prescribing a tea made from Chinese ephedra for colds, asthma, and hay fever around 3000 B.C. The Indian and Pakistani species of the herb have been used medicinally for almost as long.

When the Mormons reached Utah in 1847, local Native Americans introduced them to American ephedra, a piney-tasting tonic beverage. The Mormons adopted it as a substitute for coffee and tea, and around the West it became known as Mormon tea, a name that survives today.

American ephedra is a mild diuretic. In the Old West, it developed a reputation as a cure for syphilis and gonorrhea. It was served in many Western brothels, hence another of its common names, whorehouse tea, and the Latin name for one species, *Ephedra antisyphilitica.*

Contemporary herbalists recommend ephedra just as the ancient Chinese did, to treat asthma, hay fever, and the nasal and chest congestion of colds and flu.

Therapeutic Uses

American ephedra is simply a refreshing beverage. It contains none of the pharmacologically active compounds (ephedrine, pseudoephedrine, and norpseudoephedrine) found in Chinese ephedra, which is the plant used in herbal medicine.

When people say "ephedra," they're usually referring to the Chinese variety, ma huang (*E. sinica*). Some herb marketers mistakenly refer to American ephedra as ma huang and the Chinese herb as Mormon tea.

Worldwide, there are about 40 species of ephedra. If you're interested in using the herb medicinally, look for a product that's identified by species on the label and be sure that it says *Ephedra sinica* or *E. sinica*.

The active compounds in Chinese ephedra are strong central nervous system stimulants, more powerful than caffeine but less potent than amphetamine. All three open the bronchial passages (meaning that they're bronchodilators). They also stimulate the heart and uterine contractions; increase blood pressure, metabolic rate, and perspiration and urine production; and reduce the secretion of both saliva and stomach acid.

Respiratory problems. From the late 1920s through the 1940s, ephedrine was added to cold, asthma, and hay fever products as a decongestant and bronchodilator. Ephedrine was generally effective and reasonably safe, but it was known to cause potentially hazardous side effects, including increased blood pressure and rapid heartbeat (palpitations). It was eventually replaced with a close chemical substitute, pseudoephedrine, which is also an active compound in ma huang.

Scientists consider pseudoephedrine just as effective as ephedrine but with less problematic side effects. Pseudoephedrine is the active ingredient in many over-the-counter cold and allergy products, most notably Sudafed, whose name is derived from its active ingredient.

Ephedra continues to be used in herbal cold, flu, allergy, and decongestant products. Chinese physicians prescribe it to treat asthma. Commission E, the expert panel that evaluates herbal medicines for the German counterpart of the FDA, endorses ma huang for the treatment of bronchial congestion.

Overweight. Ma huang increases metabolic rate, the speed at which the body burns calories. It also depresses appetite somewhat. This combination of effects led to studies of the herb (actually chemically isolated ephedrine) for weight control, usually in combination with another stimulant, caffeine.

In physician-supervised weight-loss programs that include a low-fat diet and regular exercise, treatment with a combination of ephedrine and caffeine has increased weight loss by about an additional 5 percent.

One 3-month study conducted by Danish researchers showed that compared with overweight women taking medically inactive placebos, those taking oral ephedrine (20 milligrams three times a day) lost somewhat more weight. And in their own 2-month study, Italian researchers found that overweight women lost more weight if they supplemented their low-calorie diets with oral ephedrine (50 milligrams three times a day).

To experience ephedra's weight-reduction benefits, you must be clinically obese—that is, at least 20 percent heavier than your recommended weight. Ephedrine has shown no effect in moderately overweight people who simply want to lose 5 to 10 pounds.

Keep in mind that pounds lost with the help of ephedra may not be gone permanently, especially once you stop using the herb. What's more, routine use of ephedra for weight control typically causes side effects that may be unpleasant (more on this later).

Experts generally agree that the keys to permanent weight loss are a low-fat, high-fiber diet and regular aerobic exercise. Nonetheless, ephedra is an ingredient in many herbal weight-loss formulas sold in health food stores and drugstores.

Women's health concerns. Ephedrine causes uterine contractions in laboratory animals. Women may want to try ephedra to initiate menstruation; those who are pregnant or trying to conceive should not use it.

Medicinal Myth

Although American ephedra was popular in the Old West as a remedy for syphilis and gonorrhea, in reality, the herb has no effect on either disease. Anyone who develops a genital sore or discharge should consult a physician.

Rx Recommendations

To take advantage of ephedra's potent healing benefits as a decongestant or a menstruation promoter, you'll want to use a decoction or tincture. You'll find the taste pleasantly piney.

For a decoction, use 1 teaspoon of dried herb per cup of water. Bring it to a boil, then simmer for 10 to 15 minutes. Drink up to 2 cups a day.

As a homemade tincture, take ¼ to 1 teaspoon up to three times a day.

When using commercial preparations, follow the package directions and be alert for possible side effects.

Do not give ephedra to children under age 2. For older children and adults over age 65, start with low-strength preparations and increase the strength if necessary.

The Safety Factor

At the time of this writing, ephedra is at the center of a regulatory storm. Starting in the mid-1990s, very large doses of the herb were included in products that promised a legal high similar to that provided by methamphetamine ("speed"). Brand names of these products included Herbal Ecstasy, Cloud 9, and Ultimate X-phoria.

Irresponsibly large doses of ephedra can indeed produce effects similar to those of methamphetamine. In such enormous doses, however, the herb may also cause serious—even fatal—heart problems and stroke in healthy people.

In one study, researchers at the New England Medical Center in Boston used data supplied by the FDA to document 14 cardiac arrests, 13 strokes, 9 heart attacks, and more than 900 other adverse reactions associated with ephedra. The people who suffered harm were typically either dieters using ephedra to lose weight or young people seeking intoxication.

Subsequently, however, an audit of the FDA's ephedra database by the General Accounting Office (GAO), the investigative arm of Congress, accused the FDA of using "questionable" science and unsubstantiated information to compile its statistics. The GAO concluded that the FDA's database of adverse reactions was "open to question."

Despite the GAO's criticism, in 1997 the FDA announced its intention to regulate ephedra more closely. At this time, final regulations have not been announced, but the FDA has hinted that it will require marketers to reduce the amount of ephedra in products containing the herb and require labeling that warns of possible heart problems and stroke from overdose.

Assuming that you steer clear of irresponsibly large doses of ephedra, it's important to understand that even recommended doses can have a powerful stimulant effect. They may also cause nervousness, jitters, irritability, anxiety, insomnia, dizziness, heart palpitations, and skin flushing.

Some compounds in ma huang have been shown to raise blood pressure and blood sugar levels. Other compounds have been shown to lower them. People with diabetes or high blood pressure should err on the side of caution and not use the herb. Nor is ephedra appropriate for people with heart disease, glaucoma, or kidney conditions, because of the risk of elevated blood pressure.

People with overactive thyroid (hyperthyroidism or Graves' disease) should avoid all stimulants, including ephedra.

Likewise, ephedra constricts the urethra and can lead to difficulty urinating. For this reason, men with benign prostate enlargement, which also causes urinary problems, should not use the herb.

In addition, ephedra often causes insomnia. People who have difficulty sleeping should avoid taking the herb late in the day.

Ephedra can lead to dry mouth, so if you're using the herb, be sure to increase your intake of nonalcoholic liquids.

Finally, if you're a competitive athlete, you need to think twice about taking ephedra. It is on the United States Olympic Committee's list of banned substances, for example.

Wise-Use Guidelines

You should use medicinal amounts of ephedra only in consultation with your doctor. If it causes insomnia, nervousness, or stomach upset, reduce the dosage or stop using it altogether. Let your doctor know if you experience any unpleasant effects or if the symptoms for which you're taking the herb do not improve significantly within 2 weeks.

Growing Information

Ephedra is not a garden herb. It is an odd-looking, botanically primitive, almost leafless shrub that resembles horsetail. It has tough, jointed, barkless stems and branches, with small scalelike leaves and tiny yellow-green flowers that appear in summer. Male and female flowers appear on different plants. The seeds develop in cones.

Eucalyptus

Family: Myrtaceae; other members include myrtle, tea tree, and clove

Genus and species: *Eucalyptus globulus*

Also known as: Gum tree, blue gum, and Australian fever tree

Parts used: Leaves

If you've ever used Listerine mouthwash or a decongestant such as Vicks VapoRub, you're undoubtedly familiar with the unique, refreshing scent of eucalyptus. And if you've ever seen a koala, you've probably seen eucalyptus, because the plant's long, scythe-shaped leaves are the sole food source for the cute, furry marsupial.

Eucalyptus is also Australia's contribution to herbal healing. The herb has even won FDA approval as a treatment for colds and flu.

Healing History

Eucalyptus roots hold an astonishing amount of water. Australia's aborigines chewed them for water in the dry outback. They also drank eucalyptus leaf tea for fevers.

In the 1780s, when England declared Australia a penal colony and started shipping con-

victs to what is now Sydney, it took a while for the new immigrants to catch on to eucalyptus as a water source. Many early outback explorers died of thirst within sight of eucalyptus stands.

Around 1840, crew members on a French freighter anchored off Sydney developed a disease involving high fever. They were cured with eucalyptus tea. Reports of similar incidents slowly made their way back to Europe, and the herb became known as "Australian fever tree."

By the 1860s, eucalyptus leaves and oil were being used around the Mediterranean area to treat intermittent fever (what we now know as malaria), which had plagued the area since ancient times. Some physicians reported curing malaria with eucalyptus, but others dismissed the herb as worthless.

Today, we understand that eucalyptus has no direct effect on the protozoan that causes malaria. Ironically, however, the eucalyptus tree was responsible for virtually eradicating the devastating disease in much of Italy, Sicily, and Algeria, where it had raged unchecked for thousands of years. Malaria is transmitted by mosquitoes that live in swampy areas. Europeans planted eucalyptus trees in the marshlands bordering the Mediterranean, and as the trees grew, their roots soaked up water and drained the swamps, eliminating malarial mosquitoes' habitat—and the disease they carried.

Eucalyptus oil was used as an antiseptic on urinary catheters in 19th-century British hospitals, where it became known as catheter oil. In America, 19th-century Eclectic physicians, forerunners of today's naturopaths, used eucalyptus oil as an antiseptic on wounds and medical instruments. They also recommended inhaling the vapors in steam to treat bronchitis, asthma, whooping cough (pertussis), and emphysema.

Contemporary herbalists recommend eucalyptus as a topical antiseptic, a gargle for sore throat, and a treatment for the nasal and chest congestion of colds, flu, bronchitis, croup, and asthma.

Therapeutic Uses

Eucalyptus leaf oil contains eucalyptol, a compound that gives the herb its pleasant aroma and healing value.

Colds and flu. Eucalyptol loosens phlegm in the chest so it's easier to cough up. That's why so many cough lozenges are flavored with eucalyptus.

Eucalyptus is one of the few traditional herbal medicines approved by the FDA. Commission E, the expert panel that evaluates herbal medicines for the German counterpart of the FDA, also endorses the herb as a cold and flu treatment.

In Russia, animal studies have shown that eucalyptol kills influenza A, the virus that causes the most serious form of flu. It also kills certain bacteria. Inhaling the vapors of a strong eucalyptus infusion may help prevent bacterial bronchitis, a possible complication of colds and flu.

Wounds. The antibacterial action of eucalyptol makes it an effective treatment for minor cuts and scrapes.

Headaches. In two very similar studies, German researchers treated people who were prone to tension headaches with either medically inactive placebos or different combinations of eucalyptus and peppermint oils. Participants rubbed the preparations on their foreheads and temples. The herb treatments produced more significant relief. The formula that was mostly eucalyptus oil produced the greatest muscle relaxation, while the formula that was mostly peppermint oil yielded the greatest pain relief. The researchers suggested trying an herbal treatment instead of or in addition to an over-the-counter pain reliever.

Insect repellent. Eucalyptol repels cockroaches, according to a report in *Science News*.

Rx Recommendations

To make a eucalyptus inhalant, boil a handful of leaves or a few drops of essential oil in water.

For minor cuts and scrapes, thoroughly wash the wound with soap and water, then apply a drop or two of eucalyptus oil.

To relieve headaches, rub the oil on your forehead and temples.

To prepare a eucalyptus bath, wrap a handful of leaves in a cloth and run the bath water over it.

For a cool, spicy, refreshing infusion to treat colds and flu, use 1 to 2 teaspoons of dried, crushed leaves per cup of boiling water. Steep for 10 minutes. Drink up to 2 cups a day. You can also make an infusion by using 1 to 2 drops of eucalyptus oil.

When using commercial preparations, follow the package directions.

Do not give eucalyptus to children under age 2. For older children and adults over age 65, start with low-strength preparations and increase the strength if necessary.

If your home is infested with cockroaches and you don't want to use insecticides, try soaking small cloths in eucalyptus oil and placing them around your cabinets.

The Safety Factor

Used externally, eucalyptus oil is considered nonirritating, but it may cause a rash in people who are unusually sensitive to it. Anyone who does not develop a rash may use eucalyptus preparations externally, although infants and children may rebel against the pungent aroma.

For internal use, eucalyptus leaf is considered safe for use by healthy adults who are not pregnant or nursing.

If you use eucalyptus oil, be very careful not to ingest more than a drop or two. It is highly poisonous, and fatalities have been reported from ingestion of as little as a teaspoon.

Wise-Use Guidelines

You should use medicinal amounts of eucalyptus only in consultation with your doctor. If it causes minor discomfort, such as stomach upset or diarrhea, reduce the dosage or stop using it altogether. Let your doctor know if you experience unpleasant effects or if the symptoms for which you're using the herb do not improve significantly within 2 weeks.

Growing Information

The more than 500 species of eucalyptus account for three-quarters of the native vegetation in Australia. Eucalyptus varies from 5 foot shrubs to the tallest trees on Earth—up to 475 feet, the size of a 40-story building.

Eucalyptus grows anywhere with loamy soil and adequate water, as long as the temperature does not dip below freezing. Plant saplings obtained at a nursery. If the leaves begin to blister, cut back on watering.

Eucalyptus often kills surrounding vegetation (except other Australian plants), which is why the trees are usually found in stands with little between them. They grow extremely rapidly, up to several feet per year, and their trunks eventually attain enormous girth. If you plant a eucalyptus, be prepared for it to dominate your yard.

Horticulturists discourage planting eucalyptus. The plant's roots break up water and sewer lines, its trunks buckle sidewalks, and its limbs have a tendency to break off in gusting winds, damaging property and endangering lives.

Evening Primrose

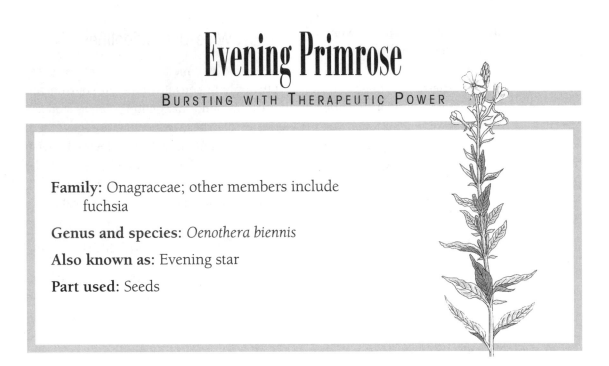

Family: Onagraceae; other members include fuchsia

Genus and species: *Oenothera biennis*

Also known as: Evening star

Part used: Seeds

Have you ever seen an evening primrose bloom? It's one of the most beautiful sights in the plant kingdom.

Each flower opens for only one night. Just before dusk, all that's visible is the ripe, unopened bud. As the light of day begins to fade, the bud starts quivering. All of a sudden, the four green sepals flick out perpendicular to the flower stem, revealing a tight bundle of dainty yellow petals. The petals tremble as they emerge from their tight cocoon. With jerky, dancing contortions that take about a minute, the golden petals spread out, 2 inches across, radiant in the sunset. By morning, the flower withers and dies.

Fortunately, the healing power of evening primrose's seed oil is much longer lasting than the plant's flowers. Evening primrose oil (EPO) began attracting research attention only in the 1970s. Since then, many studies have shown that it helps treat cardiovascular disease, premenstrual syndrome, rheumatoid arthritis, eczema, and possibly even breast cancer, multiple sclerosis, and a complication of diabetes.

Healing History

Evening primrose is native to North America. Native Americans used the plant as both a food and a medicine. Many tribes boiled the roots and ate them; others ate the young leaves and seeds.

Medicinally, Native Americans applied the whole evening primrose plant externally to control the swelling and inflammation of wounds. They also drank root tea to treat coughs.

Early colonists adopted evening primrose enthusiastically. They, too, boiled the roots as food and used the seeds to garnish breads. They also adopted the Native American practice of applying the plant to treat wounds.

The Shakers, whose enormous herb gardens supplied many early Americans with medicinal herbs, used a tea made from evening primrose seeds to treat indigestion and other digestive problems.

America's 19th-century Eclectic physicians, forerunners of today's naturopaths, picked up on the Native American and Shaker recommendations. They advised mixing a strong tea with lard and applying it to wounds and other skin conditions. They also prescribed the tea for digestive upsets and suggested evening primrose for "sallow skin when the patient's mentality is of a gloomy and despondent character."

Until the 1980s, evening primrose was a minor medicinal herb. Herbalists recommended it mostly for indigestion. But since researchers discovered a key essential fatty acid in the herb's seed oil, evening primrose has become much more widely studied and recommended.

Therapeutic Uses

Evening primrose seeds contain an oil that has a high concentration of a compound rarely found in plants: gamma-linolenic acid (GLA), which is an essential fatty acid, or EFA. Essential fatty acids play many important roles in the body. They are involved in the synthesis of prostaglandins, compounds that regulate dozens of bodily functions. They also act as anti-inflammatory agents and help to regulate metabolism.

EFA cannot be synthesized by the body and must be obtained from diet. Fish—especially cold-water fish such as salmon—contain these fatty acids, most notably the omega-3's. We Americans, who eat meat-dominated diets, tend to have low EFA intakes.

When laboratory animals have been placed on diets devoid of EFA, they have exhibited a number of health problems: eczema-like skin conditions, immune suppression, cardiovascular disease, poor wound healing, liver abnormalities, and infertility. This finding has led researchers to give EFA supplements to people with conditions linked to EFA deficiencies. The results have been remarkably positive.

The *Review of Natural Products,* a scientific publication that monitors research on herbal medicines, has concluded that for conditions related to EFA deficiencies, the value of evening primrose oil "cannot be overstated [and produces] excellent results."

Heart disease and stroke. The GLA in evening primrose oil can lower cholesterol substantially. In one Scottish study, 79 people with high cholesterol took 4,000 milligrams of evening primrose oil every day for 3 months. Their average cholesterol levels fell 31.5 percent. Cardiologists believe that for every 1 percent decrease in total cholesterol, the risk of heart attack drops 2 percent. So in the Scottish study, the participants' risk of heart attack plummeted more than 60 percent.

Other research has shown that evening primrose oil lowers blood pressure and reduces the likelihood of the blood clots that lead to heart attacks and most strokes.

Premenstrual syndrome (PMS). The current research goes both ways on the use of evening primrose oil as a treatment for the mood swings, fluid retention, and breast tenderness of PMS. Some studies show benefit, while others do not. Those that show benefit generally are of longer duration, lasting five cycles or more.

In one of these studies, 19 women took evening primrose oil for the 2 weeks before their menstrual periods for 5 months. Their PMS symptoms declined significantly, with the greatest benefit occurring during the final month.

Breast pain. PMS may trigger breast pain or tenderness, but other conditions unrelated to the menstrual cycle may also cause it. In one study, which spanned 17 years and involved more than 400 women, researchers at the University of Wales prescribed either one of two standard drugs (Danazol or bromocriptine) or evening primrose oil. All three treatments produced similar results: significant relief for about 90 percent of the women whose pain came and went with their menstrual cycles as well as for 60 percent of the women with constant breast pain.

Rheumatoid arthritis. Several studies have shown that evening primrose helps relieve the joint pain, swelling, and tenderness of rheumatoid arthritis. At the University of Pennsylvania, researchers gave 37 people with rheumatoid arthritis either GLA or medically inactive placebos. After 6 months, those receiving placebos experienced no change in their symptoms, while those taking GLA reported 36 percent fewer tender joints and 45 percent less joint pain. What's more, the GLA caused no side effects.

Two British studies came up with similar results. In one, 40 people with rheumatoid arthritis added either evening primrose oil or placebos to their routine drug regimens. After 6 months, those on the placebos reported no change in their symptoms, while those taking evening primrose oil noted significant improvement.

Eczema and other skin conditions. Finnish researchers gave 25 people with eczema either evening primrose oil or placebos for 3 months. The participants taking the evening primrose oil showed a significantly greater decrease in the amount and severity of their skin inflammation. Several other studies confirmed this finding, recording significant relief from inflammation and itching after treatment with evening primrose oil.

Intriguing Possibilities

Animal studies have shown that evening primrose oil reduces the size of breast tumors when injected under the skin. Pilot trials with humans hint that the oil may improve some symptoms of multiple sclerosis. It has also been used successfully to treat diabetic nerve damage (neuropathy) and alcohol-related liver damage.

Rx Recommendations

Evening primrose oil is sold commercially in 500-milligram capsules containing 320 to 480 milligrams of GLA. Studies that showed benefit from evening primrose oil supplementation used 3 to 12 capsules a day. Take the product you choose according to the package directions.

Do not give evening primrose oil to children under age 2. For older children and adults over age 65, start with a small number of capsules and increase the number if necessary.

The Safety Factor

No significant side effects from evening primrose oil have been documented in the medical literature. Still, allergic reactions and mild digestive upsets are possible.

You should use medicinal amounts of evening primrose oil only in consultation with your doctor. If it causes minor discomfort, such as stomach upset or diarrhea, reduce the dosage or stop using it altogether. Let your doctor know if you experience any side effects or if the symptoms for which you're using the oil do not improve significantly within 2 weeks (or, in the case of PMS, 6 months).

Growing Information

Evening primrose is an annual or biennial that grows throughout the United States and is very popular with gardeners. Botanically, it is not a true primrose.

Depending on conditions, the plants reach from 3 to 9 feet. Flowers bloom from June through September for one night each.

The medicinal uses of evening primrose have led to its commercial farming in the United States and Canada, which together produce about 400 tons of seed annually. In this country, most commercial production is centered in California, the Carolinas, Oregon, and Texas.

Fennel

Family: Umbelliferae; other members include carrot, parsley, celery, dill, and angelica

Genus and species: *Foeniculum vulgare* and *F. vulgare dulce*

Also known as: Finocchio, carosella, and Florence fennel

Parts used: Fruits (seeds); stalks and bulbs are used in cooking

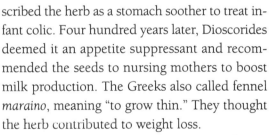

Bulb

New England's Puritans referred to fennel as "meeting seeds." The meetings were their endless church services, and some experts believe that they used fennel as an appetite suppressant. Others theorize that many Puritans steeled themselves for church with whiskey and then chewed fennel seeds to mask the odor.

The Puritans also used fennel as a digestive aid. This has been the herb's primary purpose in herbal healing from the time of the Pharaohs to the present day.

Healing History

In Greek mythology, humanity received knowledge from Mount Olympus as a fiery coal encased in a fennel bulb.

The ancient Greeks had several different ideas about the medicinal value of fennel. During the 3rd century B.C., Hippocrates prescribed the herb as a stomach soother to treat infant colic. Four hundred years later, Dioscorides deemed it an appetite suppressant and recommended the seeds to nursing mothers to boost milk production. The Greeks also called fennel *maraino*, meaning "to grow thin." They thought the herb contributed to weight loss.

The Roman naturalist Pliny loved fennel and included the plant in 22 medicinal recipes. He noted that some snakes rubbed against the plant after shedding their skins and that soon after, their glazed eyes cleared. Pliny took this as a sign that fennel could cure human eye problems, including blindness.

Ancient India's Ayurvedic physicians revered fennel as a digestive aid.

Under the medieval Doctrine of Signatures—the notion that plants' physical characteristics revealed their medicinal value—fennel's yellow flowers were linked to the liver's yellow bile. Thus, the herb was recommended for jaundice.

The emperor Charlemagne ordered that fennel be cultivated in all of his imperial "physic" or medicinal gardens. And the household of King Edward I of England consumed more than 8 pounds of the herb a month. The Church permitted the seeds to be nibbled on fast days as an appetite suppressant.

Fennel was one of Hildegard of Bingen's favorite herbs. The 12th-century German abbess/herbalist recommended it for colds, flu, the heart, and to "make us happy, [with] good digestion . . . and good body odor."

The Anglo-Saxons who settled England around the 5th century used fennel as both a spice and a digestive aid. They also hung fennel over their doors to protect against witchcraft.

By the 17th century, fennel was a mainstay of herbal healing and a standard seasoning for fish. Seventeenth-century English herbalist Nicholas Culpeper, apparently not a fish lover, wrote that fennel "consumes the phlegmatic humour which fish . . . annoys the body with." Culpeper also echoed the ancient recommendations, prescribing fennel to "break wind, increase milk, cleanse the eyes from mists that hinder sight, take away the loathings which oftentimes happen to stomachs of sick persons . . . [and] in drink or broth to make people lean that are too fat." He claimed that it "brought women's courses" (menstruation).

Folk herbalists often mixed fennel with strong laxative herbs, such as buckthorn, senna, rhubarb, and aloe, to relieve the intestinal cramps that the laxatives often caused.

Colonists brought fennel to North America. Henry Wadsworth Longfellow alluded to Pliny when he wrote:

Above the lower plants it towers
The Fennel with its yellow flowers;
And in an earlier age than ours
Was gifted with wondrous powers
Lost vision to restore.

America's 19th-century Eclectic physicians prescribed fennel as a digestive aid, milk and menstruation promoter, and flavoring agent to "conceal the unpleasantness of other medicines." Latin Americans still boil the seeds in milk as a milk promoter for nursing mothers. Jamaicans use fennel to treat colds. And Africans take the herb for diarrhea and indigestion.

Contemporary herbalists recommend fennel as a digestive aid, milk promoter, expectorant, eyewash, and buffer in herbal laxative blends.

Therapeutic Uses

Fennel won't cure blindness, but science has supported some of its other traditional uses.

Digestive problems. Like most other aromatic herbs, fennel relaxes the smooth muscle lining the digestive tract, meaning that it's an antispasmodic. It also expels gas and promotes the secretion of bile, which helps in the digestion of fats. And European research shows that fennel kills some bacteria, lending some support to its traditional role in treating diarrhea.

In Germany, where herbal medicine is more mainstream than it is in the United States, fennel is used like caraway as a treatment for indigestion, gas pains, irritable bowel syndrome, and infant colic. And many Indian restaurants keep a bowl of candied fennel seeds by the door as a digestive aid for departing diners.

German researchers gave either a standard pharmaceutical stomach-settler (metoclopramide) or a combination of herbs (fennel, peppermint, caraway, and wormwood) to 60 people ages 18 to 85, all of whom had complained of indigestion, heartburn, nausea, or unusual belching or fullness. The participants were instructed to take their medicine 20 minutes before meals. After two weeks of treatment, those taking the herbal combination reported significantly greater relief from their symptoms, and with fewer side effects.

Commission E, the expert panel that evaluates herbal medicines for the German counterpart of the FDA, endorses fennel for the treatment of digestive upsets.

Women's health concerns. Antispasmodics soothe not only the digestive tract but also other smooth muscles, including the uterus. Fennel, however, was traditionally used not to relax the uterus but to stimulate it into menstruation. It's possible that high doses of fennel provide sufficient stimulation to promote menstruation.

One study suggests that the herb has a mild estrogenic effect, meaning that it acts like the female sex hormone estrogen. This action may have something to do with its traditional use as a milk and menstruation promoter.

Some women may try fennel to help start their periods or increase milk production. Older women might use it to relieve the discomforts of menopause.

Overweight. Animal studies show that fennel has diuretic action. This probably accounts for the herb's traditional role in weight control.

Keep in mind that diuretics of any kind eliminate only water weight. For this reason, weight-loss experts discourage the routine use of diuretics for weight management. The keys to permanent weight loss are a low-calorie, low-fat, high-fiber diet and regular exercise.

Prostate cancer. Female sex hormones are often prescribed for prostate cancer. All forms of cancer require professional care. Try fennel in addition to conventional therapies only with the supervision of your physician.

Rx Recommendations

To use fennel as a digestive aid, either chew a handful of seeds or try an infusion or tincture. You can also use an infusion or tincture to attempt to bring on menstruation or (while under the care of a physician) as a complementary therapy in treating prostate cancer.

To make a pleasant, licorice-flavored infusion, steep 1 to 2 teaspoons of bruised seeds in 1 cup of boiling water for 10 minutes. Drink up to 3 cups a day.

As a homemade tincture, take ½ to 1 teaspoon up to three times a day.

When using commercial preparations, follow the package directions.

You may give weak fennel preparations cautiously to children under age 2, in consultation with a physician, for colic. For older children and adults over age 65, start with low-strength preparations and increase the strength if necessary.

The Safety Factor

At best, fennel has only a mild estrogenic effect. But estrogen, a key ingredient in birth control pills, has many effects on the body. Women advised by their doctors not to take the Pill should not use medicinal amounts of fennel. The same is true for anyone with a history of abnormal blood clotting or estrogen-dependent breast tumors.

Pregnant women should not use medicinal amounts of fennel.

Fennel seeds are safe, but fennel oil may cause skin rash in people who are sensitive to it. When taken internally, even small amounts of the oil—a teaspoon or so—may cause nausea, vomiting, and possibly seizures. Don't ingest it.

Wise-Use Guidelines

Fennel is included in the Food and Drug Administration's list of herbs generally regarded as safe. For adults who are not pregnant or nursing, fennel is safe when used in the amounts typically recommended.

Medicinal amounts of fennel should be taken only in consultation with your doctor. If the herb causes minor discomforts, such as stomach upset or diarrhea, reduce your dosage or stop using it altogether. Let your doctor know if you experience unpleasant effects or if the symptoms for which you're taking the herb do not improve significantly in two weeks.

Growing Information

Native to southern Europe and Asia Minor, fennel is a striking 6-foot perennial with feathery leaves and tall stalks capped by large umbrella-like clusters of tiny yellow flowers. The tiny oval-shaped fruits (seeds) are ribbed and greenish gray. All parts of the plant have the herb's characteristic anise/licorice fragrance.

Fennel grows easily from seeds sown in rich, moist soil in fall or after the danger of frost has passed. Germination takes about two weeks. Thin seedlings to 12-inch spacing. Do not overwater the seedlings, but as plants develop, extra water increases stem succulence. The leaves may be harvested once plants are established.

When the stems are about an inch thick, hill the soil over them to cause blanching, which results in milder flavor. Harvest about ten days after hilling.

Harvest the seeds in late summer as they turn greenish gray.

Fennel may damage some neighboring plants: bush beans, tomatoes, caraway, and kohlrabi. If coriander is planted nearby, fennel will not fruit.

Warning: In the wild, fennel may be confused with poison hemlock, which has caused fatalities. Don't gather wild fennel unless you're sure you've identified it correctly.

Fenugreek

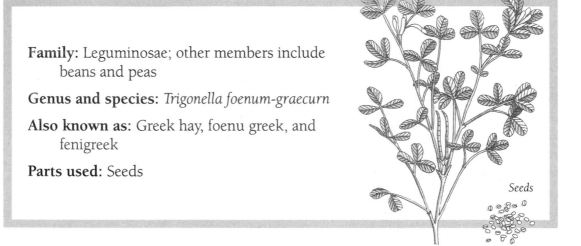

Family: Leguminosae; other members include beans and peas

Genus and species: *Trigonella foenum-graecurn*

Also known as: Greek hay, foenu greek, and fenigreek

Parts used: Seeds

Seeds

From ancient times through the late 19th century, fenugreek played a major role in herbal healing. It was even found in the tomb of King Tut (Tutankhamen), who died in 1323 B.C. Then it fell by the wayside.

Lately, however, things are looking up for the herb with a taste that is an odd combination of bitter celery and maple syrup. Fenugreek helps reduce cholesterol levels, as well as blood sugar levels in people with diabetes.

Healing History

Fenugreek plants were used to help sick animals long before the seeds became a popular remedy for human ills. Early Greeks mixed the plant into moldy or insect-damaged animal forage to make it more palatable. In the process, they discovered that sick horses and cattle would eat fenugreek when they wouldn't eat anything else. The Egyptians and Romans subsequently adopted "Greek hay." The name in Latin, *foenum graecum*, evolved into "fenugreek."

Today fenugreek is widely used to flavor horse and cattle feed. Some veterinarians still rely on it to encourage sick livestock to eat.

As fenugreek spread around the Mediterranean, ancient physicians learned that its seeds contain a great deal of a special type of fiber called mucilage. When mixed with water, mucilage becomes gelatinous and soothes inflamed or irritated tissue. Egyptian physicians put fenugreek into ointments to treat wounds and abscesses. They also recommended using the herb internally to treat fevers and respiratory and intestinal complaints. Hippocrates and other ancient Greek and Roman physicians used the herb similarly.

Ancient Chinese healers recommended

fenugreek to treat fevers, hernias, gallbladder problems, muscle aches, and even impotence.

In India, where the herb is an ingredient in curry spice blends, Ayurvedic physicians prescribed it to treat arthritis, bronchitis, and digestive upsets.

Indian women ate fenugreek seeds to increase their milk production. Arab women from Libya to Syria ate the roasted seeds to help them gain weight, enlarge their breasts, and attain the Rubenesque proportions that were synonymous with beauty from ancient times through the 19th century.

Fenugreek is the only healing herb ever used as a weapon of war. During the Roman siege of Jerusalem (A.D. 66–70), general and future emperor Vespasian ordered his troops to scale the city's imposing walls. The standard defense against this kind of attack was to pour boiling water or oil on the attackers and their ladders. According to *The History of the Jewish War* by Jewish traitor Flavius Josephus, Jerusalem's defenders added fenugreek to their oil, making it more slippery and hindering the Romans as they tried to climb their ladders.

Around the 9th century, the Benedictine monks, who were avid herb gardeners and creators of fine liqueurs, popularized fenugreek throughout Europe. From that time on, the herb was widely used in folk medicine as it had been by the ancients—to treat wounds, fevers, and digestive and respiratory ailments.

Early settlers brought fenugreek to North America and used it as forage and in folk medicine, where it gained a reputation as a treatment for menstrual complaints and the discomforts of menopause. The herb became a key ingredient in Lydia E. Pinkham's Vegetable Compound, one of 19th-century America's most popular patent medicines for "female weakness" (menstrual and menopausal discomforts). The manufacturer proclaimed her compound "the greatest medical discovery since the dawn of history." Health authorities were outraged, and their outcry played a part in creating the FDA, which regulates drug claims.

Modern herbalists recommend fenugreek poultices and plasters to treat wounds, boils, and rashes. They say that a warm fenugreek gargle soothes a sore throat. They also recommend using the herb internally to treat coughs, bronchitis, and menstrual and menopausal complaints. Some are even convinced that eating fenugreek—especially its sprouts—enlarges women's breasts.

Today, fenugreek is most widely used in the United States as a source of imitation maple flavor.

Therapeutic Uses

Some of fenugreek's traditional uses have been supported by modern science, but the herb's most important potential benefit has only recently come to light.

High cholesterol. Researchers at the S. N. Medical College in Agra, India, measured the cholesterol levels of 60 people who were not taking any cholesterol-lowering medications. Then the participants were instructed to eat a bowl of soup containing about 1 ounce of powdered fenugreek seed before lunch and dinner each day.

After 4 weeks of consuming about 2 ounces of powdered fenugreek seed daily in this way, the participants saw their cholesterol levels begin to decline. After 24 weeks, their average total cholesterol dropped 14 percent. For every

1 percent decrease in total cholesterol, the risk of heart attack risk drops about 2 percent, so in this study, the participants' risk of heart attack plummeted by about 28 percent.

In another study lasting 3 months, 2 teaspoons (5 grams) of powdered fenugreek seed a day produced no changes in the cholesterol levels of 30 people with normal readings. In 30 people with elevated cholesterol, however, the same dose for the same period of time reduced levels significantly.

Diabetes. In the same Indian study, all of the participants had Type 2 (non-insulin-dependent) diabetes. Besides lowering their cholesterol levels, daily consumption of about an ounce of powdered fenugreek seed lowered their blood sugar levels. Another Indian study produced the same results. These trials corroborate animal research showing that fenugreek reduces blood sugar levels.

Sore throat. Fenugreek's soothing mucilage may help relieve sore throat pain and cough, as well as mild indigestion.

Wounds. Fenugreek's mucilage also soothes minor wounds. Commission E, the expert panel that evaluates herbal medicines for Germany's counterpart of the FDA, approves fenugreek as an external wound treatment.

Women's health concerns. Fenugreek seeds contain diosgenin, a compound that's similar to the female sex hormone estrogen. Estrogen causes fluid retention and stimulates breast tissue growth, which is why many women who take estrogen-based birth control pills report weight gain and breast swelling.

The discovery of a plant estrogen in fenugreek suggests that the herb may be used as a natural form of hormone replacement therapy to treat the hot flashes associated with menopause. Fenugreek's phytoestrogen content also supports the age-old practice among Arab women of eating the seeds to gain weight, as well as the American folk practice of eating the seeds to enlarge the breasts.

James A. Duke, Ph.D., retired USDA herbal medicine authority and author of several highly regarded herbal medicine references, has observed that fenugreek sprouts contain much more diosgenin than the unsprouted seeds. He has recommended the sprouts to women interested in nonsurgical breast augmentation, and he says that he has received several thank-you notes from satisfied users.

Arthritis. Belgian researchers have discovered that fenugreek has mild anti-inflammatory action. This lends some credence to the herb's traditional role in treating arthritis, wounds, and other inflammatory conditions.

Rx Recommendations

Use a fenugreek decoction to take advantage of the herb's many potential healing benefits—to soothe a sore throat, relieve menstrual or menopausal discomforts, or possibly relieve arthritis pain. You might also try the herb to lower your cholesterol or to help control blood sugar levels, in conjunction with conventional therapy and under the supervision of your physician.

For a bitter, maple-flavored decoction, gently boil 2 teaspoons of crushed seeds in 1 cup of water, then simmer for 10 minutes and strain. Drink up to 3 cups a day. To improve the flavor, add sugar, honey, lemon, anise, or peppermint.

As a homemade tincture, use $1/4$ to $1/2$ teaspoon up to three times a day.

When using commercial preparations, follow the package directions.

Do not give medicinal fenugreek preparations to children under age 2. For older children and adults over age 65, start with low-strength preparations and increase the strength if necessary.

The Safety Factor

Because fenugreek may be a uterine stimulant, pregnant women should not take it.

Wise-Use Guidelines

Fenugreek is included in the FDA list of herbs generally regarded as safe. For adults who are not pregnant or nursing, fenugreek is safe when used in the amounts typically recommended.

You should take medicinal amounts of fenugreek only in consultation with your doctor. If the herb causes minor discomfort, such as stomach upset or diarrhea, reduce the dosage or stop using it altogether. Let your doctor know if you experience any unpleasant effects or if the symptoms for which you're taking the herb do not improve significantly within 2 weeks.

Growing Information

Fenugreek is an annual that reaches 18 inches and resembles a large clover. It has three-lobed leaves and white, triangular, pealike flowers, which produce the long seed pods characteristic of the bean family. Fenugreek's seed pod is sickle-shaped and 2 inches long, containing 10 to 20 hard, smooth, oblong, somewhat flattened seeds.

After the danger of frost has passed and the soil temperature has reached 55°F, sow seeds in almost any soil in an area that receives full sun. Germination typically takes only a few days. To prevent root rot, do not overwater the plants.

The plants flower in about 3 weeks and produce seeds in another 3 weeks. Harvest the pods when they're fully formed but before they begin to crack. Remove the seeds and dry them in the sun.

Feverfew

Family: Compositae; other members include daisy, dandelion, and marigold

Genus and species: *Chrysanthemum parthenium*; *Matricaria parthenium*; *Tanacetum parthenium*

Also known as: Febrifuge plant, wild quinine, and bachelor's button

Parts used: Leaves

From the 19th century well into the late 1970s, feverfew was largely washed up as a healing herb. In 1974, in *The Herb Book*, noted herbalist John Lust summarized most of his colleagues' feelings: "Feverfew has fallen into considerable disuse. It is also hard to find, even at herb outlets."

Shortly after Lust penned this obituary, however, feverfew experienced something of a renaissance. It became clear that the herb is remarkably effective at preventing migraines.

Healing History

Many sources claim that the herb's name comes from the Latin *febrifugia*, meaning "driver-out of fevers." They also say that the herb has been used since ancient times to treat fever.

They're wrong on both counts. The plant was never called febrifugia. Ancient physicians, including Dioscorides and Galen, referred to it by its Greek name, *parthenion*, and prescribed it for menstrual and childbirth-related problems, not fever.

During the Middle Ages, the name parthenion faded, and the plant was renamed featherfoil because of its feathery leaf borders. "Featherfoil" evolved into "featherfew" and eventually into "feverfew."

Once the name feverfew became popular, herbalists decided that it was, in fact, a fever treatment. They planted the strong-smelling herb around their homes in hopes of purifying the air to ward off malaria, which they mistakenly believed was caused by bad air (the word *malaria* comes from the Italian *mala*, "foul," and *aria*, "air").

Malaria had plagued Europe since prehistoric times. It was untreatable until Spanish explorers returned from Peru with cinchona bark and early chemists isolated the bark's anti-malarial constituent, quinine. Quinine proved so successful at curing malaria that for a brief period, other herbs prescribed for fever basked in its reflected glow. That's how feverfew became known as wild quinine. But the name didn't stick. Quinine proved so superior as a malaria treatment that feverfew was all but abandoned for this purpose.

For a while, some herbalists recommended feverfew for ailments other than fever, particularly for headache. In the 17th century, England's John Parkinson described feverfew as "very effectual for all paines in the head." More than 100 years later, John Hill wrote, "In the worst headache, this herb exceeds whatever else is known."

Most herbalists stuck with feverfew's traditional gynecological uses, however. Seventeenth century English herbalist Nicholas Culpeper called it a "general strengthener of wombs" and prescribed it in tea form for colds and chest congestion. Culpeper also recognized the herb's decline, declaring it "not much used in present practice."

Early colonists introduced feverfew into North America, where malaria was also a major problem. But as the herb fell from fashion in England, it stopped being used here as well.

America's 19th-century Eclectic physicians, forerunners of today's naturopaths, prescribed feverfew mainly as a menstruation promoter and as a treatment for "female hysteria" (menstrual discomforts) and some fever-producing diseases.

Therapeutic Uses

In the late 1970s, a chance meeting between two migraine sufferers made earlier observations about feverfew's benefit for "paines in the head" appear prophetic.

Migraines. The wife of the chief medical officer of Britain's National Coal Board was prone to chronic migraines. A miner heard about her problem. When she accompanied her husband on a visit to his mine, the miner told her that he'd also been a longtime migraine sufferer—until he started chewing a few feverfew leaves every day. Upon trying the herb, the woman noticed immediate improvement. Fourteen months later, she was free of her searing headaches.

The medical officer brought his wife's experience to the attention of Dr. E. Stewart Johnson of the City of London Migraine Clinic. In a pilot study, Dr. Johnson gave feverfew leaves to 10 of his patients. Three pronounced themselves cured, and the other 7 reported significant improvement in their symptoms.

Next, Dr. Johnson gave feverfew to 270 of his migraine patients. Seventy percent reported significant relief—and for many of them, standard medical treatment had done nothing at all.

Finally, Dr. Johnson arranged a scientifically rigorous double-blind, placebo-controlled trial in which some of the participants took feverfew, while others took medically inactive placebos. Neither the participants nor the researchers knew who got what until after the trial had ended. (This is what's meant by "double-blind.") Feverfew significantly outperformed the placebos.

Soon after Dr. Johnson completed his research, the British medical journal *Lancet* reported the results of an even more rigorous experiment. Seventy-two people with chronic migraines were randomly assigned to take either placebos or capsules of powdered, freeze-dried feverfew (85 milligrams, the equivalent of two medium-size leaves) every day. Neither the participants nor the researchers knew who was using which treatment. After 2 months, the groups switched treatments, so those who had been taking placebos were given feverfew and vice versa (a "crossover trial"). The results were striking: Feverfew cut migraine episodes by 24 percent, and the headaches that did occur were comparatively mild, with significantly less nausea and vomiting.

Since then, several other studies have shown feverfew to be effective for migraine prevention. In 1996, however, one highly publicized study by Dutch researchers found that the herb had no benefit. As it turned out, this trial used a tincture (alcohol extract) of feverfew, not the leaves that had proven effective in all the other studies.

In 1998, British researchers reviewed five studies of feverfew for migraine prevention, using sophisticated statistical techniques to combine the studies as though they were all arms of one big trial (called a meta-analysis). The researchers' conclusion: Feverfew works.

Digestive problems. Like chamomile, its close botanical relative, feverfew contains chemicals that calm the smooth muscles of the digestive tract, making the herb an antispasmodic. Try feverfew after meals to protect against digestive upset.

Women's health concerns. Antispasmodic herbs soothe not only the digestive tract but also other smooth muscles, such as the uterus. In addition, feverfew has the ability to neutralize certain prostaglandins, substances that have been linked to pain and inflammation. (This may be another reason that feverfew helps prevent migraines.) Prostaglandins also play a role in menstrual cramps. Feverfew's possible antispasmodic and anti-prostaglandin actions support its traditional use in treating menstrual discomforts.

Intriguing Possibilities

One animal study suggests that feverfew has a mild tranquilizing effect. Taken before bedtime, the herb just might help bring on sleep.

Another report hints at feverfew's tumor-fighting properties. It's much too early to deem the herb a cancer treatment, but that day may come.

Rx Recommendations

To control the frequency and severity of migraine attacks, chew two fresh (or freeze-dried) leaves a day or take a pill or capsule containing 85 milligrams of whole-leaf material. Since feverfew is quite bitter, most people prefer the pills or capsules to chewing the leaves.

If feverfew doesn't seem to be helping within a few weeks, try changing brands before you decide to give up on the herb. A report in *Lancet* showed that some "feverfew" pills and capsules actually contain only trace amounts.

To improve digestion or promote menstruation, take feverfew as an infusion. Use ½ to 1 teaspoon of herb per cup of boiling water, steep for 5 to 10 minutes, then strain. Drink up to 2 cups a day.

Do not give feverfew to children under age 2. For older children and adults over age 65, start with low-strength preparations and increase the strength if necessary.

The Safety Factor

While feverfew suppresses migraines, it does not cure them. When treatment with the herb is suspended, the headaches typically return, which means that migraine sufferers might wind up taking feverfew for a long time. The herb has been used in migraine prevention for about 20 years with no reports of significant problems, but there is no research examining the herb's longer-term effects.

Feverfew has not been shown to cause uterine contractions, but it has a long folk history as a menstruation promoter. Pregnant women should err on the side of caution and not take it.

Chewing fresh feverfew leaves may cause mouth sores. Some people also report abdominal pain from using the herb.

Feverfew may inhibit blood clotting. People with clotting disorders and those who are taking anticoagulant (blood-thinning) medications or supplements (vitamin E, for example) should consult a physician before using it.

Wise-Use Guidelines

For adults who are not pregnant or nursing, don't have clotting disorders, and are not taking anticoagulants, feverfew is considered safe in the amounts typically recommended.

You should use medicinal amounts of feverfew only in consultation with your doctor. If it causes mouth sores or stomach upset, reduce the dosage or stop using it altogether. Let your doctor know if you experience any unpleasant effects or if the symptoms for which you're taking the herb do not improve significantly within 2 weeks.

Growing Information

Feverfew is a perennial that reaches 3 feet and has lovely daisylike flowers with yellow centers and up to 20 white rays. For personal migraine prevention, a few plants should suffice.

Feverfew grows from seeds, but most authorities recommend planting root cuttings when the temperature reaches 70°F. Space plants 18 inches apart.

Feverfew does best in partial shade. Compost stimulates better growth. Pinch back the flower buds to encourage bushiness. Harvest the leaves when they mature.

Bees dislike feverfew and generally avoid the plant, so don't plant it around other plants that require bee pollination. Feverfew can also be grown indoors year-round as a houseplant.

Garlic

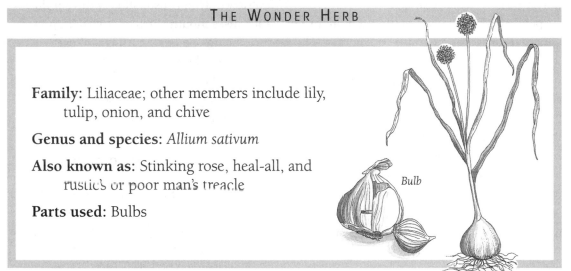

Family: Liliaceae; other members include lily, tulip, onion, and chive

Genus and species: *Allium sativum*

Also known as: Stinking rose, heal-all, and rustics or poor man's treacle

Parts used: Bulbs

Bulb

If the term *wonder drug* can be applied to any healing herb, garlic deserves the honor. It is one of the world's oldest medicines and is still among the best.

Within the genus *Allium*, garlic is the most powerful (and most thoroughly researched) healer. But traditional herbalists also valued garlic's close botanical relatives—onions, scallions, leeks, chives, and shallots—although they were considered less medicinally potent. Modern research bears this out. While onions have almost as much therapeutic value as garlic, scallions, leeks, chives, and shallots have less.

Healing History

Remains of garlic have been found in caves inhabited 10,000 years ago, but the first prescription for the herb, chiseled in cuneiform on a Sumerian clay tablet, dates from 3000 B.C.

Garlic also appears prominently in the world's oldest surviving medical text, the *Ebers Papyrus*, which dates to about 1500 B.C. The herb was an ingredient in 22 remedies for headache, insect and scorpion bites, menstrual discomforts, intestinal worms, tumors, and heart problems.

The entire ancient world from Spain to China loved garlic. No people enjoyed the herb more, however, than the Egyptians, who were called "the stinking ones" by Greek writers because of their garlic breath. Egyptians taking solemn oaths swore on garlic in the same way that we swear on the Bible. The herb was found in the tomb of King Tut. For 15 pounds of it, Egyptians could buy a healthy male slave.

Speaking of slavery, garlic played a major role in the lives of the slaves who built Egypt's pyramids. The Egyptians believed that the herb prevented illness and increased strength and endurance. They gave their slaves a daily ration, and over time, the slaves came to revere garlic just as their masters did.

Legend has it that during the construction of one pyramid, a garlic shortage forced the Egyptians to cut the slaves' ration. The result was a labor revolt that led to the world's first recorded strike.

Around 1200 B.C., soon after Moses led the Hebrew slaves out of Egypt, they complained of missing the finer things of life in bondage. As the Bible relates, "We remember the fish we ate in Egypt, and the cucumbers, melons, leeks, onions, and garlic" (Numbers 11:5).

For Combat and Competition

Greek athletes ate garlic before races, and Greek soldiers munched the herb before battle. In his play *Knights*, Aristophanes wrote: "Now bolt down garlic. You will have greater mettle for the fight."

In Homer's *Odyssey*, Ulysses turns to garlic for strength against the sorceress Circe, who had turned Ulysses' men into swine and planned to do the same to him. But Hermes, the god of science (whose symbol, the serpent-wrapped staff, came to symbolize medicine), gave Ulysses garlic, which thwarted Circe's spells.

Greek midwives hung garlic cloves around birthing rooms to safeguard newborns from disease and witchcraft. As the centuries passed, Europeans fastened braided garlic plants to their doorposts to keep evil spirits at bay, a custom that survives today in the garlic braids hung in many kitchens.

Greek and Roman physicians loved garlic. Hippocrates recommended it for infections, wounds, cancer, leprosy, and digestive problems. Dioscorides prescribed it for heart problems. And Pliny listed it in 61 remedies for ailments ranging from the common cold to epilepsy and

from leprosy to tapeworm. Many of these uses have been supported by modern science.

Upper-class Greeks and Romans came to hate the stinking rose, however. They viewed garlic breath as a sign of low social ranking. Antipathy to garlic breath is with us today.

Garlic may have been unfashionable among the well-to-do, but many Roman emperors couldn't eat enough. The ancients considered the herb to be an antidote to poisons, which were popular in ancient Rome, where political rivals were known to taint each other's food. In fact, many Roman herbalists specialized in poisons and in elaborate antidotes that usually included garlic.

Like the Greeks, ancient India's Ayurvedic healers prescribed garlic for leprosy, a practice that continued for thousands of years. In fact, when India became a British colony and adopted English, leprosy became known as "peelgarlic" because lepers spent so much time peeling cloves and eating them. The Indians also used garlic to treat cancer. Modern research supports garlic's ability to treat leprosy and prevent certain cancers.

Tenth-century Arab physicians inherited the Greco-Roman ambivalence toward garlic. One Persian herbal of that time said that the herb should be "despised because of its unpleasant odor," then affirmed that it "acts as an antidote to deadly poisons. It drives away toothache if you bruise it and lay it upon the tooth. We should not be without it in any kitchen."

The same ambivalence persisted in medieval Europe. While the well-to-do shunned garlic, the peasantry consumed huge amounts, viewing the herb as an all-purpose preventive medicine and cure-all—hence one of its names, heal-all. By the Elizabethan era, the Latin term for antidote, *theriaca*, had evolved into the English word *treacle*, meaning "panacea." Garlic was commonly called the poor man's treacle.

From Social Scourge to Saving Grace

As the centuries passed, the upper class returned to using garlic, but only medicinally and even then, sparingly. The 17th-century English herbalist Nicholas Culpeper endorsed the herb as "a remedy for all diseases and hurts. . . . It helpeth the biting of mad dogs and other venomous creatures, killeth worms in children, cutteth tough phlegm, purgeth the head . . . and is a good remedy for any plague."

As an affluent, educated man, though, Culpeper also embraced upper-class disdain for garlic and criticized folk healers for "quoting many diseases this [herb] is good for, but concealing its vices." Culpeper warned against garlic's "offensiveness on the breath" and wrote, "Its heat is very vehement, [and it] sends up ill-favoured vapours to the brain. Therefore, let it be used inwardly with great moderation."

Culpeper's call for moderation fell on deaf ears. As a Welsh rhyme advised, "Eat leeks in March, and garlic in May / And all the year after, physicians may play."

During Culpeper's time, the typical breakfast for French peasants consisted of dark bread and garlic. French folk healers considered the herb a strengthener and cure-all.

In 1721, French reverence for garlic soared to new heights when a plague struck Marseilles, killing most of the city's inhabitants. Legend has it that convicted thieves were assigned to bury the dead, a task that was certain to infect them with the fatal disease and thus save the government the bother of executing them. But four enterprising thieves drank a mixture of garlic and wine and survived the plague. They not only escaped the guillotine, they grew rich robbing all the bodies.

This tale is more myth than history, but to this day, southern Europeans drink a garlic/wine medicine called Four Thieves Vinegar (*Vinaigre des Quatre Voleurs*).

America's 19th-century Eclectic physicians, forerunners of today's naturopaths, shared the Victorian prejudice against garlic's "strong, offensive smell . . . and acrimonious, almost caustic taste." But they conceded that the herb is effective in treating colds, coughs, whooping cough, and other respiratory ailments. They also believed that fresh garlic juice applied to the ear could cure deafness.

During World War I, British, French, and Russian army physicians used garlic juice to treat infected battle wounds. They also prescribed the herb to prevent and treat amoebic dysentery.

Alexander Fleming's discovery of penicillin in 1928 launched the age of antibiotics. By World War II, penicillin and sulfa drugs had largely replaced garlic as the treatment of choice for infected wounds. In Russia, however, the needs of more than 20 million World War II casualties overwhelmed its antibiotic supply. Red Army physicians relied heavily on garlic, which came to be called Russian penicillin.

Modern herbalists recommend garlic (as well as other allium vegetables) for colds, coughs, flu, fever, bronchitis, ringworm, intestinal worms, and cardiovascular disease.

Therapeutic Uses

Garlic does not cure epilepsy or deafness, but an enormous amount of scientific evidence proves beyond doubt that the "poor man's treacle" is an herbal wonder drug.

Infections. During World War I, garlic's success in treating infected wounds and amoebic dysentery (caused by the protozoan *Entamoeba histolytica*) showed that the herb has potent antibacterial and anti-protozoan properties, validating thousands of years of healing tradition. But garlic's antibiotic constituent remained a mystery until the 1920s, when researchers at Sandoz Pharmaceuticals in Switzerland isolated a compound called alliin (pronounced *AL-lee-in*).

Alliin by itself has no medicinal value, but when garlic is chewed, chopped, bruised, or crushed, the alliin comes in contact with the enzyme allinase. This transforms alliin into allicin, a chemical that's a powerful antibiotic.

Since the 1920s, garlic's broad-spectrum antibiotic properties have been confirmed in literally dozens of animal and human studies. Garlic kills the bacteria that cause tuberculosis (*Mycobacterium tuberculosis*), food poisoning (salmonella), and women's bladder infections (*Escherichia coli*). The herb may also fend off the influenza virus

Chinese researchers report success in using garlic to treat 21 cases of cryptococcal meningitis, an often fatal fungal infection. Several studies have also shown the herb to be effective in treating the fungi that cause athlete's foot (*Trichophyton mentagrophytes*) and vaginal yeast infections (*Candida albicans*).

Commission E, the expert panel that evaluates herbal medicines for the German counterpart of the FDA, recognizes garlic's antibiotic value.

Ulcers. Most ulcers are caused by the bacterium *Helicobacter pylori*. In one study, garlic significantly inhibited the germ's growth. The researchers estimate that two cloves of garlic a day may provide significant protection against *H. pylori* infection.

Heart attack and stroke. No standard medication can match garlic when it comes to acting on so many cardiovascular risk factors at the same time. Some drugs lower cholesterol. Others rein in blood pressure. Still others reduce the likelihood of the blood clots that trigger heart attacks and most strokes. But garlic does all of these things, thanks to allicin and another chemical, called ajoene.

More than a dozen journal reports document garlic's ability to reduce cholesterol. In one study published in the British medical journal *Lancet*, researchers had volunteers eat a meal containing about 4 ounces of butter, which raises cholesterol. Half of the volunteers also ate about nine cloves of garlic. After 3 hours, the average cholesterol level among those who didn't consume garlic increased by 7 percent. Among those who did consume garlic, average cholesterol *decreased* by 7 percent. The researchers concluded that "garlic has a very significant protective action [against high cholesterol]."

Two groups of researchers—one Australian, the other American—have published analyses of a selection of garlic-cholesterol studies. The Australian team reviewed 16 trials involving 952 people with high cholesterol. They concluded that a daily dose of either 10 fresh cloves or 1 gram of a dried high-allicin preparation can reduce total cholesterol levels by about 12 percent.

Meanwhile, the American team reviewed five rigorous trials involving 365 people. They concluded that a daily dose of either one fresh clove or 1 gram of a dried high-allicin preparation can lower total cholesterol levels by about 9 percent.

Experts estimate that for every 1 percent decrease in total cholesterol, the risk of heart attack drops 2 percent. Going by the results of the Australian and American analyses, daily garlic consumption may reduce heart attack risk by as much as 24 percent.

Over the years, a few highly publicized studies have shown that garlic has no effect on cholesterol. These reports have been criticized for poor methodology. The scientific consensus is that garlic lowers cholesterol, and Commission E endorses it for that purpose.

Several studies dating back to the Sandoz Pharmaceuticals experiments confirm garlic's ability to reduce blood pressure in animals and humans. It also helps prevent the blood clots that trigger heart attack and most strokes. One researcher describes the herb as "at least as potent as aspirin," a standard anti-clotting heart attack preventive.

More recently, researchers at Humboldt University in Berlin demonstrated that garlic not only helps prevent heart disease but can also treat the condition, even when it's quite advanced. They gave 152 people with advanced heart disease either medically inactive placebos or 900 milligrams of a standardized powdered garlic preparation (Kwai). Four years after starting the study, those taking the placebos had 16 percent more arterial narrowing. Among those taking the garlic, however, arterial blockages actually receded by 3 percent.

Cancer. In addition to being an antibiotic, the allicin in garlic is a potent antioxidant. It helps prevent the cell damage that can set the stage for cancer. Many cell culture, animal, and human studies have shown that garlic helps protect against various cancers, especially those of the digestive tract.

In the Iowa Women's Health Study, researchers have been tracking the diet, lifestyle, and health status of 41,387 middle-aged Iowa women for many years. They have found that the women who eat the most garlic are the least likely to develop colon cancer. Eating just a few cloves a week has cut their risk by 35 percent. Greater consumption lowers their risk even more.

Generally, eating fruits and vegetables helps protect against cancer, but in this study, of all the plant foods analyzed, garlic yielded the greatest preventive benefits.

In the Netherlands Cohort Study, Dutch researchers have been following a group of more than 120,000 middle-aged men and women for many years. The research has shown that as the participants' consumption of garlic's close relative, onion, increases, their risk of stomach cancer significantly decreases.

Meanwhile, a study of 1,800 Chinese found that those most likely to develop stomach cancer eat the least garlic. The researchers concluded that a diet high in garlic "can significantly reduce risk of stomach cancer."

Diabetes. Garlic reduces blood sugar levels in both laboratory animals and humans. Diabetes is a serious condition that requires professional treatment, but if you have it, there's no harm in increasing your garlic consumption in combination with your standard therapy.

Lead poisoning. European studies show that garlic helps eliminate lead and other toxic heavy metals from the body. Lead interferes with thinking and causes other serious medical problems. Children are particularly susceptible to its effects. Add liberal amounts of garlic to spaghetti sauces and other foods that kids enjoy.

Leprosy. Ancient Ayurvedic healers were onto something when they used garlic to treat leprosy, now called Hansen's disease. In one study, Indian researchers gave people with

Hansen's an ointment made with garlic as well as foods containing large amounts of the herb. Compared with people in the study who did not receive garlic treatment, those who did showed significant improvement.

AIDS. Studies that examine garlic as a treatment for AIDS are preliminary but exciting. In one of them, seven patients with AIDS who took a clove of garlic a day for 3 months experienced significant increases in the immune functions normally destroyed by the disease. What's more, two of the seven saw chronic herpes sores clear up during treatment, while two others with chronic diarrhea—a common AIDS symptom—also reported improvement in their symptoms.

Rx Recommendations

For minor skin infections, garlic juice applied externally may prove sufficient. Unless you're working with an experienced herbalist, however, you shouldn't rely exclusively on garlic to treat infectious diseases. No antibiotic, including garlic, kills all disease-causing microorganisms.

The standard medical approach is to conduct a "sensitivity test," in which several antibiotics are pitted against the germ. The doctor then prescribes the antibiotic that works best. You might ask your physician to include garlic in a sensitivity test, or simply take it in addition to standard medication.

Researchers have found that one medium garlic clove packs the antibacterial punch of about 100,000 units of penicillin. Depending on the type of infection, oral penicillin doses typically range from 600,000 to 1.2 million units. The equivalent in garlic would be about 6 to 12 cloves. It's best to chew 3 cloves at a time two to four times a day.

To help reduce blood pressure, cholesterol, and the likelihood of blood clots, experts recommend eating 3 to 10 fresh cloves of garlic a day. The herb must be chewed, chopped, bruised, or crushed to transform its medicinally inert alliin into antibiotic allicin. Using fresh garlic is most medicinally effective, but the herb does retain some of its healing benefits when lightly cooked.

Raw garlic has a sharp, biting flavor, which cooking eliminates. Use it in foods to taste. (The cloves' papery skins peel easily if you smash them with the flat side of a cleaver.)

To prepare an infusion, put six chopped cloves in 1 cup of cool water and steep for 6 hours.

For a tincture, soak 1 cup of crushed cloves in 1 quart of brandy. Shake the mixture daily for 2 weeks, then take up to 3 tablespoons a day

When using commercial preparations, follow the package directions.

You may give garlic cautiously to children under age 2.

What About the Smell?

Since 3000 B.C., the main issue with garlic has been its odor. The stinking rose continues to bother some people.

In recent decades, however, garlic-rich Italian and Asian cuisines have become increasingly popular. Some of the nation's finest restaurants now proudly serve dishes heavily flavored with garlic. We may well be entering the age of garlic chic.

In Gilroy, California, near Monterey, garlic is already the height of fashion. Gilroy is the garlic capital of America, and every year garlic lovers gather for the annual Garlic Festival, which features delights such as garlic soup, garlic cake, and garlic ice cream. A popular festival bumper sticker proclaims "Fight Mouthwash. Eat Garlic."

Still, we're probably a long way from cultivating garlic breath. To eliminate it, try chewing a traditional herbal breath freshener such as parsley, fennel, or fenugreek.

Today, deodorized medicinal garlic preparations are available in health food stores and some drugstores. Many scientists believe that the herb's medicinal value comes from its odor-causing sulfur compounds, which has raised doubts about the medicinal effectiveness of deodorized garlic. Still, some studies have shown that even without the stink, garlic retains its healing benefits.

The Safety Factor

Garlic's anti-clotting action may help prevent heart attacks and some types of stroke, but medicinal amounts could conceivably cause problems for people with clotting disorders. If you have this type of disorder, or if you take any anticoagulant (blood-thinning) medication or supplement (vitamin E, for example), consult your physician before using garlic in medicinal amounts.

Garlic's genus name, *Allium*, comes from the Celtic word *all*, meaning "burning." Fresh garlic can cause a burning sensation in the mouth that some people find unpleasant.

Allergic reactions are possible. Rashes have been reported from touching or eating the herb. If garlic gives you a rash, don't eat it. Garlic-induced stomach upset has also been reported.

Garlic enters the milk of nursing mothers and may cause colic in infants. The herb has never been implicated in miscarriage or birth defects.

Wise-Use Guidelines

For adults who are not nursing and do not have clotting disorders or take anticoagulants, garlic is considered safe in the amounts typically recommended.

You should use medicinal amounts of garlic only in consultation with your doctor. If it causes minor discomfort, such as stomach upset, reduce the dosage or stop using it altogether. Let your doctor know if you experience unpleasant effects or if the symptoms for which you are using the herb do not improve significantly within 2 weeks.

Growing Information

Garlic grows easily from seeds or cloves. It's easier to start with cloves. Plant them 2 inches deep and 6 inches apart in early spring for harvesting in fall.

Garlic is cold-tolerant and can be planted up to 6 weeks before the final frost date. It thrives best in rich, deeply cultivated, well-drained soil. Do not overwater. Full sun produces the largest bulbs, but garlic tolerates some shade. During summer, cut back the flower stalks so the plant devotes all its energy to producing fat, aromatic bulbs.

Harvest bulbs in late summer and store them in a cool, dark place.

Take care not to bruise the bulbs, as bruising invites mold and insects. You can braid the leaves into a wreath or rope and display it in your kitchen, removing bulbs as needed.

Gentian

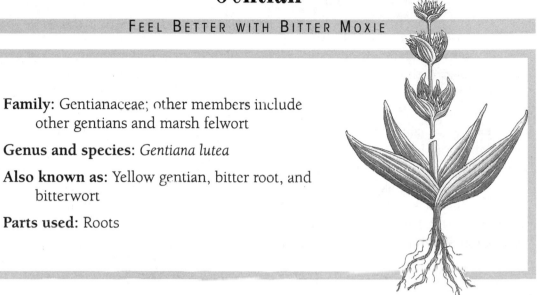

Family: Gentianaceae; other members include other gentians and marsh felwort

Genus and species: *Gentiana lutea*

Also known as: Yellow gentian, bitter root, and bitterwort

Parts used: Roots

In Depression-era slang, "moxie" meant courage tinged with recklessness. Teddy Roosevelt, Charles Lindbergh, Al Capone—all of them had moxie. The term comes from Moxie, a bitter soft drink available only in New England since the 1890s.

Moxie owes its bite to gentian root, a healing herb with a 3,000-year history as a digestive "bitter." Modern research shows that gentian does indeed stimulate digestion.

Healing History

Gentian was used by the ancient Egyptians, Greeks, and Romans as an appetite stimulant and antiseptic wound wash. The herb also served as a treatment for intestinal worms, digestive disorders, liver ailments, and "female hysteria" (menstrual discomforts).

Sixth-century Arab physicians adopted gentian from the Greeks and introduced its medicinal uses to Asia. Since then, Chinese physicians have prescribed the herb to treat digestive disorders, sore throat, headache, and arthritis. India's Ayurvedic physicians have recommended it for fevers, venereal diseases, and jaundice and other liver problems.

During the Middle Ages, European herbalists prized gentian because it caused less intestinal irritation than other digestive bitters.

Seventeenth-century English herbalist Nicholas Culpeper wrote that gentian "strengthens the stomach exceedingly, helps digestion, comforts the heart, helps agues [fevers] of all sorts, kills worms, and preserves against fainting and swooning. It provokes urine and terms [menstruation] exceedingly; therefore, let it not be given to women with child."

When colonists arrived in Virginia and the Carolinas, they were greeted by Native Americans who applied a root decoction of American gentian (*Gentiana puberula*) to relieve back pain.

America's 19th-century Eclectic physicians, forerunners of today's naturopaths, considered gentian a powerful tonic and prescribed it to "improve appetite and stimulate digestion." But their text *King's American Dispensatory* (1898) warned, "When taken in large doses, it is apt to oppress the stomach, irritate the bowels, and produce nausea, vomiting, and headache."

Gentian was listed in the *U.S. Pharma-copoeia*, a standard drug reference, from 1820 to 1955 as a digestive stimulant.

Before the introduction of hops, gentian root was an ingredient in beer brewing. The herb is still used in liqueurs, vermouths, and many digestive bitters popular in Europe.

In 1885, Augustin Thompson of Union, Maine, introduced his beverage Moxie Nerve Food, made with gentian. The original label proclaimed that the bitter brew cured "brain and nervous exhaustion, loss of manhood, help-lessness, imbecility, and insanity"—claims that took a lot of moxie even in the pre-FDA heyday of patent medicines.

Thompson peddled Moxie on the road in classic patent-medicine style, and eventually it caught on—not as a medicine but as a beverage. That was fine with Thompson, who backed off from his medicinal claims and repositioned Moxie as a soft drink. For years, Moxie outsold Coca-Cola in New England. It's still available there, and gentian is still one of its ingredients.

In the 1930s, in her *Modern Herbal*, Maude Grieve called gentian "one of our most useful bitter tonics, especially in general debility, weakness of the digestive organs, or want of ap-petite. It is one of the best strengtheners of the human system." Contemporary herbalists echo Grieve. One suggests chewing gentian root as a substitute for smoking cigarettes.

Therapeutic Uses

While you can forget gentian for "loss of man-hood, helplessness, imbecility, and insanity," the bitter root lives up to its ancient reputation as a digestive aid.

Digestive problems. Gentian contains gen-tianine, a bitter-tasting compound that stimu-lates salivation and the secretion of stomach acid, lending credence to the herb's 3,000-year history as a digestive aid. Try some before meals.

Commission E, the expert panel that evalu-ates herbal medicines for the German counter-part of the FDA, endorses gentian for loss of appetite and digestive complaints.

Arthritis. One Chinese study found that gentian has strong anti-inflammatory proper-ties, suggesting that traditional Chinese physi-cians may have been on the right track when they prescribed the herb for arthritis. Try it if you have arthritis or any other inflammatory condition.

Women's health concerns. Gentian has never been shown to stimulate the uterus, but for hundreds of years, herbalists have consid-ered gentian a powerful menstruation promoter. Pregnant women should err on the side of cau-tion and not use it. Other women may try it to stimulate their periods.

Rx Recommendations

Use a decoction or tincture of gentian to stimu-late digestion. Either form is also appropriate for treating arthritis or bringing on menstruation.

To make a decoction, boil 1 teaspoon of powdered root in 3 cups of water for 30 minutes, then strain if you wish and let cool. Take 1 tablespoon before meals. Gentian tastes very bitter, so you may want to add sugar or honey.

As a homemade tincture, take ¼ to 1 teaspoon before meals.

When using commercial preparations, follow the package directions.

Do not give gentian to children under age 2. For older children and adults over age 65, start with low-strength preparations and increase the strength if necessary.

The Safety Factor

Gentian digestive bitters are popular in Germany, where herbal medicine is considerably more mainstream than in the United States. German physicians discourage the herb's use by people with high blood pressure. They also echo the Eclectics' warning that large amounts may cause stomach irritation, with possible nausea and vomiting.

The FDA has approved gentian as an ingredient in foods and alcoholic beverages.

Wise-Use Guidelines

For adults who are not pregnant or nursing and do not have high blood pressure or chronic gas-trointestinal conditions, gentian is considered safe in the amounts typically recommended.

You should use medicinal amounts of gentian only in consultation with your physician. If the herb causes minor discomfort, such as stomach upset or nausea, reduce the dosage or stop using it altogether. Let your doctor know if you experience any unpleasant effects or if the symptoms for which you're using the herb do not improve significantly within 2 weeks.

Growing Infomation

Gentian is a striking 6-foot perennial with branching medicinal roots; deeply veined, pointed oval leaves; and large, beautiful yellow flowers.

Once established, the plant requires little care other than abundant water and shelter from wind and excessive sun. But establishing gentian can be a problem. The seeds need frost to germinate, and even with frost, germination may take a year, if it occurs at all. Most authorities recommend using root cuttings instead.

Gentian prefers rich, loamy, slightly acidic soil. An annual dressing of peat moss helps. Harvest the roots in late summer. Desirable roots are dark reddish brown, tough, and flexible, with a strong, unpleasant odor. They should taste rather sweet initially, then very bitter. Dry the roots, then powder them.

Ginger

Family: Zingiberaceae; other members include turmeric and cardamom

Genus and species: *Zingiber officinale*

Also known as: Jamaican, African, and Cochin (Asian) ginger

Parts used: Rhizomes (commonly called roots)

An old Indian proverb says, "Every good quality is contained in ginger." That's not much of an exaggeration.

Fleshy and aromatic, ginger has played a role in cooking and healing since the dawn of history. Modern science has supported some of its traditional medicinal uses, most notably its remarkable ability to prevent the nausea of motion sickness and morning sickness. Researchers have discovered that the herb has other therapeutic benefits as well.

Healing History

Ancient Indians used their native ginger in cooking, to preserve food, and to treat digestive problems. They also considered the herb a physical and spiritual cleanser. Indians shunned strong-smelling garlic and onions before religious celebrations for fear of offending their deities, but they ate lots of ginger because it left them smelling sweet and therefore presentable to the gods.

Ginger figured prominently in China's first great herbal, the *Pen Tsao Ching* (*Classic of Herbs*), which was reportedly compiled by the mythical emperor-sage Shen Nung around 3000 B.C. As the story goes, the wise herbalist tested hundreds of medicinal herbs on himself—until he took a little too much of a poisonous herb and died.

Shen Nung recommended ginger for colds, fever, chills, tetanus, and leprosy. The *Pen Tsao Ching* also echoed Indian practice, saying that fresh ginger "eliminates body odor and puts a person in touch with the spiritual [realm]."

Over time, Chinese women began taking ginger for menstrual discomforts. Then they noticed that the herb relieved the nausea of morning sickness. Chinese sailors adopted ginger to prevent seasickness by chewing the root while at sea. Chinese physicians prescribed it to treat arthritis, ulcers, and kidney problems.

The Chinese also consider ginger an antidote to shellfish poisoning. This is why Chinese fish and seafood dishes are often seasoned with the herb.

Ancient Greek traders learned of the Asian practice of using ginger as a nausea-preventing digestive aid. They took the herb with them to Greece, where, after big meals, it was wrapped in sweetened bread and eaten as a stomach settler. Eventually, the Greeks began baking the herb into the sweet bread, and thus the herbal remedy evolved into the world's first cookie, gingerbread.

The Romans also used ginger as a digestive aid. After the fall of Rome, however, the herb became scarce in Europe and quite costly.

Once renewed Asian trade made ginger more available, European demand proved almost insatiable. The ancient Greeks' modest gingerbread cakes evolved into sugary gingerbread men and elaborate confections like the witch's gingerbread house in *Hansel and Gretel*.

In England and her American colonies, ginger was incorporated into a stomach-soothing drink called ginger beer, the forerunner of today's ginger ale. Ginger ale is still a popular home remedy for diarrhea, nausea, and vomiting.

America's 19th-century Eclectic physicians, forerunners of today's naturopaths, prescribed ginger powder, tea, wine, and beer for infant diarrhea, indigestion, nausea, dysentery, flatulence, fever, headache, toothache, and "female hysteria" (menstrual complaints).

Contemporary herbalists recommend ginger for colds, flu, and motion sickness and as a digestive aid.

Therapeutic Uses

Break out the gingerbread and ginger ale. Scientific research has lent support to some of ginger's traditional uses—and has revealed several more benefits.

Motion sickness and morning sickness. The ancient Chinese were right. Ginger does indeed prevent the nausea associated with seasickness and other types of motion sickness, as well as the morning sickness of pregnancy.

Ginger's anti-nausea action first received scientific validation in 1982 in a study conducted by researchers at Brigham Young University and published in the British medical journal *Lancet*. The researchers gave 36 volunteers with a history of motion sickness either 100 milligrams of the popular anti-motion sickness drug dimenhydrinate (Dramamine) or 940 milligrams of ginger powder. A short time later, the participants were seated in a computerized rocking chair programmed to move in such a way that it would trigger motion sickness. The chair was equipped with a switch that allowed its riders to stop the movement when they began to feel nauseated.

Compared with the people who had taken Dramamine, those who had taken ginger were able to stay in the chair 57 percent longer. Based on their finding, the researchers also recommended ginger capsules, ginger tea, or ginger ale for morning sickness.

Since that study, many others have confirmed ginger's value for the prevention of motion and morning sickness. Here's a small sampling.

• Swedish Navy researchers gave ginger to 80 naval cadets who were sailing in turbulent seas. Compared with a group that took medically inactive placebos, those who took ginger experienced 72 percent less seasickness.

• British surgeons gave 60 women about to have gynecological surgery either ginger or the prescription antinausea drug metoclopramide (Reglan). Those who received ginger experienced significantly less postsurgical nausea and vomiting.

• Danish researchers gave 30 pregnant women, all battling morning sickness, either ginger or placebos for 4 days. Then the women switched treatments for 4 days. While taking ginger, 70 percent of the study participants reported significant relief from nausea. Doctors discourage moms-to-be from taking any drugs, including anti-nausea medications, but ginger is safe to use during pregnancy.

• Italian researchers asked all of the passengers boarding a cruise ship if they were prone to seasickness. Sixty reported a history of the condition. The ship's doctor gave these people either a standard dose of Dramamine or ginger (500 milligrams before embarking and 500 milligrams every 4 hours during 2 days of rough seas). Among those taking Dramamine, 50 percent reported "very good" or "excellent" results. Among those taking ginger, that figure rose to 70 percent.

• Another group of Italian researchers studied 28 children—18 boys and 10 girls between the ages of 4 and 8—who took a 2-day class trip that involved travel by car, boat, and airplane. All were given either a standard children's dose of Dramamine or ginger (for those younger than 6, 250 milligrams before departure and every 4 hours thereafter; for those 6 and older,

500 milligrams). A physician rated their motion sickness symptoms. Among those who took Dramamine, 31 percent showed "good" benefits, while 69 percent demonstrated "modest" benefits. Among those who took ginger, 100 percent had "good" results.

Commission E, the expert panel that evaluates herbal medicines for the German counterpart of the Food and Drug Administration, endorses ginger for the prevention and treatment of motion sickness. In addition, many cancer specialists recommend it for the nausea associated with chemotherapy.

Digestive problems. Ginger is a gastrointestinal antispasmodic. It prevents indigestion and abdominal cramping by soothing the muscles that line the intestines. It also contains some compounds similar to digestive enzymes that break down proteins. Commission E approves ginger to prevent and treat indigestion.

Heart disease and stroke. Few people in the ancient world lived long enough—or combined a high-fat diet with a sedentary lifestyle—to develop heart disease or stroke. Today, these conditions account for half of all deaths in the United States.

Ginger may help prevent heart disease and stroke by controlling three key risk factors. The herb helps reduce cholesterol, according to a study published in the *New England Journal of Medicine*. It also helps lower blood pressure, and it prevents the blood clots that trigger heart attacks and most strokes.

Ulcers. Research confirms the ancient Chinese practice of using ginger to treat ulcers. In experiments involving animals that were given drugs known to produce ulcers, pre-treatment with a ginger preparation acted as a preventive.

Ginger does not cure ulcers, nor has it been well-researched in humans. But a small pilot study, in which 10 people with ulcers took 6 grams of ginger a day, showed that the herb can help relieve symptoms.

Arthritis. Studies have identified anti-inflammatory substances in ginger, lending support to the herb's traditional use in treating arthritis.

Women's health concerns. Antispasmodics soothe not only the digestive tract but also other smooth muscles, such as the uterus. As an antispasmodic, ginger may help ease menstrual cramps.

Colds and flu. Chinese studies show that ginger helps kill influenza virus, and an Indian report found that the herb increases the immune system's ability to fight infection. These findings lend some support to ginger's traditional role in treating colds, flu, and other infectious illnesses.

Intriguing Possibilities

In animal studies, ginger reduces blood sugar levels, suggesting that the herb may help control diabetes.

Other animal studies have shown that ginger promotes the shrinkage of tumors. While these findings don't necessarily apply to humans, ginger may someday find a role in the treatment of cancer. And if you have cancer, there's no harm in using ginger in consultation with your doctor.

Rx Recommendations

Use ginger to taste in cooking to create warm, spicy, aromatic dishes.

For motion sickness, the recommended dose of ginger is 1,000 milligrams approximately 30 minutes before travel. Commercial capsules are usually most convenient, but a 12-ounce container of ginger ale also provides the proper amount, provided that it's made with real ginger and not artificial flavor. Check the label to be sure.

You can also drink 2 cups of ginger infusion. To make it, use 2 teaspoons of powdered or fresh grated root per cup of boiling water, steep for 10 minutes, and strain if you wish.

To ease other digestive upsets or to treat colds or flu, make an infusion. To help relieve arthritis or prevent heart disease and stroke, use the herb in cooking or drink ginger ale or ginger tea.

You may give weak ginger preparations to children under age 2 for colic.

The Safety Factor

Ginger's anti-nausea effects may prevent morning sickness, but the herb has a long history as a menstruation promoter. Might it cause miscarriage? One study suggests that its uterine effects depend on the amount used.

In the study published in *Lancet* that was previously mentioned, less than 1 gram of ginger was needed to prevent nausea. To trigger menstruation, Chinese physicians recommend 20 to 28 grams. A strong cup of ginger tea contains about 500 milligrams, and an 8-ounce glass of ginger ale contains approximately 1,000 milligrams. None of these come close to the amount that promotes menstruation.

There have been no reports in the scientific literature of ginger triggering abortion or causing birth defects. Pregnant women with no history of miscarriage should feel free to try modest amounts of ginger tea or ginger ale to treat morning sickness.

Although ginger generally relieves indigestion, some people who take it to prevent motion sickness report heartburn.

Wise-Use Guidelines

Ginger is on the FDA list of herbs generally regarded as safe. For adults, ginger is safe when used in the amounts typically recommended.

You should use medicinal amounts of ginger only in consultation with your physician. If the herb causes minor discomfort, such as heartburn, reduce the dosage or stop using it altogether. Let your doctor know if you experience any unpleasant effects or if the symptoms for which you're taking the herb do not improve significantly within 2 weeks.

Growing Information

Ginger is a tropical perennial that grows from a tuberous underground stem, or rhizome. Each year, the plant produces a round, 3-foot stem with thin, pointed, lance-shaped, 6-inch leaves and a single, large, yellow and purple flower.

Ginger grows outdoors in Hawaii, Florida, southern California, New Mexico, Arizona, and Texas. It does best when well-watered in partial shade in raised beds deeply cultivated with composted manure and kelp.

Ginger is propagated from young fresh roots, which contain eyes similar to those in potatoes. The ginger root sold in most supermarkets, with tough, tan skin, is neither young nor fresh, so its propagation potential is low. The best place to obtain growable ginger root is at an Asian specialty market, although some nurseries carry it as well. Look for roots with light green skin.

Plant the roots about 3 inches deep and 12 inches apart. After 12 months, uproot the plant, harvest some roots, and replant the rest.

You can also grow ginger indoors in deep pots with a soil mixture of loam, sand, compost, and peat moss. Indoors, it needs warmth, plenty of water, and high humidity. A greenhouse environment is best.

Ginkgo

Family: Ginkgoaceae; no other members

Genus and species: *Ginkgo biloba*

Also known as: Maidenhair tree

Parts used: Leaves

Ginkgo is the oldest surviving tree on earth, a relic of the dinosaur age that first appeared some 200 million years ago. Individual trees can survive for up to 1,000 years.

Appropriately enough, as a healing herb, ginkgo aids the oldest surviving people. It helps prevent and treat many conditions associated with aging, including Alzheimer's disease, stroke, heart disease, impotence, deafness, blindness, and memory loss.

Healing History

The ginkgo tree is considered sacred throughout Asia, where it is often planted around Buddhist temples. Ginkgo was deemed "good for the heart and lungs" in China's first great herbal, the *Pen Tsao Ching* (*The Classic of Herbs*), attributed to the mythical emperor-sage Shen Nung around 3000 B.C.

Traditional Chinese physicians used ginkgo to treat asthma and chilblains, swelling of the hands and feet due to damp cold. The ancient Chinese and Japanese ate roasted ginkgo seeds as a digestive aid and to prevent drunkenness. Even today, some bars in Japan serve the roasted seeds to prevent intoxication.

India's traditional Ayurvedic healers associated ginkgo with long life. They reportedly used the herb as an ingredient in soma, a longevity elixir.

Ginkgo trees were introduced into Europe in 1730. Today, they're popular street and park trees throughout the temperate world. But even though 18th-century horticulturists planted them throughout Europe, herbalists of that time ignored them. As a result, ginkgo's fan-shaped leaves have no history in Western herbal medicine.

Thanks to recent research, however, ginkgo has become one of the top-selling medicinal herbs in the United States and Europe, with sales approaching an estimated $1 billion annually. It is particularly popular in Europe, where it ranks among the most widely prescribed medications. An increasing number of older Americans take it as well.

Therapeutic Uses

There are two reasons for the medical excitement over ginkgo. First, the herb contains potent antioxidant compounds called ginkgo flavone glycosides and terpene lactones. Antioxidants help prevent and reverse the cell damage that scientists believe is behind many of the degenerative conditions associated with aging, including heart disease, stroke, and many cancers.

In addition, ginkgo interferes with the action of a substance called platelet activation factor (PAF) that's produced by the body. Discovered in 1972, PAF is involved in an enormous number of biological processes, including arterial blood flow, asthma attacks, organ graft rejection, and the blood clots involved in heart attacks and most strokes.

Alzheimer's disease and multi-infarct dementia. In the United States, ginkgo made its biggest splash in 1997, when the *Journal of the American Medical Association* published a study by researchers at Albert Einstein College of Medicine in the Bronx. It showed that ginkgo not only slows mental deterioration in people with Alzheimer's disease but, in some cases, also improves their cognitive abilities.

For the study, the researchers gave 202 people in various stages of Alzheimer's either a medically inactive placebo or 120 milligrams of a standardized ginkgo extract every day for 1 year. Compared with the patients who received the placebo, those who received ginkgo retained significantly more mental function.

Several other studies have corroborated ginkgo's effectiveness for slowing the progression of Alzheimer's. Here's a sampling of the research to date.

• German researchers gave 20 people with mild to moderate Alzheimer's either a placebo or 240 milligrams of ginkgo a day. After 3 months, the 10 patients taking the placebos showed significant progression of Alzheimer's. Among the 10 people taking ginkgo, one showed progression, two stayed the same, and seven experienced improvement in mental function.
• A group of European researchers gave 60 people with Alzheimer's either placebos or 120-milligram or 240-milligram doses of ginkgo every day. After 3 months, both groups taking ginkgo performed better on cognitive tests than the group taking the placebos.
• Another European team gave 156 people with either Alzheimer's or multi-infarct dementia (MID, an Alzheimer's-like condition caused by mini-strokes) either placebos or 240 milligrams of ginkgo a day. Six months later, the group receiving ginkgo retained greater cognitive function.

In all of these studies, the response rate to ginkgo was similar to what would be expected from the pharmaceuticals currently approved to slow the progression of Alzheimer's or MID. It is not clear exactly how ginkgo affects these conditions, but both of the herb's medicinal properties—it's an antioxidant, and it improves blood flow through the brain—appear to play roles.

Commission E, the expert panel that evaluates herbal medicines for the German counterpart of the FDA, approves ginkgo for the treatment of Alzheimer's disease and MID.

It should be noted that as of this time, no

treatment, either pharmaceutical or herbal, permanently halts or reverses the progression of Alzheimer's disease or MID. Ginkgo slows the conditions significantly, however, and causes very few, if any, side effects.

Cerebral insufficiency. As people get older, blood flow through the brain tends to decline, a condition known as cerebral insufficiency. This slows reaction time and impairs memory, concentration, and problem-solving ability—the effects that Americans increasingly refer to as "senior moments." Many studies show that ginkgo improves blood flow through the brain and, as a result, lessens symptoms of cerebral insufficiency.

Memory loss. Animal studies have found that ginkgo improves memory. Human trials have shown similar results.

• A team of European researchers gave 241 otherwise healthy elderly people who had memory problems either medically inactive placebos or ginkgo. After 6 months, those taking gingko showed improvement in some areas of mental sharpness, especially memory.
• British researchers gave 31 middle aged people who reported memory problems either placebos or 120 milligrams of ginkgo a day. After 6 months, the ginkgo group showed significant improvement in memory and reaction time.
• In another British study, researchers tested the short-term memory skills and reaction times of eight women in their twenties and thirties before and after they were given either placebos or 600 milligrams of ginkgo. Both measurements improved "very significantly" when the women took the herb.

Commission E approves ginkgo as a treatment for memory problems.

Stroke. As people grow older and blood flow to the brain decreases, there are less food and oxygen for brain cells. If blood flow becomes blocked, the result is a stroke, the third leading cause of death in the United States.

In Europe, ginkgo is widely prescribed to support recovery from stroke. Commission E also approves it for the treatment of stroke.

Heart disease. Ginkgo improves blood flow not only through the brain but also through the heart muscle. It contains antioxidants that help prevent heart disease, and it helps prevent the blood clots that trigger heart attacks.

A French study hints that treating heart patients with ginkgo may speed their recovery from coronary artery bypass surgery.

Intermittent claudication. When cholesterol deposits narrow the arteries in the legs, the result is intermittent claudication, which causes pain, cramping, and weakness, particularly in the calves. Ginkgo improves blood flow through the legs, thus relieving symptoms.

In one year long German study of 36 people with intermittent claudication, ginkgo produced significantly greater pain relief than standard treatment. In another study, German researchers measured how far people with intermittent claudication could walk before developing leg pain. Then the participants began taking either placebos or ginkgo. After 6 months, those in the placebo group showed scant improvement, while those in the ginkgo group were able to walk 50 percent farther before developing leg pain.

Commission E approves ginkgo as a treatment for intermittent claudication.

Impotence. A study published in the *Journal of Urology* concluded that ginkgo helps relieve impotence caused by narrowing of the arteries that supply blood to the penis. In the study, 60 men with erection problems caused by impaired penile blood flow were instructed to take 60 milligrams of ginkgo a day. After 1 year, half of the men had regained their ability to have erections.

Antidepressant-related sexual problems. Pharmaceutical antidepressants work. Unfortunately, however, some drugs often cause problems: loss of libido and difficulty with orgasm in both sexes, impotence in men, and loss of vaginal lubrication in women.

At the University of California, San Francisco, Medical Center, an elderly man who was taking ginkgo for his memory told his doctor that the herb seemed to give him a little sexual boost. This comment led to a study of ginkgo's effects in 63 people who were experiencing sexual problems while on antidepressants. In addition to their medications, the patients took 207 milligrams of ginkgo a day. Ninety-one percent of the women and 76 percent of the men reported improvement: enhanced sexual desire, greater ability to have erections or produce lubrication, and generally more pleasurable sex.

Because the researchers didn't test ginkgo against placebos, the study can't be regarded as scientifically rigorous. Placebos usually benefit about one-third of those who use them. The positive response rate in this study was much greater than a typical placebo response, suggesting that ginkgo has real ability to relieve these types of sexual problems.

Macular degeneration. Macular degeneration is the leading cause of blindness in adults. It involves the deterioration of the macula, an area of the eye's nerve-rich retina that's responsible for central vision and fine detail. In one small French study, people with macular degeneration who took ginkgo experienced "significant improvement" in their vision.

Cochlear deafness. Researchers believe that cochlear deafness results from decreased blood flow to the nerves involved in hearing. One French study that compared ginkgo with standard therapy for cochlear deafness showed significant recovery in both groups, but distinctly better improvement in the ginkgo group.

Chronic ringing in the ears (tinnitus). A 13-month French study involving 103 people deemed ginkgo "conclusively effective" for chronic tinnitus. According to the researchers, the herb improved all the patients who took it. Commission E also approves ginkgo as a treatment for tinnitus.

Chronic dizziness (vertigo). In one French study, 70 people with chronic vertigo were treated with either a ginkgo extract or placebos for 3 months. At the conclusion of the trial, 18 percent of the placebo group no longer felt dizzy, compared with 47 percent of the ginkgo group. Statistically, this is a highly significant difference. Commission E approves ginkgo as a treatment for vertigo.

Intoxication. There may be some truth to the age-old Asian belief that ginkgo helps prevent drunkenness. Japanese researchers have discovered an enzyme in ginkgo seeds that accelerates the body's metabolism of alcohol. Faster metabolism means less alcohol in the bloodstream and less likelihood of intoxication.

It's not clear whether ginkgo speeds the metabolism of alcohol in humans, and, of course, consuming roasted ginkgo seeds is no substitute for responsible drinking.

Intriguing Possibilities

Preliminary reports suggest that ginkgo may help prevent the rejection of transplanted organs. It may also be effective against allergies, altitude sickness, high blood pressure, migraines, and kidney problems.

Rx Recommendations

The medicinal compounds in ginkgo leaves occur in concentrations too dilute for infusions or tinctures to provide any benefit. Commercial preparations use a concentrated 50:1 extract; in other words, 50 pounds of leaves are processed to provide 1 pound of standardized extract containing 24 percent ginkgo flavone glycosides and 6 percent terpene lactones.

Buy a commercial ginkgo product and take it according to the package directions. Most studies have used doses of 120 or 240 milligrams a day, typically divided into three doses—40 or 80 milligrams three times a day.

Do not give ginkgo to children under age 2.

The Safety Factor

No serious side effects have been associated with ginkgo in any study to date, but mild side effects such as stomach upset, headache, and rash are possible. Some people who take large doses have reported irritability, restlessness, diarrhea, nausea, and vomiting.

Platelet activation factor plays a key role in blood clotting. Ginkgo's PAF-inhibiting action may cause problems for people with clotting disorders and those taking anticoagulant (blood-thinning) medications.

Wise-Use Guidelines

For adults who are not pregnant or nursing, do not have clotting disorders, and are not taking anticoagulant (blood-thinning) medications or supplements (vitamin E, for example), ginkgo is considered safe in the amounts typically recommended.

You should use medicinal amounts of ginkgo only in consultation with your doctor. If it causes minor discomfort, such as nausea or diarrhea, reduce the dosage or stop using it altogether. Let your doctor know if you experience unpleasant effects or if the symptoms for which you're using the herb do not improve significantly within 2 weeks.

Growing Information

Ginkgo is a stately, deciduous tree that reaches 100 feet with a 20-foot girth. Its flat, fan-shaped leaves have two lobes, hence its Latin species name, *biloba*. Ginkgoes are dioecious—that is, male and female flowers appear on different trees. The females produce apricot-size, orange-yellow fruits that contain edible seeds.

Ginkgoes are attractive street or yard trees that can be grown throughout much of the United States. If you'd like to plant them for ornamental purposes, obtain saplings from a nursery in your area. Plant only males, however, since the fruits produced by female trees are messy and foul-smelling.

Plant saplings in well-drained soil and stake them to ensure straight growth. Young trees are oddly proportioned and often look gawky, but they become stately with age. Water regularly until the trees are about 20 feet tall. After that, they are self-sufficient.

Ginkgoes are resistant to insects and disease and grow up to 2 feet per year. In autumn, the leaves turn a beautiful gold color before they fall.

Ginseng

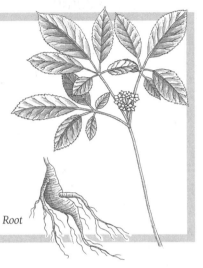

Family: Araliaceae; other members include ivy

Genus and species: *Panax ginseng* (Chinese/ Korean/Japanese); *Panax quinquefolius* (American); *Eleutherococcus senticosus* (Siberian)

Also known as: Man root, life root, root of immortality, Tartar root, heal-all, 'seng, and 'sang

Parts used: Roots

Root

Ginseng is as fascinating as it is controversial. The root of an unassuming, ivy-like groundcover, the herb has been the subject of more than 1,500 books and scientific papers, yet its effects continue to be hotly debated.

Advocates call ginseng the ultimate tonic, a Chinese medical term that means a general overall strengthener. They say the herb boosts well-being, immune function, athletic performance, and liver function. It also helps treat high blood pressure, diabetes, cancer, emphysema, impotence, low sperm count, loss of appetite, and possibly heart disease.

Critics of ginseng counter that the herb does little, if anything, except cause a potentially hazardous "abuse syndrome." Even the latest scientific research has done little to bring the two sides closer together.

Healing History

Ginseng is not one herb but three: Chinese, Korean, or Japanese (*Panax ginseng*); American (*P. quinquefolius*); and Siberian (*Eleutherococcus senticosus*). The Siberian variety is not a true ginseng, but it contains similar active chemicals, and studies have shown that it has similar effects. As a result, all three species are grouped together as ginseng and used interchangeably in the West (although Chinese physicians make subtle distinctions among them).

Ginseng has a fleshy, multibranched root. If you stretch your imagination, some roots resemble the human form, with limblike branches suggesting arms and legs. The ancient Chinese called the plant man root, or *jen shen*, which eventually entered English as "ginseng."

Ginseng figured prominently in the first great Chinese herbal, the *Pen Tsao Ching* (*The*

Classic of Herbs), reportedly compiled by the mythical emperor-sage Shen Nung around 3000 B.C. Shen Nung recommended the herb for "enlightening the mind and increasing wisdom," and noted that "continuous use leads to longevity."

The Doctrine of Signatures, the belief that a plant's physical characteristics reveal its healing virtues, did not exert as much influence in China as it did in medieval Europe. Nonetheless, ginseng's fancied resemblance to the human form led to the belief that the herb was a whole-body tonic, particularly for the elderly. It was widely used to treat infirmities of old age, such as lethargy, impotence, arthritis, senility, menopausal complaints, and loss of sexual interest. The Chinese, Koreans, and Japanese still consider ginseng the best health promoter, although calling it the root of immortality stretches things a bit.

As the popularity of ginseng spread throughout ancient Asia, demand soared and rapacious collection decimated the wild supply. Chinese ginseng became increasingly rare and more valuable than gold. Unscrupulous merchants sold other roots as ginseng (adulteration is still a problem today).

Unlike other Asian herbs that became favorites in the West (ginger and cinnamon, for example), ginseng remained relatively unknown in Europe until the 18th century, when missionaries informed early European botanists of ginseng's reputation as a longevity herb. Europeans scoffed at Asian claims, but those familiar with Asia, particularly the Jesuits, who had many missions in China, appreciated the herb's great value there.

In 1704, a French explorer returned to Paris with a sample of what turned out to be American ginseng from southern Canada. Jesuits in France alerted their brethren in Canada to its enormous value in China. Jesuits in Mon-

treal shipped a boatload to Canton, where other Jesuits sold it to the Chinese for what was then a king's ransom, $5 a pound.

Immediately, the Jesuits in Canada began shipping to China as much ginseng as their Indian collectors could find. They made a fortune while keeping the lucrative trade a secret for many years. Eventually, word leaked out that the celibate fathers seemed to take an unusual interest in a certain low-growing herb that was rumored to be an aphrodisiac in far-off Cathay.

Once ginseng's reputation spread, the herb was discovered growing as far south as Georgia. It enjoyed a brief burst of popularity among American colonists who were interested in sexual stimulation. Most were disappointed. Virginia plantation owner William Byrd wrote that ginseng "frisks the spirits" but causes none "of those naughty effects that might make men too troublesome and impertinent to their wives."

America's "Ginseng Rush"

By the 1740s, few Americans were consuming ginseng, but news of the herb's incredible value in China hit the 13 colonies like news of the California gold strike 100 years later. Shipping agents circulated handbills offering to buy the herb for the then-fabulous sum of $1 a pound. Foragers scoured the countryside, and frontier scouts, surveyors, and fur trappers collected ginseng as a sideline to their other work. Ginseng quickly became the colonies' most valuable export—more precious pound for pound than even the rarest furs.

By the 1770s, ginseng fever had wiped out the plant along the eastern seaboard, forcing collectors into the trackless wilderness across the Appalachians. The search for ginseng played a significant role in the exploration of western Pennsylvania, West Virginia, Kentucky, and Tennessee. One intrepid pioneer who combined trapping and scouting with ginseng collecting was none other than Daniel Boone. According to Scott Persons, author of *American Ginseng: Green Gold*, in 1788, Boone lost 12 tons of wild ginseng when his boat capsized in the Ohio River.

Native Americans learned about ginseng from the Jesuits and used it to combat fatigue, stimulate appetite, and aid digestion. Some tribes mixed it into love potions.

America's 19th-century Eclectic physicians, forerunners of today's naturopaths, called ginseng a stimulant for "mental exhaustion from overwork" and prescribed it for loss of appetite, indigestion, asthma, laryngitis, bronchitis, and tuberculosis. The Eclectic textbook *King's American Dispensatory* (1898) added that the herb "invigorates the virile powers."

Contemporary herbalists echo the Chinese, recommending ginseng as a tonic stimulant that promotes vitality, longevity, virility, and resistance to stress and illness. Various experts estimate that Americans currently spend $120 to $400 million a year on ginseng products.

American ginseng is no longer plentiful in the wild, but in Appalachia, collectors still forage for the herb. In 1997, wild ginseng reportedly brought foragers $500 per pound. Most collectors never use the herb themselves. In the words of Georgia ginseng trader Jake Plott, "I never found it worth a damn for anything but to get money out of."

Plott's comment aptly sums up how many Western scientists feel about Asia's most revered herb. Critics dismiss its purported benefits as folklore of the Far East and insist that the studies supporting the herb's therapeutic effects are seriously flawed. They also charge that ginseng causes serious side effects, including ner-vousness, insomnia, diarrhea, high blood pressure, and hormonal disturbance—symptoms collectively known as ginseng abuse syndrome.

Therapeutic Uses

In defiance of the critics' charges, the scientific literature shows that ginseng is reasonably safe and beneficial for many ailments. The herb owes its healing value to several compounds collectively known as ginsenosides.

The ginsenosides are not fully understood, and their effects can be downright confusing. For example, some stimulate the central nervous system, while others depress it. Some raise blood pressure, while others lower it. These observations need to be clarified through additional study, but researchers have already learned a great deal about the herb and its many effects.

Among the first Western scientists to investigate ginseng, notably *Eleutherococcus* (Siberian ginseng), was pharmacologist Israel I. Brekhman, Ph.D., of the Academy of Sciences of the former Soviet Union. He popularized the term *adaptogen*, which indicates that the herb helps the body adapt to physical and emotional stresses, increases resistance to disease, and exerts subtle but real generalized strengthening effects.

Beginning in 1960 and continuing for the next 30 years, hundreds of studies conducted by Dr. Brekhman and his colleagues showed that ginseng combats fatigue (without caffeine), improves physical stamina, counteracts the damage caused by physical and emotional stress, prevents the depletion of stress-fighting adrenal hormones, and enhances memory. Basically, Dr. Brekhman concurred with what Asian herbalists had been saying for thousands of years—that ginseng is a tonic. More recent research from around the world bears this out.

Improved general well-being. At the Medical School of the National Autonomous University of Mexico, researchers gave 500 people questionnaires asking about their health, well-being, occurrence of pain, mood, energy level, sex life, sleep quality, and personal satisfaction. Then 162 members of the group were given a daily multivitamin/mineral supplement, while 338 were given the same supplement plus ginseng (80 milligrams of a standardized extract). Four months later, the participants completed the questionnaires again. Both groups reported better quality of life, but those taking ginseng claimed significantly greater improvement.

Increased energy. Ginseng is a noncaffeine stimulant that helps counteract fatigue. European researchers studied 232 people between the ages of 25 and 60 who complained of persistent fatigue. Half were given daily doses of a medically inactive placebo, while the rest received a formula containing 80 milligrams of ginseng plus nine vitamins and eight minerals. After 7 weeks, all of the participants were evaluated using standard tests of fatigue. The group taking the ginseng formula showed significantly less lethargy. The study authors concluded that ginseng combats fatigue by supporting the adrenal glands.

Enhanced athletic performance. For decades, Russian, Chinese, and Korean Olympic athletes have used ginseng in their training. They take the herb before events in the belief that it improves stamina and performance, much like coffee (see page 144).

Some American athletes have also adopted ginseng. Research shows that the herb does indeed enhance athletic performance.

Italian researchers gave 50 male physical education teachers between the ages of 21 and 47 either placebos or a combination of ginseng, vitamins, and minerals, then had the men run on treadmills. Subsequently, the two groups switched treatments, so the men who had taken the placebos received the ginseng formula, and vice versa. While they were using the ginseng, the men's stamina increased significantly because their hearts and lungs worked more efficiently.

Improved mental function. Ginseng may enhance memory and other aspects of mental acuity. In one study, a team of Danish researchers gave 112 healthy middle-aged adults a battery of tests that assessed their memory skills, reaction times, and ability to learn, concentrate, and reason abstractly. The researchers then gave the study participants either placebos or 400 milligrams of ginseng extract daily for 9 weeks. When re-examined, those taking the ginseng showed significant improvement in two of the tests: reaction time and abstract thinking.

Enhanced immunity. In animal studies, Chinese researchers have found that ginseng revs up certain white blood cells (macrophages and natural killer cells) that devour disease-causing microorganisms. Meanwhile, researchers at the University of Southern California in Los Angeles have demonstrated that ginseng spurs the production of interferon, the body's own virus-fighting compound. It also increases the synthesis of antibodies, another component of the immune system.

In their own study, German researchers concluded that ginseng enhances immune function in humans. They gave 36 healthy volunteers either placebos or ginseng (about 2 teaspoons of tincture) three times a day for 4 weeks. Those taking the ginseng showed increased activity in their T-lymphocytes (T-cells), another kind of infection-fighting white blood cell.

Italian researchers gave people with chronic bronchitis either placebos or ginseng (100 milligrams of extract) every 12 hours for 8 weeks. Periodically, the researchers took respiratory mucus samples and analyzed them for macrophages, the white blood cells that engulf and devour invading germs. By the end of the study, the white blood cells of the people taking ginseng were significantly more active and killed more germs when tested.

Enhanced immune function means greater resistance to illness, speedier recovery, and improved general well-being, all of which support the Chinese belief that ginseng is a tonic. Commission E, the expert panel that evaluates herbal medicines for the German counterpart of the FDA, approves ginseng for invigoration, convalescence, and support of work capacity and concentration.

More Than a Tonic

In addition to its tonic-adaptogen benefits, ginseng has been shown to help prevent and treat several specific conditions.

High blood pressure. At Seoul National University College of Medicine, Korean researchers gave 34 middle-aged men and women with high blood pressure either placebos or 1.5 grams of ginseng three times a day. Eight weeks later, those taking the placebos showed no change in blood pressure, while those taking ginseng registered a significant decrease in their readings.

Some of the study participants took their ginseng in combination with mainstream blood pressure medication (a beta-blocker or calcium channel-blocker). Compared with ginseng alone, the addition of the pharmaceutical did not produce greater declines in blood pressure.

Despite this study, there have been scattered reports of ginseng raising blood pressure. If you have high blood pressure and want to include ginseng in your treatment program, work closely with your physician and monitor your pressure regularly. If it rises, stop taking ginseng.

Diabetes. In a Finnish study, 36 people newly diagnosed with Type 2 (non-insulin-dependent) diabetes received either placebos or 100 or 200 milligrams of a ginseng extract every day. Compared with those in the placebo group, the people in both ginseng groups reported greater improvement in mood, enhanced performance on physical and psychological tests, and lower blood sugar levels. Those taking 200 milligrams of ginseng experienced more benefit than those taking the lower dose.

Diabetes is a serious condition that requires professional treatment. If you'd like to try ginseng in addition to your standard treatment regimen, consult your physician.

Cancer. In the battle against cancer, ginseng may prove a worthy preventive weapon. Korean researchers added a number of supplements, including ginseng, to the drinking water of mice. Then they exposed the animals to tobacco smoke. Compared with the mice that drank plain water, those that drank water containing an extract of 6-year-old ginseng root developed significantly fewer lung tumors. (Four-year-old ginseng root had no effect.)

Ginseng may also support cancer treatment. Chinese researchers gave a large number of mice a toxic chemical that causes liver cancer. Subsequently, some of the mice received no treatment, some were given radiation, some were given ginseng, and some received a combination of radiation and ginseng. Compared with the untreated mice, those treated with radiation alone survived 17 percent longer, those treated with ginseng survived 20 percent longer, and the group that received a combination of radiation and ginseng survived 82 percent longer.

Of course, the results of studies involving animals don't always apply to humans. If you'd like to try ginseng as a complement to mainstream cancer therapy, consult a cancer specialist.

Emphysema. Israeli researchers asked 15 people with emphysema (average age, 67) to undergo tests of lung function and then walk as far as they could in 6 minutes. Subsequently, all 15 patients were instructed to take two 100-milligram capsules of ginseng every day. Three months later, the researchers repeated the tests. The participants' lung function improved significantly, meaning that more oxygen entered their bloodstreams. This increased their work capacity, as demonstrated by the fact that the distance they could walk in 6 minutes increased by 42 percent, from 600 meters to at least 854 meters.

Impotence and low sexual desire. Korean researchers gave 90 men with erectile dysfunction one of three treatments: placebos, an antidepressant (trazodone), or ginseng. Those in the placebo and antidepressant groups showed 30 percent improvement in erection rigidity and girth and sexual desire, but those in the ginseng group experienced 60 percent improvement. This study supports the traditional Chinese belief that ginseng is a mild aphrodisiac.

Male infertility. Italian researchers at the University of Rome gave 4,000 milligrams of ginseng extract daily to 30 men between the ages 26 and 41 who were infertile because of low sperm counts, as well as to 20 men with normal sperm counts. After 3 months, the sperm counts in the infertile men rose 93 percent, from 15 million to 29 million per milliliter. The men with initially normal sperm counts showed a 9 percent increase, from 85 million to 93 million per milliliter.

Liver damage. Ginseng protects the liver from the harmful effects of drugs, alcohol, and other toxic substances. In one experiment, researchers gave what should have been fatal doses of various narcotics to experimental animals pretreated with ginseng extract. Most of the animals survived. And in a pilot human study, ginseng improved liver function in 24 elderly people with alcohol-induced cirrhosis.

Radiation therapy. Ginseng can minimize the cell damage from radiation. In two studies, experimental animals were injected with various protective agents, then subjected to doses of radiation similar to those used in treating cancer. Ginseng did the best job of protecting healthy cells against harm, suggesting that the herb may be beneficial during cancer radiation therapy.

Appetite loss. Asians have long considered ginseng particularly helpful for the elderly. As people age, their senses of taste and smell deteriorate, leading to reduced appetite. In addition, the intestine's ability to absorb nutrients declines. As a result, some older people suffer malnutrition, which reduces their energy and alertness and increases their risk of illness.

Ginseng enjoys a thousand-year-old reputation as an appetite stimulant. One study showed that it increases the ability of the intestine to absorb nutrients, thus helping to prevent malnutrition.

Intriguing Possibilities

According to Japanese animal studies and one small human trial, ginseng appears to reduce cholesterol and helps prevent the blood clots that trigger heart attack and most strokes.

Rx Recommendations

Many studies of ginseng have produced impressive evidence of the herb's therapeutic benefits. But critics cite other studies that have found ginseng to have no benefit at all. Why are there such disparate results? Adulteration appears to be a big part of the answer.

Because of ginseng's rarity and enormous value, adulteration has been a problem for centuries—and still is. It's quite possible that some researchers have used "ginseng" that in fact contained little or none of the herb.

One study from the mid-1980s evaluated 54 ginseng products sold in health food stores in the United States. The researchers judged 60 percent of the products worthless because they contained too little of the herb to have any biological effect. Twenty-five percent contained no ginseng at all.

The health food industry denounced the study, and the health food trade journal *Whole Foods* commissioned an independent test. It produced essentially the same results.

The most notorious of the nonginseng "ginsengs" is wild red American ginseng or wild desert ginseng, which appeared in health food stores during the late 1970s. Although ginseng is a shade-loving, moisture-demanding plant, which means that desert ginseng is a botanical impossibility, many consumers fell for the fraud. The phony ginseng was actually red dock, a laxative plant.

Although an outcry from responsible herbalists forced most wild desert ginseng off health food store shelves by the early 1980s, problems with adulteration and fraud persist. That's why the American Herbal Products Association, an herb trade group, and the American Botanical Council, a nonprofit research and education organization, both periodically analyze ginseng products to help ensure quality, a program that's rarely undertaken with other herbs.

Even if you start with real ginseng, it may not provide medicinal benefits if it's not mature. Ginseng roots should not be harvested until they are 6 years old, but sometimes younger roots are mixed in to stretch the amount—a form of adulteration that may render a ginseng product useless. Processing can also decrease the herb's quality.

Unfortunately, the only way to be absolutely certain of ginseng's purity and age is to grow it yourself, which is much easier said than done. If you buy ginseng, read labels carefully. Look for products that are identified by species and made with whole, unprocessed, 6-year-old roots.

Ginseng tastes sweetish and slightly aromatic. To take advantage of its many therapeutic powers, use root powder, teas, tinctures, capsules, or tablets. All of these forms are available in health food stores, herb shops, supplement centers, and some drugstores. You can even buy ginseng-containing soft drinks that promise a lift similar to that of caffeinated sodas.

To prepare a tea, use $\frac{1}{2}$ to 1 teaspoon of powdered root per cup of boiling water, simmer for about 15 minutes, and strain if you wish. Drink up to 2 cups a day.

When using a tincture or any other commercial preparation, follow the package directions.

If you plan to use ginseng over the long term, most herbalists recommend taking it daily for 1 month, then stopping for a month before resuming treatment.

The Safety Factor

Problems with ginseng are rare, but the medical journals contain a few dozen reports of adverse reactions. The herb may cause insomnia, breast medicine fell from fashion by [the] Civil War, but America's 19th-[century eclec]tic physicians, forerunners of [naturop]paths, adopted goldenseal. They [called it h]ydrastis, after its Latin name, and [ex]panded its uses. They prescribed it ex[ternally] to relieve hemorrhoids, rectal fissures, [pink ey]e (conjunctivitis), eczema, boils, and [woun]ds. They also recommended it internally [as a] treatment for colds, tonsillitis, diphtheria, [ut]erine problems, postpartum hemorrhage, and digestive ailments and as a tonic during convalescence from any major illness.

After the Civil War, the golden herb enjoyed a golden age. Goldenseal was an ingredient in many patent medicines, notably Dr. Pierce's Golden Medical Discovery, a popular tonic. Demand for the herb soared. Its price jumped to $1 a pound, making it almost as costly as America's most expensive healing herb, ginseng.

While ginseng was being exported to China, goldenseal remained in the United States. But like ginseng, goldenseal was collected to the point of near extinction.

Over time, goldenseal acquired some of ginseng's medicinal reputation as a panacea and ginseng's medicinal reputation as a panacea and longevity tonic, hence another of its popular names, poor man's ginseng. The herb was listed as an astringent and antiseptic in the *U.S. Pharmacopoeia*, a standard drug reference, from 1831 to 1936, and in the *National Formulary*, the pharmacists' reference, from 1936 to 1960, when modern antibiotics pushed it aside.

Still, goldenseal has remained a favorite among herbalists. In the late 1940s, in *Back to Eden*, Jethro Kloss described the herb as "one of the most wonderful remedies in the entire herb kingdom. . . . A real cure-all."

Modern herbalists recommend goldenseal externally as an antiseptic to clean wounds and as a treatment for eczema, ringworm, athlete's foot, itching, and conjunctivitis. They prescribe it internally for digestive upset and colds, as a douche, and to stop excessive menstrual flow and postpartum uterine bleeding—although most also caution that the herb may trigger uterine contractions and "overstimulate the nervous system."

Goldenseal is a favorite of homeopaths, who prescribe microdoses for alcoholism, asthma, indigestion, cancer, hemorrhoids, and liver ailments. The herb remains a popular folk medicine as well. In *Hoosier Home Remedies*, a 1985 survey of Indiana folk medicine, Varro E. Tyler, Ph.D., reported that goldenseal was used extensively as an astringent and antiseptic to treat canker sores, chapped lips, and many other external problems.

Therapeutic Uses

In the late 1970s, heroin addicts came to believe that goldenseal tea could prevent the detection of opiates in urine specimens. Much to their chagrin, they were wrong. Goldenseal absolutely does not prevent the detection of opiates, or any other drugs, in urine. Nor is it a cure-all.

Scientists have determined that goldenseal contains two active constituents: berberine and hydrastine. Berberine, the more important, is also the active chemical in barberry. As a result, barberry and goldenseal have similar uses (and similar hazards), although goldenseal is more popular—and more expensive. Those who are interested in a "poor person's goldenseal" should try barberry.

soreness, allergy symptoms, asthma attacks, increased blood pressure, and heart rhythm disturbances (cardiac arrhythmias). People with insomnia, fibrocystic breasts, or hay fever should use ginseng only with caution. Anyone with asthma, high blood pressure, cardiac arrhythmia, or fever shouldn't take it at all.

Because of ginseng's anti-clotting action, it should be considered off-limits to people who have clotting problems or are taking anticoagulant (blood-thinning) medications.

If you have diabetes, check with your physician before taking ginseng. The herb has been shown to lower blood sugar levels.

In Asia, ginseng is viewed as an herb for the elderly. Do not give it to children. While Asian studies have concluded that ginseng does not cause birth defects in the offspring of rats, rabbits, or lambs, women who are pregnant or nursing should err on the side of caution and not use it.

Abuse of "Abuse"

Ginseng may not be completely harmless, but the study that found the herb to have serious side effects, dubbed ginseng abuse syndrome, was badly flawed.

The term *ginseng abuse syndrome* was coined in a 1979 article published in the *Journal of the American Medical Association*—an old study to be sure, but one that's still cited as evidence of alleged ginseng hazards.

For the study, a researcher assessed 133 psychiatric patients who claimed to use ginseng. He said that 14, or about 10 percent, had developed ginseng abuse syndrome. Since his subjects were psychiatric patients, they presumably had mental health problems. The researcher never bothered to identify those problems, but he freely applied his findings to the general population.

The patients revealed their ginseng use in a survey. The researcher later admitted that he never attempted to verify that their "ginseng" was, in fact, the real herb. He acknowledged that many used wild desert ginseng, which, as we have seen, is not ginseng at all.

What's more, the patients consumed up to 15 grams of the herb a day, which is many times the usual recommended dosage. And some inhaled and injected it, methods that are unheard of in traditional ginseng therapy—and that strongly suggest that the people also abused illicit drugs. The researcher never discussed whether his subjects had taken other drugs, except to mention that many consumed caffeine regularly throughout his 2-year study.

According to the researcher, ginseng abuse syndrome included symptoms such as nervousness, sleeplessness, and increased blood pressure. In rare cases, ginseng may cause sleep problems or raise blood pressure, but the same symptoms are normal side effects of caffeine. With the study's results polluted by caffeine, unusually large doses of ginseng, and quite possibly illicit drugs, it's impossible to say what caused the so-called abuse syndrome.

Another hallmark of ginseng abuse syndrome was "morning diarrhea." This may well have been caused by the wild desert ginseng, which is a laxative. Real ginseng is not known to cause diarrhea.

Finally, the researcher charged that ginseng abuse syndrome mimics corticosteroid poisoning. Even at their worst, the purported symptoms of ginseng abuse syndrome are nothing like corticosteroid poisoning, a complex condition characterized by acne, unusual hair growth, fluid retention (edema), increased blood pressure and blood sugar, increased susceptibility to infection, and rounding of the face (moon face).

Nevertheless, ever since the publication of this seriously flawed paper, reports on ginseng in medical journals and the popular press often mention ginseng abuse syndrome and corticosteroid poisoning. For the record, ginseng has never been shown to cause either one.

Wise-Use Guidelines

The FDA includes ginseng on its list of herbs generally regarded as safe. For adults who are not pregnant or nursing and do not have any of the conditions that make using ginseng inadvisable, the herb is safe when used in the amounts typically recommended.

You should use medicinal amounts of ginseng only in consultation with your doctor. If the herb causes minor discomfort, such as allergy symptoms or insomnia, reduce the dosage or stop using it altogether. Let your doctor know if you experience any unpleasant effects or if the symptoms for which you're using the herb do not improve significantly within 2 weeks.

Keep in mind that ginseng is a stimulant. People who take large doses have reported nervousness and restlessness, symptoms similar to those experienced by people who drink more coffee than they're accustomed to. Ginseng may also enhance the effects of other stimulants, such as ephedra and caffeine, thus setting the stage for overstimulation.

Growing Information

Ginseng is extremely difficult and expensive to grow. Prospective ginseng gardeners should heed the words of one frustrated horticulturist:

"God and the growers know what they're doing, but neither one is talking."

Today, an estimated 80 percent of the United States' 1,200-ton annual ginseng crop is grown in Marathon County, Wisconsin. In Canada, the herb is largely a product of British Columbia. The plants require shade, so growers drape nylon mesh over frames constructed along their rows.

Ginseng is prone to several fungal infections; it's a struggle to keep the young plants alive. Also, since the roots should be 6 years old at harvest, growers must be extremely patient.

When it's time to harvest the roots, the process is painstaking. Their value in the Orient depends in part on the arrangement of their limbs. The more humanlike the root, the higher the price. Breaking off an "arm" or "leg" during harvesting or drying lowers the price.

Root cuttings are often diseased, so most growers start with seeds, which are costly. Before planting, the seeds must be disinfected in a solution of one part chlorine bleach and nine parts water for 10 minutes.

If you want to try your hand at growing ginseng, plant the seeds in early autumn in well-prepared, humus-rich beds at a depth of ½ inch and 6-inch spacing. Ginseng grows poorly in sandy or clay soils. Maintain soil pH in the range of 5.0 to 6.0.

Germination of the seeds can take up a year. The plants must be shaded, ideally under trees, although the covered frames work, too.

Harvest roots after 6 years, digging carefully to avoid breaking the root limbs. Dry them for 1 month.

Goldenseal

A POTENT ANTIB

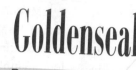

Family: Ranunculaceae; other members include buttercup, larkspur, and peony

Genus and species: *Hydrastis canadensis*

Also known as: Yellow root, yellow puccoon, Indian turmeric, Indian dye, Indian paint, jaundice root, eye balm, eye root, golden root, and poor man's ginseng.

Parts used: Rhizomes and roots

Goldenseal is both popular and powerful. This combination virtually guarantees controversy. Thus, it should come as no surprise that many contemporary herbalists view goldenseal as one of our most useful herbs, while several scientific authorities continue to quote a pharmacologist who, in 1948, wrote that the herb has "few, if any, rational indications" and may cause "death from respiratory paralysis or cardiac arrest."

On balance, there's no cause for alarm. Goldenseal may be beneficial, although harmful effects are possible. Informed home herbalists who use it safely and carefully can take advantage of its many therapeutic powers.

Healing History

The Native Americans of the northeastern United States pounded goldenseal's yellow roots (the source of most of its names) and used the yellow juice as a dye. They also used the herb medicinally as an eyewash (hence the names eye balm and eye root), as a treatment for skin wounds, sore throat, and digestive complaints, and as an aid to recovery from childbirth. The Cherokees mixed the herb with bear grease to make an insect repellent.

American colonists adopted the plant but didn't do much with it until the early 19th century, when Samuel Thomson, founder of Thomsonian herbal medicine, popularized it as an antiseptic. Thomson disliked the herb's Indian name, yellow root. So he changed it to goldenseal, combining *golden* from its color and *seal* from the circular scars left on the plant by each year's stems. Thomson thought the scars resembled the circular wax seals that were used to keep correspondence private in the days before glued envelopes.

Infections. The berberine in goldenseal kills many of the bacteria that cause diarrhea (*Escherichia coli*, salmonella, shigella, klebsiella, and even *Vibrio cholerae*, which causes cholera). In one study, 165 adults with diarrhea resulting from either *E. coli* or cholera were given either medically inactive placebos or 400-milligram oral doses of berberine. After 24 hours, among those with *E. coli* diarrhea, 43 percent of the berberine group were cured, compared with just 20 percent of the placebo group. Among those with cholera, berberine also produced significant benefit. These results support goldenseal's long history as a treatment for infectious diarrhea.

Goldenseal has also shown benefit against the protozoa that cause amoebic dysentery (*Entamoeba histolytica*) and giardiasis (*Giardia lamblia*). In addition, it kills the protozoan that causes trichomoniasis (*Trichomonas vaginalis*) and the fungus that causes yeast infections (*Candida albicans*). This lends credence to goldenseal's traditional topical application as a treatment for fungal infections.

In recent years, goldenseal has come to be viewed as a treatment for all manner of infectious diseases. Many people take it to treat colds and flu, in part because it is often paired with echinacea in commercial tinctures.

There is no evidence that goldenseal is effective against the viruses that cause colds and flu. In traditional herbal folklore, goldenseal was used almost exclusively as an oral treatment for digestive tract infections or topically for bacterial and fungal infections. Modern research validates these benefits, but goldenseal should not be expected to shorten the duration of colds or flu.

Enhanced immunity. In addition to killing germs, some research shows that berberine boosts the immune system by revving up macrophages, the white blood cells that devour disease-causing microorganisms.

Women's health concerns. In some animal studies, berberine calms the uterus, supporting its traditional use in stopping excessive menstrual flow and postpartum hemorrhage. Other studies, however, show that it stimulates uterine contractions. For this reason, women who are pregnant or trying to conceive should not take goldenseal. Women troubled by heavy menstrual flow might try the herb to see if it helps.

Postpartum hemorrhage is a potentially serious condition that requires prompt professional attention. If you'd like to try goldenseal in addition to standard therapy, discuss it with your obstetrician or midwife.

Digestive problems. Goldenseal stimulates bile secretion in humans, which means that it helps digest fats.

Intriguing Possibilities

Some naturopaths claim that goldenseal helps restore digestive and liver function in people with alcoholism.

Several cell culture studies have shown that the herb helps kill tumor cells, lending support to its traditional role as a cancer treatment. In the future, it may serve as a complement to cancer chemotherapy.

Rx Recommendations

To take advantage of goldenseal's possible antibiotic or immune-stimulating properties or to help ease heavy menstrual flow, prepare the herb as an infusion or tincture.

For an infusion, use ½ to 1 teaspoon of powdered root per cup of boiling water, steep for 10 minutes, and strain if you wish. Drink up to 2 cups a day. Goldenseal tastes bitter; you may add honey, sugar, or lemon or mix it with a beverage tea to improve its flavor.

As a homemade tincture, take ½ to 1 teaspoon up to twice a day.

When using a commercial preparation, follow the package directions.

Do not give goldenseal to children under age 2. For older children and adults over age 65, start with low-strength preparations and increase the strength if necessary.

The Safety Factor

The active chemicals in goldenseal have opposite effects on blood pressure: Berberine may lower it, but hydrastine may raise it. People with high blood pressure, heart disease, diabetes, glaucoma, kidney disease, or history of stroke should exercise caution and not take goldenseal. If you have a home blood pressure monitor, though, you might try goldenseal to see how it affects you. If it doesn't raise your blood pressure, feel free to use it in recommended amounts in consultation with your physician.

Because of goldenseal's high cost and scarcity, adulteration has been a problem for more than 100 years. One traditional adulterant is bloodroot (*Sanguinaria canadensis*). When fresh, bloodroot is red, but when dried, it turns yellow like goldenseal and tastes equally bitter.

Bloodroot has a powerful laxative action. In high doses, it also causes dizziness, gastrointestinal burning, intense thirst, and vomiting. If your "goldenseal" causes purging or any of these other symptoms, stop using it. It's probably bloodroot.

Large doses of goldenseal may irritate the skin, mouth, and throat and cause nausea and vomiting. Goldenseal douches may cause vaginal irritation.

The medical literature contains no reports of serious harm resulting from goldenseal, but hydrastine stimulates the central nervous system, and in animals, unusually large doses have caused death from respiratory paralysis and cardiac arrest. Do not use more than recommended amounts.

Wise-Use Guidelines

The FDA lists goldenseal as an herb of undefined safety. For adults who are not pregnant or nursing and do not have high blood pressure, glaucoma, diabetes, kidney disease, or a history of heart disease or stroke, goldenseal may be used safely in the amounts typically recommended.

You should take medicinal amounts of goldenseal only in consultation with your doctor. If it causes minor discomfort, such as stomach upset or mouth irritation, reduce the dosage or stop using it altogether. Let your doctor know if you experience unpleasant effects or if the symptoms for which you're using the herb do not improve significantly within 2 weeks.

Growing Information

A 1997 report in the *Endangered Species Bulletin* described wild goldenseal as critically imperiled. Today, the herb is farmed but still costly, and adulteration continues to be a problem.

Goldenseal is a small, erect perennial with a hairy, purplish, annual stem that rises from a short, knotty rhizome with yellow-brown bark and bright yellow pulp. The herb has lobed leaves somewhat similar to raspberry leaves and small, greenish white flowers that bloom in spring and produce orange-red berries. It grows wild from Vermont to Arkansas, if you're fortunate enough to find it.

Goldenseal is difficult to raise in a garden. Plants may be started from seeds, but it takes 5 years for the roots to become medicinally mature. Most authorities recommend buying 2-year-old rhizomes from specialty nurseries so you can harvest the roots 3 years later.

Viable rhizomes should have a sweet, licorice-like aroma. Plant them in early fall at a depth of 1 inch with 8-inch spacing. The soil should be amended with compost, leaf mold, sand, and bone meal. Frequently, top-growth will not appear until the second summer.

Goldenseal requires moisture with good drainage and about 70 percent shade. It grows best under tree cover or shade frames.

Harvest the rhizome and roots in late fall, after frost has killed the topgrowth. Clean the roots and dry them until they become brittle, then powder them and store the powder in air-tight containers.

Gotu Kola

Family: Umbelliferae; other members include carrot, parsley, celery, fennel, dill, and angelica

Genus and species: *Centella asiatica* or *Hydrocotyle asiatica*

Also known as: Sheep rot, Indian pennywort, marsh penny, water pennywort, and hydrocotyle

Parts used: Leaves

Long ago, the native Sinhalese of Ceylon (now Sri Lanka) noticed that elephants, renowned for their longevity, loved the rounded leaves of the diminutive gotu kola. The herb gained a reputation as a longevity promoter, and a Sinhalese proverb advised, "Two leaves a day keep old age away."

While you can't expect gotu kola to add years to your life, it may stimulate your immune system, accelerate wound healing, relieve psoriasis, and improve circulation in the legs, which may help prevent varicose veins.

Healing History

India's Ayurvedic herbalists first used gotu kola in the same way as ginseng to promote longevity and mental acuity and to treat problems associated with aging. Over time, however, the herb became popular as an internal and external treatment for skin diseases, including leprosy.

Philippine healers prescribed gotu kola to treat wounds and gonorrhea. Chinese physicians recommended it for fever and colds.

Gotu kola got a bum rap in Europe, where several species grow. Europeans believed that the herb caused foot rot in sheep (hence its once-popular name, sheep rot). There's no evidence to support this claim.

Close relatives of gotu kola also grow in the United States. America's 19th-century Eclectic physicians, forerunners of today's naturopaths, were well-aware of the herb's use as a treatment for leprosy in Asia. According to one report, "In 1852, Dr. Boileau of India, having been for many years afflicted with leprosy . . . experimented with [it] and recovered."

The Eclectics considered gotu kola safe and effective when used externally to treat skin problems. They deemed the herb a poison when taken internally, however, asserting that large doses produce "headache, dizziness, stupor, itching, and bloody passages from bowels."

Gotu kola wasn't very prominent during the early 20th century, but after World War II, it surfaced in an herbal tea blend called Fo-Ti-Tieng, which was touted to boost longevity—a claim that revived the ancient Sinhalese belief. The legend was that one Li Ching Yun, an ancient Chinese herbalist, had taken the blend regularly and lived for 256 years, surviving 23 wives. The tea caught on, and gotu kola re-emerged from obscurity as an herbal tonic.

Contemporary herbalists recommend gotu kola externally as a poultice for wounds. For internal use, they prescribe small doses as a tonic stimulant and large doses as a sedative.

Therapeutic Uses

Any longevity claims for gotu kola are as far-fetched as the tale of Li Ching Yun. But modern science has found support for other traditional therapeutic powers of this ancient herb.

Wounds. One compound in gotu kola, asiaticoside, supports wound healing. Another, madecassoside, is an anti-inflammatory. According to a study published in *Annals of Plastic Surgery*, gotu kola accelerates the healing of burns and minimizes scarring. Other studies have shown that the herb accelerates the healing of skin grafts and surgical enlargement of the vagina during childbirth (episiotomy).

Psoriasis. Validating gotu kola's traditional role as a treatment for skin diseases, one small study found that a cream made with the herb can help relieve the painful, scaly red welts of psoriasis. For the study, seven people with psoriasis were instructed to apply the cream. In five of the participants, the welts healed within 2 months. Only one of the five experienced any recurrence within 4 months after the treatment ended.

Gotu kola cream is not available commercially. You can use a compress of gotu kola infusion to help treat psoriasis.

Varicose veins. Gotu kola may help promote blood circulation in the lower limbs. In one study, 94 people with swelling, heaviness, and pain from poor circulation in the legs (venous insufficiency) were given either 60 milligrams of gotu kola or medically inactive placebos. After 2 months, those taking the herb showed significantly improved circulation and less swelling. The researchers concluded that the herb strengthened veins. Weak veins, along with poor circulation through the legs, contributes to varicose veins.

High blood pressure. In one study, researchers gave either placebos or gotu kola extract to 89 people with high blood pressure. Those taking the herb experienced a significant drop in their blood pressures.

Leprosy. Gotu kola's traditional use in treating leprosy (now called Hansen's disease) was supported by a study published in the British journal *Nature*. The bacteria that cause leprosy have a waxy coating that protects them against attack by the immune system. The asiaticoside in gotu kola dissolves the waxy coating, allowing the immune system to destroy the bacteria.

Intriguing Possibilities

There may be something to the ancient Ayurvedic belief that gotu kola improves memory. One Indian study found that treatment with the herb improves the intellectual performance of mentally challenged children.

A cell-culture study, also by Indian researchers, concluded that gotu kola extract destroys cancer cells without toxic effects on other cells. While the results of laboratory studies don't always apply to humans, at some time in the future, gotu kola may be included in cancer treatment regimens.

Rx Recommendations

Use an infusion of gotu kola to improve circulation in your legs. To prepare it, steep ½ teaspoon of herb in a cup of boiling water for 10 to 20 minutes, then strain. Drink up to 2 cups a day. Gotu kola tastes bitter and astringent; adding sugar or honey and lemon or mixing it into an herbal beverage blend will improve its flavor.

To help treat wounds or psoriasis topically, apply compresses made from a gotu kola infusion. If the results are disappointing, try a stronger infusion.

When using commercial preparations, follow the package directions.

Anyone may use gotu kola externally, but do not give it internally to children under age 2. For older children and adults over age 65, start with low-strength preparations and increase the strength if necessary.

The Safety Factor

The only confirmed side effect of gotu kola is skin rash in people who are sensitive to it.

In laboratory animals, gotu kola acts as a sedative. Large doses are narcotic, causing stupor and possibly coma. Sedation has never been reported in humans, but some scientists claim that it's possible. They echo the Eclectics, who advised against ingesting the herb.

Ironically, reports have appeared claiming that gotu kola causes restlessness and insomnia, which is rather odd for a purported "narcotic." Apparently, these cases involved the caffeine-containing herb kola, which was mislabeled as gotu kola.

Wise-Use Guidelines

The FDA considers gotu kola an herb of undefined safety. For adults who are not pregnant or nursing and are not taking tranquilizers or sedatives, gotu kola is considered safe when used in the amounts typically recommended.

You should use medicinal amounts of gotu kola only in consultation with your doctor. If it causes minor discomfort, such as a rash or headache, reduce the dosage or stop using it altogether. Let your doctor know if you experience unpleasant effects or if the symptoms for which you're using the herb do not improve significantly within 2 weeks.

Growing Information

Gotu kola is not related to true kola (*Cola nitida*), the caffeine-containing nut used in cola drinks. Nor is it cultivated in North America, although several related species grow wild.

As a member of the Umbelliferae family, gotu kola is related to carrot, parsley, dill, and fennel, but it has neither the characteristic feathery leaves nor the umbrella arrangement (umbel) of tiny flowers. Instead, gotu kola's creeping stem grows in marshy areas and produces fan-shaped leaves about the size of an old British penny—hence its names Indian pennywort, marsh penny, and water pennywort. A cuplike clutch of inconspicuous flowers develops near the ground. Leaves are harvested throughout the year.

Hawthorn

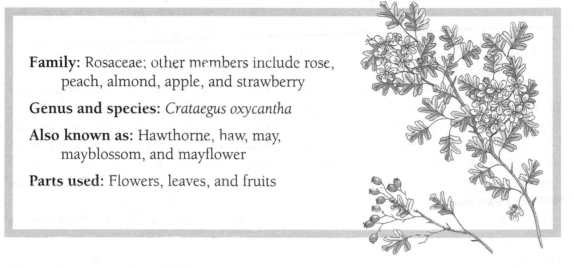

Family: Rosaceae; other members include rose, peach, almond, apple, and strawberry

Genus and species: *Crataegus oxycantha*

Also known as: Hawthorne, haw, may, mayblossom, and mayflower

Parts used: Flowers, leaves, and fruits

Every American schoolchild learns that the Pilgrims' ship was called the *Mayflower*. Few if any Americans, however, know that the name refers to hawthorn, which, in England, flowers in May. Even fewer know that the herb is very beneficial to the heart.

Today, hawthorn is widely used in Europe as a treatment for heart disease, especially congestive heart failure, which involves fatigue of the heart muscle, fluid buildup around the body, and shortness of breath after mild exertion. Now hawthorn is starting to catch on in this country as well.

Healing History

Archeologists have discovered the seeds of hawthorn fruits at Neolithic sites, suggesting that the fruits were used for food.

To the ancient Greeks and Romans, haw-thorn was rich in symbolism, linked to hope, marriage, and fertility. Greek bridesmaids wore fragrant hawthorn blossoms, and brides carried a hawthorn bough. The Romans placed hawthorn leaves in babies' cradles to ward off evil spirits.

The arrival of Christianity changed haw-thorn's image dramatically. Christ's crown of thorns was reputedly made of hawthorn, and as a result, the herb became a symbol of bad luck and death.

The hawthorn-death association was bolstered by the unpleasant aroma of the flowers of some European species. These trees are pollinated by carrion-eating insects, and to attract them, their flowers emit the odor of rotting meat. A similar odor was associated with bubonic plague. (Because the disease killed so many so quickly, bodies often remained unburied for quite a while.) As a result, hawthorn came to be associated with plague, and it was shunned.

As time passed, hawthorn shed its bad reputation and was embraced as a medicinal herb. Seventeenth-century English herbalist Nicholas Culpeper praised it as "a singular remedy for the stone [kidney stones], and no less effectual for dropsy [congestive heart failure]."

Despite the influential Culpeper's endorsement, hawthorn was not widely recommended to treat heart problems until the very end of the 19th century, when it was popularized by an Irish doctor who used it to treat congestive heart failure. In 1896, an article touting the Irish physician's work appeared in a medical journal for Eclectic physicians, forerunners of today's naturopaths. The Eclectics began prescribing hawthorn for congestive heart failure and the chest pain of angina.

Modern herbals echo these recommendations. Most would agree with David Hoffmann's *Holistic Herbal*: "Hawthorn [is] one of the best tonic remedies for the heart. . . . It may be used safely in long-term treatment for heart weakness or failure . . . palpitations . . . angina pectoris . . . and high blood pressure."

Therapeutic Uses

A great deal of research supports the traditional role of hawthorn as a heart stimulant.

Heart disease. Hawthorn supports the heart in several ways. It opens (dilates) the coronary arteries, improving the blood supply to the heart muscle. This strengthens the heart and helps it to beat more forcefully and efficiently. As a result, the herb boosts the heart's blood-pumping force, which is vital in congestive heart failure.

In addition, hawthorn dilates blood vessels elsewhere around the body, which allows blood to circulate more freely with less strain on the heart. The herb helps counteract some types of heart rhythm disturbances (arrhythmias), and it reduces cholesterol and blood pressure, both important risk factors for heart disease.

Many studies provide important evidence of hawthorn's benefits in treating heart disease, particularly congestive heart failure. Here's a sampling of the research to date.

• German researchers gave heart function tests to 3,664 people with congestive heart failure. Then all of the study participants were instructed to take hawthorn (one 300-milligram tablet, standardized to contain 2.2 percent flavonoids, three times a day). After 2 months, the participants were tested again. Their heart function improved significantly, about as much as would be expected from standard pharmaceuticals. In addition, the proportion of participants experiencing heart palpitations dropped from 40 percent to 18 percent. Leg swelling declined 37 percent. And work capacity, measured as the ability to expend effort by riding a stationary cycle, increased 15 percent.

• In another study, German researchers gave 136 people with congestive heart failure either medically inactive placebos or 80 milligrams of hawthorn twice a day. After 8 weeks, those taking the placebos had gotten worse, while those taking hawthorn had improved significantly.

• A third German trial involved 78 people with congestive heart failure. They took work-capacity tests on a stationary cycle, then began taking either placebos or 600 milligrams of hawthorn a day. After 2 months, the work capacity of those in the placebo group improved slightly. Among those in the hawthorn group, work capacity increased almost six times as much.

Hawthorn caused no significant side effects in any of these studies.

Commission E, the expert panel that evaluates herbal medicines for the German counterpart of the FDA, approves hawthorn as a treatment for congestive heart failure. German doctors are permitted to prescribe any of several hawthorn-based heart medicines. According to noted German medical herbalist Rudolph Fritz Weiss, M.D., the herb "has become one of [our] most widely used heart remedies." German physicians rely on hawthorn to normalize heart rhythm, reduce the likelihood and severity of angina attacks, and prevent cardiac complications in elderly patients with influenza and pneumonia.

Dr. Weiss cautions, however, that hawthorn is no quick fix. "One cannot expect rapid improvement in cardiac function," he states. "[Hawthorn] has a long term, sustained effect. . . . Hawthorn is not for cutting short angina attacks—nitroglycerin continues to be the drug of choice here."

Although hawthorn is considered safe and may be effective in the treatment of congestive heart failure, angina, and cardiac arrhythmias, these are serious, potentially life-threatening conditions that require professional medical care. Consult your physician if you'd like to use hawthorn as part of your overall treatment plan.

Rx Recommendations

If you use a homemade tincture, German physicians recommend taking 1 teaspoon upon waking and at bedtime for periods of up to several weeks. To mask its bitter taste, you can sweeten it with sugar, honey, or lemon, or mix it with an herbal beverage blend.

To prepare an infusion, herbalists recommend using 2 teaspoons of crushed leaves or fruits per cup of boiling water. Steep for 20 minutes. Drink up to 2 cups a day.

When using commercial preparations, follow the package directions.

The Safety Factor

Large amounts of hawthorn may cause sedation and/or a significant drop in blood pressure, possibly resulting in faintness.

The FDA lists hawthorn as an herb of undefined safety. This heart stimulant should be used only by people who have been diagnosed with congestive heart failure, angina, or cardiac arrhythmias, and then only in consultation with a physician. Children and pregnant or nursing women should not take hawthorn.

Growing Information

Hawthorn is a small deciduous tree with white bark, extremely hard wood, sharp thorns, clusters of white, aromatic flowers, and brilliant red fruits that look like small apples. It blooms from April to June, depending on latitude. In England, blossoms appear in May; hence the herb's other names, may, mayblossom, and mayflower.

With approximately 900 North American species, hawthorn is well-adapted to many environments, from urban areas to windswept hillsides. The tree tolerates a variety of soils but prefers somewhat alkaline, rich, moist loam. Some species prefer full sun, while others grow well in partial shade. Consult a nursery for the species best suited to your area.

Hop

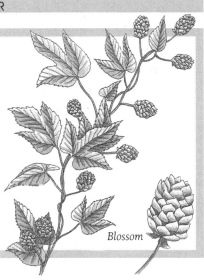

Family: Cannabaceae; other members include hemp and marijuana

Genus and species: *Humulus lupulus*

Also known as: Humulus

Parts used: Strobiles (glandular hairs of female fruits)

Blossom

Hop is best known as the bitter, aromatic ingredient in beer. It also has a long history in herbal healing, and some of its traditional uses have been supported by modern science.

Healing History

Chinese physicians have prescribed hop for centuries as a digestive aid and a treatment for leprosy, tuberculosis, and dysentery.

Ancient Greek and Roman physicians also recommended the herb as a digestive aid and as a treatment for intestinal ailments. The Roman naturalist Pliny touted hop as a garden vegetable, the young shoots of which could be eaten in spring before they matured and grew tough and bitter. (People still eat the shoots, prepared like asparagus.)

Hop was a minor herb until about 1,000 years ago. That's when brewers began using it to preserve the fermented barley beverage that we know as beer.

Actually, beer was an accidental offshoot of bread baking. As agriculture developed, late-prehistoric homemakers noticed that bread made from raw grain did not keep as well as bread made from sprouted grain. So before pounding their grain into flour, they soaked it in water to sprout it. If the water happened to become contaminated with yeast microorganisms from the skins of fruit, it fermented into a crude, sweet beer.

Ancient beers, probably undrinkable by modern standards, were nonetheless amazingly popular. Around 2500 B.C., an estimated 40 percent of the Sumerian grain crop was used in brewing. And the world's first written legal code—Babylonia's Code of Hammurabi, developed in 1750 B.C.—described punishments for ale houses that sold beer that was under strength or overpriced.

As the centuries passed, brewers used herbs such as marjoram, yarrow, and wormwood to flavor their beers. Around the 9th century, the Germans began adding hop, both for its pleasantly bitter flavor and because it preserved the brew. By the 14th century, most European beers contained hop.

A Battle Brews in England

Hop was well-known in England. The vine grew wild there, and in folk medicine, hop was a popular appetite-stimulating digestive bitter.

England's fermented beverage of choice was ale, a sweet beer that contained some other herbs, but not hop. Around 1500, British brewers began making European style bitter beer with hop. This move was a boon to brewers and innkeepers because hop's preservative action extended the shelf life of beer, but the addition of hop to English beer also provoked national outrage.

Legions of hop haters petitioned Parliament to ban the herb from beer. Henry VIII, an ale traditionalist, supported banning hop as "a wicked weed that would endanger the people." Hop remained illegal in English beer until Henry's son, Edward VI, rescinded the ban in 1552.

But the furor refused to die. A century later, English writer John Evelyn declared, "Hop transmuted our wholesome ale into beer. This one ingredient preserves the drink indeed, but repays the pleasure in tormenting diseases and a shorter life."

Beer brewing transformed hop from a spring vegetable into a cash crop, but hop farmers noticed that the herb had two odd effects on those who harvested it. They fatigued easily, and the women got their periods early. Over time, the herb gained a reputation as a sedative and menstruation promoter.

Hop has been used ever since as a sedative, not only in tea but also in pillows. The herb's warm fragrance is supposed to induce sleep.

Seventeenth-century English herbalist Nicholas Culpeper recommended hop "in opening obstructions of the liver and spleen . . . cleansing the blood . . . helping cure the French disease [syphilis], and bringing down women's courses [menstruation]." Culpeper also added his 2 pence to the lingering beer-ale controversy, writing that hop's medicinal uses made "beer . . . better than ale."

More Than a Sedative

Meanwhile, in North America, Native Americans were using the American version of hop as a sedative and digestive aid. America's 19th-century Eclectics, forerunners of today's naturopaths, deemed hop a digestive aid and a treatment for the "morbid excitement of delerium tremens." They were unimpressed with its reputation as a sedative, however, warning that it "often failed."

Still, hop was listed as a sedative in the *U.S. Pharmacopoeia*, a standard drug reference, from 1831 to 1916. Throughout the 19th century, it was a popular ingredient in many patent medicines, including Hop Bitters, a popular herb tonic with a 30 percent alcohol base. Its advertising slogan typified patent-medicine claims in the era before the FDA: "Take Hop Bitters three times a day, and you will have no doctor bills to pay."

During the 1950s, jazz musicians who smoked marijuana were called hopheads, and marijuana was said to make its users "hopped up." Hop is botanically related to marijuana, but smoking the herb does not produce intoxication.

Contemporary herbalists recommend hop primarily as a sedative, tranquilizer, and digestive aid.

Therapeutic Uses

Those old brewers knew what they were doing when they added hop to beer as a preservative. It contains two chemicals, humulone and lupulone, that kill the bacteria that cause food—and beer—to spoil.

Infections. The bacteria fighters in hop may help prevent infection in humans. Hop is not a major herbal antibiotic, but it's effective first-aid in the garden.

One laboratory study has shown hop to be effective against the bacteria that cause tuberculosis, lending some credence to one of the herb's traditional Chinese uses.

Insomnia and anxiety. For decades, scientists scoffed at hop's longstanding reputation as a sedative. Then, in 1983, they discovered a sedative chemical (2-methyl-3-butene-2-ol) in the plant. This chemical is present in only trace amounts in the fresh leaves, but its concentration increases as the herb dries and ages. If you want to try hop as a sedative, stick with the dried, aged herb.

Commission E, the expert panel that evaluates herbal medicines for the German counter-

part of the FDA, approves hop for treatment of anxiety and sleep disturbances.

Digestive problems. Hop appears to relax the smooth muscle lining the digestive tract, according to French researchers. This finding supports the herb's traditional role as an antispasmodic digestive herb.

Women's health concerns. German researchers have concluded that hop contains chemicals similar to the female sex hormone estrogen, which may help to explain some of the menstrual changes reported in women who picked hop. Other studies dispute this finding. Currently, the issue remains unresolved.

Rx Recommendations

To help protect against infection and avoid digestive upset, use the freshest hop you can find. For insomnia, use hop that has been dried and aged.

To make an infusion, use 2 teaspoons of herb per cup of boiling water and steep for 5 minutes. Drink up to 3 cups a day. Hop tastes warm and pleasantly bitter.

When using commercial preparations, follow the package directions.

To treat minor garden accidents, press some crushed flowers into cuts and scrapes until you can wash and bandage them.

Do not give hop to children under age 2. For older children and adults over age 65, start with low-strength preparations and increase the strength if necessary.

The Safety Factor

Some hop pickers develop a rash called hop dermatitis. Otherwise, there are no reports of harm from using the herb.

In case the Germans are right about hop containing chemicals similar to estrogen, women who are pregnant or who have estrogen-dependent breast cancer should not use it.

Wise-Use Guidelines

The FDA includes hop on its list of herbs generally regarded as safe. For adults who are not pregnant or nursing and are not taking other sedatives, hop is safe when used in the amounts typically recommended.

You should use medicinal amounts of hop only in consultation with your doctor. If it causes minor discomfort, such as stomach upset or diarrhea, reduce the dosage or stop using it altogether. Let your doctor know if you experience unpleasant symptoms or if the symptoms for which you're using the herb do not improve significantly within 2 weeks.

Growing Information

Hop is a resinous, hairy, climbing perennial vine that resembles grape. Grown commercially in Bavaria, Germany, and in the Pacific Northwest in pole-studded fields called hop yards, mature vines often reach 25 feet.

Hop can be raised from seeds, but most growers use root cuttings taken in spring or fall. Plant the cuttings in hills, three roots per hill, with hills 18 inches apart.

Hop needs deeply cultivated, rich, moist soil; full sun; and frequent watering.

Harvest the female flowers in fall when they feel firm, turn amber-colored, and are covered with yellow dust. Dry them immediately in an oven no hotter than 150°F.

Horehound

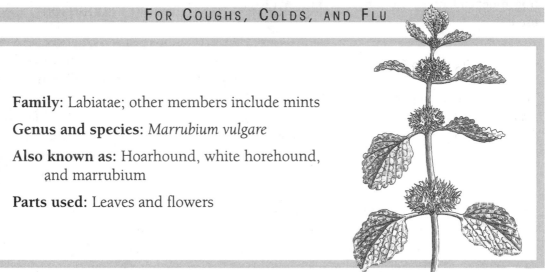

Family: Labiatae; other members include mints

Genus and species: *Marrubium vulgare*

Also known as: Hoarhound, white horehound, and marrubium

Parts used: Leaves and flowers

Horehound was a popular herbal expectorant and cough remedy for almost 2,000 years. Even skeptics of herbal medicine acknowledged its safety and effectiveness.

Then, in 1989, completely out of the blue, the FDA banned horehound from over-the-counter cough remedies, claiming that it was ineffective. The action left herbalists shaking their heads. Worse yet, the FDA decreed that another expectorant was "effective," over the objections of many scientists.

Healing History

Horehound was first used medicinally in ancient Rome as an ingredient in the multi-ingredient (and ineffective) poison antidotes known as theriaca. Medieval Europeans generalized this application and came up with the belief that the herb provided protection from witches' spells.

The Roman physician Galen was the first to recommend horehound for coughs and respiratory problems. It's been used as an expectorant ever since. The ancients also relied on it to calm upset stomachs.

The medieval German abbess/herbalist Hildegard of Bingen considered horehound one of the best herbs for colds. And England's John Gerard wrote, "Syrup made of the greene fresh leaves and sugar is a most singular remedie against cough and wheezings of the lungs."

Seventeenth-century English herbalist Nicholas Culpeper wrote that in addition to curing "those that have taken poison . . . a decoction of the dried herb taken with honey is a remedy for those that are short-winded, have a cough, or are fallen into consumption. . . . It helpeth to expectorate tough phlegm from the chest."

Early settlers introduced horehound into North America, where it became a popular cough, cold, and tuberculosis remedy. Folk herbalists also considered it to be a digestive aid, laxative, and treatment for hepatitis, malaria, intestinal worms, and menstrual problems.

America's 19th-century Eclectic physicians, forerunners of today's naturopaths, prescribed horehound for coughs, colds, asthma, intestinal worms, and menstrual complaints.

Most contemporary American herbalists recommend horehound only for minor respiratory problems such as coughs, colds, and bronchitis. In Europe, it is also used as a digestive aid.

Therapeutic Uses

The FDA order to remove horehound from cough and cold remedies may say more about the watchdog agency's shortcomings than it does about the herb's.

Coughs. Horehound contains a compound called marrubiin that Russian and German studies have found to have phlegm-loosening (expectorant) properties. In Europe, the herb has been used for decades in a large number of cough syrups and lozenges. It has been widely used in the United States as well. Even herb conservative Varro Tyler, Ph.D., coauthor of *Tyler's Honest Herbal*, describes horehound as an effective expectorant.

The FDA's horehound ban followed the recommendation of an agency advisory panel, which decreed that only one expectorant, guaifenesin, is safe and effective. Ironically, many lung experts question guaifenesin's effectiveness.

The FDA order applies only to horehound preparations marketed as cough remedies. The herb is still available in bulk and in some sore throat products.

Digestive problems. Commission E, the ex-

pert panel that evaluates herbal medicines for the German counterpart of the FDA, approves horehound for the treatment of indigestion, bloating, and flatulence.

Intriguing Possibilities

Animal studies performed in Europe show that horehound opens (dilates) blood vessels, a finding that hints at the herb's possible value in treating high blood pressure.

Other animal studies show that in small amounts, horehound helps normalize irregular heart rhythm (arrhythmia), but in large amounts, the herb can cause them.

Rx Recommendations

For an infusion to treat cough or upset stomach, use ½ to 1 teaspoon of dried leaves per cup of boiling water. Steep for 10 minutes, then strain. Drink up to 3 cups a day. To offset horehound's bitter taste, sweeten it with sugar or honey.

As a homemade tincture, take ¼ to ½ teaspoon up to three times a day.

When using commercial preparations, follow the package directions.

Do not give horehound to children under age 2. For older children and adults over age 65, start with low-strength preparations and increase the strength if necessary.

The Safety Factor

There have been no reports of adverse reactions to horehound in humans. In light of the animal studies showing that large doses of the herb may cause cardiac arrhythmias, however, people with this condition should avoid it.

Horehound's traditional use as a menstruation promoter has not been confirmed scientifically. Still, pregnant women should exercise caution and not take it.

Wise-Use Guidelines

For adults who are not pregnant or nursing and do not have arrhythmias, horehound is considered relatively safe in the amounts typically recommended.

You should use medicinal amounts of horehound only in consultation with your doctor. If it causes minor discomfort, such as stomach upset or diarrhea, reduce the dosage or stop using it altogether. Let your doctor know if you experience unpleasant symptoms or if a cough does not improve significantly within 2 weeks. If a cough brings up brown, black, or bloody phlegm, consult a physician immediately.

Growing Information

Horehound is a spreading, pleasantly aromatic perennial with square annual stems that reach about 18 inches. The leaves are rounded, wrinkled, and deeply veined, and tiny white flowers develop at the stem-leaf stalk junctions. The entire plant is covered with soft hairs, giving it a woolly appearance and a grayish white cast.

A self-seeder, horehound grows so easily that it may become a pest. It needs little water and tolerates poor soil. It thrives in full sun but tolerates partial shade.

Plant seeds just under the soil surface in either spring or fall. Thin seedlings to 9-inch spacing. Horehound does not bloom until its second year, but you can harvest the leaves and topgrowth after one growing season.

In the soil, the herb exudes a musky odor that some people dislike. As the plant dries, the odor disappears.

Horse Chestnut

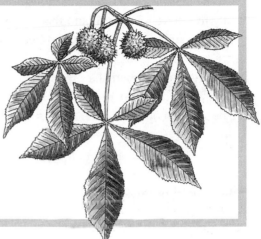

Family: Hippocastanaceae; other members include Ohio buckeye

Genus and species: *Aesculus hippocastanum*

Also known as: Chestnut and buckeye

Parts used: Seeds

Horse chestnut owes its name to the fact that the ancients thought the large seeds resembled a horse's eyes. The seeds also resembled the eyes of stags, hence buckeye, one of the herb's common names.

Healing History

Horse chestnut has had a variety of purposes since ancient times. The wood was popular in furniture-making and construction. Bark extracts produce a yellow dye that was used in weaving. Seed preparations were applied topically to treat joint aches and pains.

In 1615, a French traveler returned from a trip to Constantinople (now Istanbul) with some horse chestnut seeds. He planted them in Paris, and within 100 years, the tree had spread throughout Europe.

All parts of the horse chestnut plant are poisonous when ingested—especially the seeds, which are the parts used in modern herbal medicine. Native Americans detoxified the seeds in several ways, including burying them in the ground for many months so the soil would absorb the poisonous compounds. Then they unearthed the detoxified seeds, boiled them, and ate them as food. Some tribes combined crushed seeds with bear fat and applied the mixture to treat hemorrhoids, one type of varicose vein condition.

Native Americans in California used the fresh seeds as a poison. They crushed them and scattered them in lakes and streams to stupefy fish, making them easier to catch.

In 1896, a French researcher reported that horse chestnut seed extract helped relieve hemorrhoids. America's 19th-century Eclectic physicians, forerunners of today's naturopaths, incorporated the herb into their treatment of hemorrhoids. The Eclectic textbook *King's American Dispensatory* (1898) noted that horse chestnut helps treat "vascular fullness and capillary engorgement"—not only of hemorrhoids but of other veins as well.

The Eclectics also used horse chestnut topically to relieve joint pain, and they detoxified the seed extract for internal use to treat fevers, including malaria.

Contemporary herbalists recommend horse chestnut seed almost exclusively for varicose veins and hemorrhoids.

Therapeutic Uses

Horse chestnut seed contains aescin, a compound that helps strengthen the walls of veins and increases their elasticity. This promotes normal blood flow and helps prevent the pooling of blood that contributes to varicose veins and hemorrhoids.

Varicose veins. In one German study, 22 people with leaky veins (venous insufficiency)—an early warning sign of varicose veins—were given either medically inactive placebos or doses of horse chestnut (600 milligrams of extract containing 50 milligrams of aescin). Three hours later, fluid leakage increased in those who had taken the placebos but decreased by 22 percent in those who had taken horse chestnut. This result indicates strengthening of the veins.

Another German research team gave 240 people with venous insufficiency one of three treatments: placebos, compression therapy (using support stockings, a standard mainstream medical treatment), or horse chestnut seed extract (50 milligrams of aescin twice a day). Over the course of 3 months, leg swelling increased slightly among those taking the placebos, but it decreased significantly (by about 25 percent) in both the people wearing support stockings and those taking horse chestnut. The researchers concluded that compression therapy and herbal therapy produced equivalent benefits.

Several other studies have shown that horse chestnut has benefits equivalent to those of support stockings. Commission E, the expert panel that evaluates herbal medicines for the German counterpart of the FDA, endorses horse chestnut extract as a treatment for varicose veins.

Hemorrhoids. While more recent studies have focused on horse chestnut's effectiveness in relieving varicose leg veins, the herb's vein-strengthening action was first described as a treatment for hemorrhoids. Horse chestnut seed extract should help heal varicosities in the anal area.

Arthritis. Horse chestnut seed has anti-inflammatory action, lending credence to its traditional use as a treatment for joint pain.

Rx Recommendations

In the studies demonstrating horse chestnut's benefits as a treatment for varicose veins, the usual dose has been 50 milligrams of aescin two or three times a day.

Aescin is not recommended for internal use by women who are pregnant. If you are pregnant and you develop varicose veins, try a topical cream made with horse chestnut seed extract.

The Safety Factor

The FDA classifies horse chestnut as unsafe. No wonder: All parts of the plant are poisonous unless they're detoxified. Poisoning from the fresh, unprocessed herb causes muscle weakness and spasms, loss of coordination, pupil dilation, vomiting, diarrhea, and paralysis. Adults have become quite ill from drinking tea made from fresh leaves and twigs. Children have died.

Never ingest any part of the horse chestnut plant. Commercial medicinal preparations are detoxified, so buy one and follow the label directions.

Wise-Use Guidelines

Adults who are not pregnant or nursing may use commercial preparations of horse chestnut internally in the amounts typically recommended. Pregnant women may use topical preparations to treat varicose veins.

You should use medicinal amounts of horse chestnut only in consultation with your doctor. If it causes minor discomfort, such as stomach upset or diarrhea, reduce the dosage or stop using it altogether. Let your doctor know if you experience unpleasant effects or if the symptoms for which you're using the herb do not improve significantly within 2 weeks.

Growing Information

Native to the Balkans and the Middle East, horse chestnut trees now grow worldwide. They are majestic, climbing as high as 75 feet and producing large leaves and attractive pink and white flowers in spring or summer, depending on latitude. The fruit has a thick, leathery husk that contains from one to six seeds, or nuts.

Horsetail

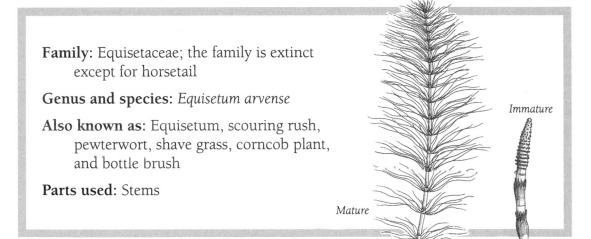

Family: Equisetaceae; the family is extinct except for horsetail

Genus and species: *Equisetum arvense*

Also known as: Equisetum, scouring rush, pewterwort, shave grass, corncob plant, and bottle brush

Parts used: Stems

Immature

Mature

All that's gold does not necessarily glitter. Take horsetail. The bamboolike marsh dweller is capable of absorbing gold dissolved in water. What makes this of interest to herbalists is that doctors often prescribe preparations containing gold for rheumatoid arthritis, and horsetail has a long history as an herbal remedy for joint pain.

Healing History

Centuries before anyone realized that horsetail contains gold, the ancients discovered its value as an abrasive cleanser. Over time, the herb was used to scour pots, polish pewter, and sand or "shave" wood—hence its popular names scouring rush, shave grass, and pewterwort (*wort* is Old English for "plant").

During ancient famines, Romans ate horse-tail shoots, which look like asparagus but are neither as tasty nor as nutritious. (Backpacking guides still recommend the tough, stringy shoots for wilderness foragers.) The Roman physician Galen claimed that horsetail healed severed tendons and ligaments and helped stop nosebleeds.

Ancient Chinese physicians recommended horsetail as a treatment for wounds, hemorrhoids, arthritis, and dysentery.

Seventeenth-century English herbalist Nicholas Culpeper called horsetail "very powerful to stop bleeding . . . [and] heal ulcers . . . the juice or decoction being drunk . . . or applied outwardly. . . . It solders together wounds and cures all ruptures."

Over the years, horsetail gained a reputation as a diuretic. America's 19th-century Eclectic physicians, forerunners of today's naturopaths, prescribed the herb for incontinence, gonorrhea, kidney stones, kidney infections, urinary complaints, and congestive heart failure, which causes fluid retention and swelling

Contemporary herbalists recommend horsetail externally for wounds and internally for urinary and prostate problems. Homeopaths prescribe microdoses of the herb for urinary problems: bladder infections, bed-wetting, incontinence, and urethritis.

Therapeutic Uses

Horsetail is not a major medicinal herb and has not been all that well researched. The available evidence suggests that it lives up to its traditional reputation, however.

Wounds. Commission E, the expert panel that evaluates herbal medicines for the German counterpart of the FDA, approves horsetail compresses as a wound treatment.

Urinary problems. Horsetail contains a weak diuretic chemical called equisetonin, which lends support to the herb's traditional use as a urinary stimulant. Commission E approves horsetail as a treatment for urinary tract infections and kidney stones.

Arthritis. Horsetail absorbs gold dissolved in water better than most plants, as much as 4 ounces per ton of fresh stalks. Of course, the amount of gold in a cup of horsetail tea is tiny, but only small amounts of the mineral are given as a treatment for rheumatoid arthritis. For this disease, the Chinese rely on horsetail. If you'd like to try the herb as part of an overall rheumatoid arthritis treatment plan, discuss it with your physician.

Medicinal Myth

Because horsetail contains nicotine, some herbalists recommend the herb as a nicotine substitute for smokers attempting to quit. But compared with cigarettes, horsetail's nicotine content is minute, only about 0.00004 percent. It's unlikely to satisfy a smoker's craving. Prescription nicotine gum (Nicorette) would be a better alternative.

Rx Recommendations

To treat a urinary tract condition, take either an infusion or a tincture. For wounds, try a topical application of either form.

To prepare an infusion, use 1 to 2 teaspoons of dried herb per cup of boiling water, steep for 10 minutes, and strain. Drink up to 2 cups a day. Horsetail has little taste.

As a homemade tincture, use ½ to 1 teaspoon up to twice a day.

When using commercial preparations, follow the package directions.

Do not give horsetail to children under age 2. For older children and adults over age 65, start with low-strength preparations and increase the strength if necessary.

The Safety Factor

Horsetail may cause rashes in people who are sensitive to it.

In addition to absorbing an unusually large amount of gold, horsetail also absorbs relatively large amounts of selenium. Selenium is an important nutrient, a potent antioxidant that has been shown to help prevent several types of cancer, but too much selenium may cause birth defects. In marshes downstream from heavily fertilized agricultural areas, horsetail may have hazardously high selenium levels. Pregnant women should not use the herb.

Horsetail contains a chemical called equisetine that in large amounts is a nerve poison. Animals that were fed the herb have experienced fever, weight loss, muscle weakness, and abnormal pulse rate. Some have even died. Children have reportedly suffered nonfatal reactions after using the hollow stems as toy blowguns and ingesting the juice. Don't let children play with the herb.

Wise-Use Guidelines

Because of the problems it has caused in animals, the FDA lists horsetail as an herb of undefined safety. For adults who are not pregnant or nursing and are not taking other diuretics, horsetail is considered safe when used cautiously for brief periods in the amounts typically recommended.

You should use medicinal amounts of horsetail only in consultation with your doctor. If it causes minor discomfort, such as stomach upset or diarrhea, reduce the dosage or stop using it altogether. Let your doctor know if you experience any unpleasant effects or if the symptoms for which you're taking the herb do not improve significantly within 2 weeks.

Growing Information

Horsetail is the sole surviving descendant of the giant fernlike plants that covered the Earth some 200 million years ago. The herb's creeping rhizome sends up hollow, jointed, virtually leafless, bamboolike stalks that reach 6 feet. At the ends of the stalks, spore-bearing structures (catkins) develop. These resemble horse tails, corncobs, or bottle brushes, hence some of the herb's names.

Horsetails may be purchased from specialty nurseries, or root cuttings may be taken from wild plants in the spring when the spearlike stems have reached a few inches in length. Set plants or cuttings just under the surface of marshy soil. Keep it wet. If you do not want the plant to spread, contain it by embedding sheet metal in the soil to a depth of 18 inches. Harvest the stalks in the fall. Make that sure children do not suck on the hollow stems.

Hyssop

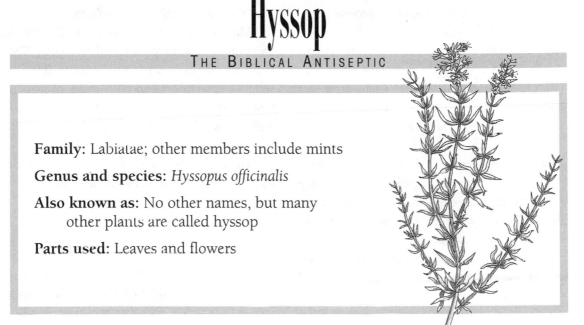

Family: Labiatae; other members include mints

Genus and species: *Hyssopus officinalis*

Also known as: No other names, but many other plants are called hyssop

Parts used: Leaves and flowers

The Book of Psalms (51:9) says, "Purge me with hyssop and I shall be clean." But the biblical herb does more than clean; it may work as an antiseptic for infections such as cold sores and genital herpes.

Healing History

Some 2,500 years ago, Jewish priests used strong-smelling hyssop to clean the temple in Jerusalem and other places of worship. Unfortunately, so many plants were called hyssop back then that we have no way of knowing if the cleanser and the medicinal herb (*Hyssopus officinalis*) were one and the same.

Despite the confusion, the Greeks adopted hyssop. The noted physician Dioscorides prescribed the herb as a tea for cough, wheezing, and shortness of breath; in plasters and chest rubs; and as an aromatic nasal and chest decongestant.

The medieval German abbess/herbalist Hildegard of Bingen wrote that hyssop "cleanses the lungs." She also recommended a meal of chicken cooked in hyssop and wine as a treatment for sadness (depression).

In 17th-century Europe, hyssop was a popular air freshener or "strewing herb." At a time when people rarely bathed and farm animals often shared human living quarters, crushed leaves and flowers were scattered around homes to mask odors. When bathing became popular and strewing ceased, hyssop was placed in scent baskets in sickrooms.

Seventeenth-century English herbalist Nicholas Culpeper echoed Dioscorides' endorsement of hyssop for chest ailments: "It expelleth tough phlegm and is effectual for all griefs of the chest and lungs." He also claimed, "It killeth worms in the belly. . . . Boiled with figs, it makes an excellent gargle for quinsey [tonsillitis] . . . Boiled in wine, it is good to wash inflammations . . . the head being anointed with the oil, it killeth lice."

Colonists introduced hyssop into North America and continued using the herb to treat chest congestion. It developed a reputation as a means of promoting menstruation and inducing abortions. (It won't do either.)

As time passed, hyssop's popularity waned. America's 19th-century Eclectic physicians, forerunners of today's naturopaths, prescribed the herb externally to relieve the pain of bruises and internally as a gargle for sore throat and tonsillitis and as a treatment for asthma and coughing.

Contemporary herbalists recommend hyssop compresses and poultices for bruises, burns, and wounds, and suggest infusions for colds, coughs, bronchitis, flatulence, indigestion, menstruation promotion, and even epileptic seizures. As proof of the herb's effectiveness for wounds and respiratory infections, some herbalists point to the fact that the microorganism that produces penicillin (*Penicillium*) grows on hyssop leaves.

Therapeutic Uses

Hyssop won't whiten your toilet bowl as modern cleansers do, but hyssop's main traditional uses have some scientific support.

Coughs. Hyssop is a member of the aromatic mint family, and its volatile oil contains several soothing camphorlike constituents, plus one expectorant chemical (called marrubiin) that loosens phlegm so it's easier to cough up. Scientific sources agree that hyssop is a "reasonably effective" treatment for the cough and respiratory irritation of colds and flu.

Herpes. Hyssop inhibits the growth of herpes simplex virus, which causes genital herpes and cold sores. Try the infusion in a compress if you have this chronic, recurring infection.

Varicose veins. Hyssop contains diosmin, a compound that helps strengthen veins. The herb can be up to 6 percent diosmin (by dry weight). It takes only about 5 grams of hyssop (approximately 2 teaspoons) to provide the 300 milligrams of disomin considered necessary to have vein-strengthening action.

Hemorrhoids. Hemorrhoids are a type of varicose vein and thus may benefit from treatment with hyssop.

Intriguing Possibility

A few laboratory studies have shown that hyssop extract exhibits potent activity against HIV, the virus that causes AIDS. It's too early to call hyssop an AIDS treatment, but the herb may be used in that capacity in the future.

Medicinal Myth

Penicillium does indeed grow on hyssop. But the assertion that hyssop heals because it carries this microorganism is nonsense.

Rx Recommendations

To make a compress for treating herpes, use 1 ounce of dried herb per pint of boiling water. Steep for 15 minutes and let cool. Soak a clean cloth in the infusion and apply it to cold sores and genital herpes sores as needed.

For an infusion to treat cough, varicose veins, or hemorrhoids, use 2 teaspoons of herb per cup of boiling water, steep for 10 minutes, and strain. Drink up to 3 cups a day. Hyssop has a strong, camphorlike smell and tastes bitter. Add sugar, honey, or lemon or mix it with an herbal beverage blend to improve the flavor.

As a homemade tincture, take 1 teaspoon up to three times a day.

When using commercial preparations, follow the package directions.

Do not give hyssop to children under age 2. For older children and adults over age 65, start with low-strength preparations and increase the strength if necessary.

The Safety Factor

Hyssop has not been shown to stimulate the uterus, but its traditional use to induce abortion should discourage pregnant women from taking it.

No reports of harm from hyssop appear in the world medical literature. Recently, however, laboratory animals injected with the herb's essential oil developed convulsions that caused some deaths. Do not exceed the recommended amounts.

In addition, make sure that the hyssop you're taking is *Hyssopus officinalis*. Several other North American plants are also called hyssop, including hedge hyssop (*Gratiola officinalis*), the giant hyssops (several species of the genus *Agastache*), and the water hyssops (several species of *Bacopa*). These plants should not be ingested. Buy hyssop only from sources that identify it by botanical name.

Wise-Use Guidelines

Hyssop is included in the FDA list of herbs generally regarded as safe. For adults who are not pregnant or nursing, hyssop is safe when used in the amounts typically recommended.

You should use medicinal amounts of hyssop only in consultation with your doctor. If it causes minor discomfort, such as stomach upset or diarrhea, reduce the dosage or stop using it altogether. Let your doctor know if you experience any unpleasant effects or if the symptoms for which you're taking the herb do not improve significantly within 2 weeks.

Growing Information

If you want bees in your garden, plant this pretty, hardy, shrubby perennial. Hyssop also has a reputation for enhancing the flavor of grapes and increasing the yield of cabbages planted nearby.

Hyssop has small, lance-shaped leaves, as well as the square stems characteristic of the mints. The plant reaches 2 feet and has a medicinal odor that becomes more mintlike when the leaves are crushed. Dense clusters of blue or violet flowers form on 6-inch spikes atop the stems in summer and early fall.

Hyssop enjoys dry, sunny locations and tolerates most soils. In partial shade, it tends to become leggy. It may be propagated from seeds, cuttings, or root divisions. Seeds should be sown ¼ inch deep after the danger of frost has passed. Cuttings and divisions may be rooted either indoors or outdoors in a cool, shady place.

Thin established plants to 12-inch spacing. Add compost each spring, and water seedlings every few days. Mature plants prefer a drier environment and require little care.

Once the plant reaches about 18 inches and exudes its characteristic aroma, cut back the tops to stimulate leaf growth. The leaves may be harvested at any time. If you don't plan to use the flowers, cut back the entire plant to 4 inches above ground just before it blooms. Dry the herb and store it in airtight containers.

Juniper

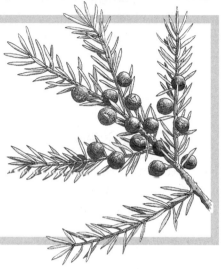

Family: Cupressaceae; other members include cypress

Genus and species: *Juniperus communis*

Also known as: Genvrier and geneva

Parts used: Berries (actually miniature female cones)

If you've ever had a martini, you know juniper. Aromatic juniper berries are the flavoring agent in gin. Juniper also increases urine production, making the herb a possible treatment for premenstrual syndrome, high blood pressure, and congestive heart failure.

Healing History

During the Middle Ages, Europeans believed that planting a juniper beside the front door kept witches out. Unfortunately, it did not provide complete protection. A witch could still enter if she correctly guessed the number of needles on the tree.

As time passed, juniper's protective reputation evolved into the belief that its smoke prevented leprosy and bubonic plague. As recently as World War II, French nurses burned juniper in hospital rooms to fumigate them.

By the 17th century, juniper was a popular diuretic, used to increase urine production. English herbalist Nicholas Culpeper wrote that the herb "provokes urine exceedingly. . . . [juniper] is so powerful a remedy against dropsy [congestive heart failure], it cures the disease." In addition, Culpeper prescribed juniper for "cough, shortness of breath, consumption [tuberculosis] . . . to provoke terms [menstruation] . . . and give safe and speedy delivery to women with child."

Native Americans independently discovered juniper's childbirth-assisting properties. In 1540, when the Spanish explorer Coronado entered what is now New Mexico looking for the mythical, gold-encrusted Seven Cities of Cibola, he found Zuni women using juniper berries to promote uterine recovery after childbirth. They also used the herb to treat wound infections and arthritis.

America's 19th-century Eclectic physicians, forerunners of today's naturopaths, dismissed juniper as a childbirth aid but strongly endorsed it for congestive heart failure. The Eclectics also prescribed juniper externally for eczema and psoriasis and internally for gonorrhea, bladder and kidney infections, and other genital and urinary problems.

Contemporary herbalists recommend juniper externally as an antiseptic and internally for bladder infections, arthritis, intestinal cramps, and gout. One herbalist suggests using the herb as a urinary deodorant in cases of chronic incontinence because it gives urine the fragrance of violets.

The medicinal claims for juniper take a back seat to its use in gin, invented in the 17th century by a Dutch professor of medicine, Franciscus Sylvius, who was interested in creating a diuretic tincture. Our word *gin* comes from the Dutch word for juniper, *geniver*. The English took to gin so enthusiastically that references to its native land still pepper the English language. Drink too much gin, and you're likely to get in trouble, or "in Dutch."

Therapeutic Uses

Juniper's aromatic oil contains terpinen-4-ol, a diuretic compound that increases the fluid-filtering rate of the kidneys. This supports the herb's traditional role as a diuretic.

High blood pressure. Physicians often prescribe diuretics to treat high blood pressure (hypertension). This is a serious condition requiring professional care. If you'd like to use juniper as part of your treatment plan, discuss it with your physician.

Congestive heart failure. Culpeper exaggerated when he said that juniper "cured" congestive heart failure. As a diuretic, however, the herb can be a part of an overall treatment plan.

Congestive heart failure is a serious condition requiring professional care. If you'd like to try juniper, discuss it with your physician.

Women's health concerns. In animal studies, juniper stimulates uterine contractions. For this reason, pregnant women should not take it (except at term under the supervision of a physician, when it may help stimulate labor). Other women might try it to help start their menstrual periods.

Since diuretics help relieve the bloated feeling caused by premenstrual fluid retention, women who are bothered by premenstrual syndrome might try juniper during the uncomfortable days right before their periods.

Arthritis. Juniper may have anti-inflammatory properties, suggesting that it may be of value in treating arthritis. Native Americans used the herb for this purpose. Likewise, in Germany, where herbal medicine is considerably more mainstream than in the United States, physicians prescribe juniper preparations for arthritis and gout.

Intriguing Possibility

Animal studies show that juniper reduces blood sugar levels. It's too early to deem the herb a treatment for diabetes, but it may play that role in the future.

Medicinal Myth

Juniper has never been shown to be effective for gonorrhea or for bladder or kidney infections.

Rx Recommendations

If you want to take advantage of juniper's diuretic properties or to try it to relieve arthritis pain or bring on your period, take it as an infusion. Use 1 teaspoon of crushed berries per cup of boiling water. Steep for 10 to 20 minutes, then strain. Drink up to 2 cups a day for no more than 6 weeks. Juniper has a strong, pleasantly aromatic taste.

When using commercial preparations, follow the package directions.

Do not give juniper to children under age 2. For older children and adults over age 65, start with low-strength preparations and increase the strength if necessary.

The Safety Factor

Diuretics deplete the body of potassium, an essential mineral. If you use juniper, be sure to eat foods rich in potassium, such as bananas and fresh vegetables.

The diuretic compound in juniper irritates the kidneys, not so much in small amounts but in high doses. It may cause kidney damage in people who are particularly sensitive to it and in those who have kidney disease.

For this reason, people with kidney infections or a history of kidney impairment should not take it. Even low doses taken over long periods may cause problems. "The rule," writes respected German medical herbalist Rudolph Fritz Weiss, M.D., "is never take juniper for longer than 6 weeks."

Symptoms of overdose include diarrhea, intestinal pain, kidney pain, protein in the urine (albuminuria), blood in the urine (hematuria), purplish urine, rapid heartbeat, and elevated blood pressure. If you notice any of these symptoms while taking juniper, discontinue use.

Since many elderly people have kidney impairment, those over age 65 should have their kidney function checked by a physician before taking juniper.

Up to one-third of people with hay fever develop allergy symptoms from exposure to juniper, according to a study in *Clinical Allergy*. If you have hay fever, you may want to avoid the herb. It may trigger other allergic reactions as well, notably rash.

Wise-Use Guidelines

Oddly enough, given its potential for kidney damage, juniper is included in the FDA list of herbs generally regarded as safe. For adults who are not pregnant or nursing, do not have kidney disease, and are not taking other diuretics, juniper is considered safe when used cautiously for short periods of time in the amounts typically recommended.

You should take medicinal amounts of juniper only in consultation with your doctor. Let your doctor know if you experience any unpleasant effects or if the symptoms for which you're using the herb do not improve significantly within 2 weeks.

Growing Information

The genus *Juniperus* contains more than 70 species of aromatic evergreens. Most are small trees, but some grow to 40 feet.

The species most widely used in herbal healing, common juniper (*J. communis*) reaches 6 to 20 feet, depending on locale. Its close, tangled, spreading branches are covered with reddish brown bark, sticky gum, and pointed 1/2-inch needles. Males produce yellow flowers and females have green flowers. The females also produce scaly, green, aromatic 1/4-inch cones (berries) that turn blue-black during their 2-year maturation. If you want berries, be sure to plant both male and female junipers, or the females will not fruit.

Junipers usually prefer sandy soil and full sun, but they adapt to many soil and climate conditions. Consult a nursery for advice specific to your locale.

Females produce immature (green) and mature (blue-black) berries simultaneously. Harvest only the mature berries in fall. Dry them in the sun. When dried, they turn a dull black. Store them in airtight containers to preserve their volatile oil.

Kava

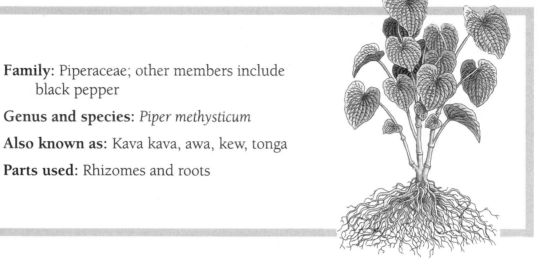

Family: Piperaceae; other members include black pepper

Genus and species: *Piper methysticum*

Also known as: Kava kava, awa, kew, tonga

Parts used: Rhizomes and roots

For centuries, the people of the South Pacific have used kava the way Americans use beer: as a social drug. Since the mid-1990s, kava has become popular in the United States as a treatment for stress and anxiety. Research shows that it is safe and effective.

Healing History

Polynesians from New Guinea to Tahiti have a longstanding tradition of enjoying kava in "kava circles." The circle begins with one or more participants placing powdered kava root in half of a coconut shell and adding about a cup of water to form a milky solution. Then everyone claps as the drinker downs the brew in one big gulp. Next, the coconut shell is passed to the next person in the circle, and the ceremony is repeated until each participant has taken several gulps of the drink. As the festivities continue, the conversation and laughter flow more easily, as it might after a few beers.

In the South Pacific, kava has been used as a treatment for headache, colds, and arthritis and as a sedative and aphrodisiac. Native Hawaiians took the herb to control asthma.

The 18th-century British explorer Captain James Cook and his crew were offered kava during their voyage among the islands of the South Pacific (1768–1771). They enjoyed the herb's peppery taste and mild intoxicating effect. They also noticed that elderly kava drinkers who had consumed large amounts of the herb over the course of many years had oddly scaly skin, the main sign of kava dermopathy (more on this later).

Around 1990, kava began attracting the attention of American herbalists. European (mostly German) studies had shown that at doses lower than those used in the South Pacific, the root produces little or no euphoria but instead acts as a mild tranquilizer.

Therapeutic Uses

The active compounds in kava, called kavalactones, have a mild tranquilizing effect similar to a low dose of diazepam (Valium). But unlike the drug, kava is much less likely to cause sedation, and it's not addictive. (The combination of kava and alcohol or other depressants is powerfully sedative, however.)

Anxiety and stress. Many recent studies, almost all German, show that kava is an effective treatment for stress and anxiety. Here's a brief overview of some of the most noteworthy research.

• German researchers gave 100 people who were complaining of nervous anxiety, agoraphobia, or social phobia either medically inactive placebos or 300 milligrams of kava extract a day. After 8 weeks, those taking kava showed measurably less anxiety and depression. The benefits continued for the 6-month duration of the study. Side effects were mild and minor, reported by only 5 of the 50 being treated with kava.

• In another German study, 58 people with anxiety disorders took either placebos or kava (100 milligrams three times a day) for a month. In the kava group, anxiety symptoms began to decline after just 1 week of treatment and continued to diminish throughout the study. The kava takers reported no side effects.

• At the Medical College of Virginia, researchers gave daily doses of either placebos or kava (240 milligrams) to 60 adults dealing with stress and anxiety. After 4 weeks, those taking the placebos showed no significant change in their anxiety symptoms, but those taking the kava reported fewer interpersonal problems, fewer anxiety symptoms, and less stress. What's more, those in the kava group experienced no side effects.

Commission E, the expert panel that evaluates herbal medicines for the German counterpart of the FDA, endorses kava as a treatment for stress and anxiety problems. The herb is best used short-term, for periods of up to a few months. If you feel that you still need anti-anxiety medication after a few months, consult your physician.

Rx Recommendations

You may be able to buy powdered bulk kava root, particularly in Hawaii, but most Americans take commercial capsules.

Look for a standardized extract that contains 60 to 75 milligrams of kavalactones per capsule. The dose used in most studies is 300 milligrams of standardized extract (the equivalent of about 200 milligrams of kavalactones), taken in divided doses. Follow the package directions.

Do not give kava to children under age 2. For older children and adults over age 65, start with a low dosage and increase it if necessary.

The Safety Factor

In unusually large doses—considerably larger than those necessary to relieve anxiety—kava causes inebriation similar to that caused by alcohol. Thinking and coordination become impaired. Walking becomes difficult, and stumbling and falling are likely. The eyes become bloodshot.

Taking unusually large doses for many years leads to the development of scaly skin, a condition called kava dermopathy. This side effect is highly unlikely in the doses recommended for anxiety. To treat kava dermopathy, experts recommend terminating use of kava.

Do not use kava at the same time as alcohol or other tranquilizing, sedative, or psychoactive medications, including antidepressants. The herb intensifies the sedative effect of other drugs.

Kava may cause some numbness of the mouth, which is harmless. Allergic reactions are also possible.

Women who are pregnant or nursing; people who have conditions that impair coordination, such as Parkinson's disease; and those taking sedative or antidepressant medications should not take kava.

Wise-Use Guidelines

For adults who are not pregnant or nursing and who do not have any of the health concerns described above, kava is considered safe in the amounts usually recommended.

You should use medicinal amounts of kava only in consultation with your doctor. If you notice any unusual symptoms after taking it, discontinue use. Let your doctor know if you experience unpleasant effects or if the symptoms for which you're using the herb do not improve significantly within 2 weeks.

Growing Information

A botanical relative of black pepper, kava is a perennial shrub with heart-shaped leaves that grows throughout the South Pacific at altitudes of 500 to 1,000 feet. It does best in stony ground with full sun exposure. Plants can climb to 20 feet, but the roots are usually harvested when the shrub reaches about 8 feet. Kava is not a garden herb in the United States.

Kola

Family: Sterculiaceae; other members include cocoa

Genus and species: *Cola nitida, C. vera,* and *C. acurninata*

Also known as: Cola

Parts used: Nuts (actually seed leaves, or cotyledons)

Nuts

Cola drinks account for a whopping 70 percent of the enormous U.S. soft drink market. Americans might consume even more if they knew that the tropical nut responsible for colas' flavor can help relieve asthma.

Healing History

West Africans have used kola since prehistoric times. They chewed the seeds for their stimulant effect and as a treatment for fever.

West African slaves introduced the kola tree into Brazil and the Caribbean. Among Caribbean natives, the herb became a favorite diuretic for water retention as well as a digestive aid and a folk remedy for diarrhea, fatigue, and heart problems. Over time, kola's stimulant properties led to the belief that it was an aphrodisiac.

Kola arrived in the United States after the Civil War. Nineteenth-century Eclectic physicians, forerunners of today's naturopaths, noted that the Caribbean people ascribed "innumerable fabulous virtues" to the herb.

The Eclectics correctly identified the stimulants in kola—notably caffeine—as the same ones in cocoa, coffee, and tea. They prescribed kola to "overcome mental depression" and prepare for "severe physical and mental exertion." They also recommended it to relieve diarrhea, pneumonia, typhoid fever, migraines, seasickness, and morning sickness and for anyone who "attempts to break the tobacco habit."

Because kola was used medicinally, it was kept in stock by 19th-century pharmacists. Legend has it that on May 8, 1886, Atlanta pharmacist John Styth Pemberton was toying with a new headache remedy. He mixed some sugar with extracts of kola and coca (the source of cocaine) in a three-legged brass pot in his backyard. He added carbonated water to his sweet syrup and created a refreshing drink that his bookkeeper dubbed Coca-Cola.

Two years later, Pemberton sold all rights to his beverage to Atlanta businessman Asa Candler for $2,300. Candler was an imaginative marketer, and by 1895, Coca-Cola had become America's first national soft drink.

Today, Coca-Cola is the best-known product in the world. People request it 250 million times a day in 80 languages and in 135 countries.

Since its development, Coca-Cola's formula has been a closely guarded secret, although it has evolved over the years. When the United States outlawed cocaine, the drug was removed from the formula. Today, Coca-Cola is known to contain decocainized coca leaf extract and a small amount of kola.

Modern herbalists recommend kola for its "marked stimulating effect on human consciousness," according to medical herbalist David Hoffmann's *Holistic Herbal*.

It's also prescribed as a treatment for diarrhea, depression, nervous debility, migraines, and loss of appetite.

Therapeutic Uses

Some herbals claim that kola contains more caffeine than coffee. Not so. A 6-ounce cup of brewed coffee contains about 100 milligrams of caffeine; a cup of instant coffee has 65 milligrams. By comparison, a 12-ounce can of a cola soft drink contains about 50 milligrams of caffeine. Most of this amount comes not from the kola nut but from added caffeine. (For more information on the health benefits of caffeine, see Coffee on page 144.)

Asthma. Coffee can help control asthma, but many children don't like the taste. That's why an article in the *Journal of the American Medical Association* recommended using cola beverages when kids start wheezing without their medicine handy or as tasty adjuncts to standard asthma medication.

Rx Recommendations

Cola beverages are the most convenient way to enjoy small amounts of this pleasant-tasting herb.

If you prefer to make a decoction, place 1 to 2 teaspoons of powdered kola nuts in 1 cup of water. Bring to a boil and simmer for 10 minutes, then strain if you wish. Drink up to 3 cups a day.

You may give small amounts of dilute cola beverages cautiously to children under age 2.

The Safety Factor

Because kola contains caffeine, pregnant women should avoid it, as should people with any of the conditions mentioned in the discussion on the safety of coffee on page 148.

Wise-Use Guidelines

Kola is currently included on the FDA list of herbs generally regarded as safe. An FDA panel has recommended removing caffeine from the safe list, however, and if this happens, kola may also be removed.

For adults who are not pregnant or nursing and do not have a history of the conditions that make coffee inadvisable, kola is considered safe in the amounts typically recommended.

You should take medicinal amounts of kola only in consultation with your doctor. If it causes minor discomfort, such as insomnia, irritability, or stomach upset, reduce the dosage or stop using it altogether. Let your doctor know if you experience any unpleasant symptoms or the symptoms for which you're using the herb do not improve significantly within 2 weeks.

Growing Information

Kola is a 40-foot tree that grows in West Africa, the Caribbean, Brazil, Sri Lanka, and Indonesia. Kolas have beautiful, purple-spotted yellow flowers that produce chocolate-colored seed pods in spring and fall.

For most plants, *nut* refers to the whole seed, but the kola nut is only part of the seed, specifically the embryonic leaves (or cotyledons) inside the seed coat. These are dried and powdered.

Lavender

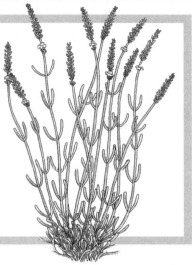

Family: Labiatae; other members include mints

Genus and species: *Lavandula angustifolia*; also known as *L. officinalis* and *L. spica*

Also known as: True lavender, spike lavender, lavandin, and aspic

Parts used: Flowers

Lavender grew in abundance around the ancient Syrian city of Nardus, near the Euphrates River. As a result, the ancient Greeks called the plant *nard*. The Bible refers to it as spikenard.

Our word *lavender* comes from the Latin *luvare*, meaning "to wash." Lavender was a frequent addition to baths and was also considered a purifier for the body and mind.

Healing History

Since ancient times, lavender has been used as a digestive aid, sleep aid, and tranquilizer for people who are anxious, restless, or emotionally troubled. Because of its mood-altering effects, lavender was also considered an antidepressant.

English farmers wore spikes of lavender flowers under their hats to prevent headache and sunstroke. The flowers were dried, powdered, and sewn into pillows as a treatment for insomnia. The herb was also considered a remedy for acne, migraines, diabetes, faintness, headache, and muscle spasms. Until World War I, lavender infusions and tinctures were used to disinfect wounds.

For centuries, lavender has been an ingredient in sachets and potpourris to freshen the air, especially in sickrooms. Sprigs were placed in wardrobes and closets to add fragrance to clothing and to repel moths.

During the Middle Ages, lavender had a reputation as an aphrodisiac that attracted lovers. Sprinkling lavender water on a lover's head was said to keep the person faithful, a reputed effect that generated great demand for the herb.

There was also a persistent rumor that the asp, a poisonous snake, nested in lavender bushes, which made people think twice about gathering the herb. This was pure fiction, apparently promoted by herbalists because it drove up lavender's price.

In his *Herball or Generall Historie of Plantes*, 16th-century British herbalist John Gerard wrote of lavender's use in treating palsy (tremors or paralysis): "It profiteth them much that have the palsy if they be washed with water of lavender flowers, or are anointed with the oil made from the flowers and olive oil."

Fifty years later, Nicholas Culpeper prescribed lavender for "all the grief and pains of the head . . . it strengthens the stomach . . . two spoonfuls of the distilled water of the flowers help them that have lost their voice. . . ."

America's 19th-century Eclectic physicians, forerunners of today's naturopaths, recommended lavender as a digestive aid. They cautioned, however, that immoderate use of lavender infusions might cause stomach upset.

The Birth of Aromatherapy

During the 1920s, French fragrance chemist Rene-Maurice Gattefosse was toiling in his laboratory, developing a new perfume. Lost in thought while blending essential oils from various herbs, he set off an explosion that burned his arm. Frantic with pain, he plunged his arm into the nearest cold liquid, which happened to be a bowl of lavender oil.

Immediately, Gattefosse felt surprising relief from his pain. Instead of the extended healing process he'd known from previous burns—accompanied by redness, heat, inflammation, blisters, and scarring—this burn healed remarkably quickly, with little discomfort and no scarring. Perhaps, the perfumer thought, he had discovered a powerful healer that had literally been right under his nose.

Gattefosse devoted the rest of his life to studying the role of essential oils in health and healing. In 1928, he published the book *Aromatherapie*, coining the term that's now used to describe the healing discipline that involves inhaling aromatic plant oils or massaging them into the skin for physical or emotional benefits.

Today, aromatherapists use dozens of essential oils, but they still consider lavender one of the best for treating anger, anxiety, burns, depression, indigestion, infection, insomnia, irritability, muscle aches, and wounds.

Lavender is grown as an ornamental all over the temperate world, but almost all of the commercial crop is used in perfumes, soaps, cosmetics, and hair care products. Some is used to flavor foods such as vinegars, vegetable oils, cheeses, and honey. Lavender scones are popular in England, and in France, lavender sorbet is considered a summer treat.

Therapeutic Uses

Lavender has never been proven either to increase sexual desire or to keep a lover faithful. But modern research has validated many of the herb's traditional medicinal uses.

The essential oil extracted from lavender flowers is chemically very complex, containing more than 150 compounds. When rubbed on the skin, the oil penetrates quickly and can be detected in the blood in as little as 5 minutes.

Anxiety. Animal studies have shown that lavender oil is calming and anticonvulsant and that it enhances the action of other sedatives. After exposure to the scent of lavender, mice become calmer.

Studies at the Smell and Taste Research

Foundation in Chicago have found that some scents, including lavender, increase the type of brain waves associated with relaxation. This lends support to the age-old practice of using lavender to treat restlessness and anxiety.

At a British hospital, researchers divided more than 90 patients in intensive care units into three groups. One group received standard care, another got standard care plus up to three massages, and the third was treated with standard care plus massages with lavender oil. All three groups experienced similar reductions in blood levels of stress-related hormones, but the people who received aromatherapy massages reported the greatest mood elevation and anxiety relief.

Commission E, the expert panel that evaluates herbal medicines for the German counterpart of the FDA, approves lavender as a treatment for anxiety and restlessness.

Insomnia. At the University of Leicester in England, researchers monitored the sleep habits of nursing home residents who had been taking sleeping pills for several years. For the first 2 weeks, the residents took their medications as usual. For the next 2 weeks, they stopped using their medications and lost sleep. For the last 2 weeks, they took no medications, but the fragrance of lavender oil was infused into the air during the overnight hours. The participants slept just as long as they had while taking medication. What's more, they slept more soundly.

This study involved only four people, but it validates lavender's traditional role as a sleep aid. Commission E endorses lavender for treating insomnia. Several British hospitals reportedly offer lavender baths or lavender pillows to help patients sleep.

Wounds. Like most aromatic herb oils, lavender oil has antimicrobial action. This means that it can protect wounds from infection and help them heal.

Digestive problems. Like its close botanical relatives, the mints, lavender helps calm the smooth muscle lining the digestive tract. It also promotes the secretion of bile, which helps digest fats. Commission E endorses lavender as a digestive aid and antiflatulent.

Women's health concerns. Herbs that soothe the digestive tract may also calm another smooth muscle, the uterus. This effect may help control menstrual cramping.

In a study of lavender as an aid to recovery from childbirth, British researchers divided 635 new mothers who had normal, uncomplicated deliveries into three groups. One group added true lavender oil to their baths, another used synthetic lavender oil, and the third was given a medically inactive placebo oil. During the 10-day study, all three groups experienced reduced pain in the genital area, and the differences in their recovery rates were not statistically significant. Nonetheless, those who used true lavender oil reported the speediest recoveries.

Insect repellent. Modern research has shown that some of the compounds in lavender oil repel insects. This validates the centuries-old practice of strewing lavender flowers for insect control.

Intriguing Possibility

According to a report in the *Journal of the National Cancer Institute*, a compound in lavender oil called perillyl alcohol has been shown to exert remarkable action against a variety of cancerous tumors in animals, notably, cancers of the breast, lung, liver, colon, and pancreas. At this time, perillyl alcohol is being tested in clinical trials as a possible cancer preventive and treatment.

Rx Recommendations

To prepare an infusion, use 1 to 3 teaspoons of lavender flowers per cup of boiling water, steep for 10 minutes, and strain. Drink up to 3 cups a day.

To treat a minor wound or burn, wash it with soap and water, then apply a compress made with a lavender infusion.

As a homemade tincture, take 1 teaspoon up to three times a day. You may also apply the tincture topically to wounds and burns.

When using commercial preparations, follow the package directions.

For a relaxing bath, place a handful of lavender flowers in a cloth bag and run water over it, or add lavender infusion, tincture, or oil to your bath.

For an aromatherapy massage, apply a few drops of lavender oil directly to the skin or blend it into a commercial massage lotion (10 drops of oil per ounce of lotion).

To make a lavender pillow, put powdered flowers into a cloth bag and place the bag inside your pillowcase.

The Safety Factor

Lavender is considered safe in the amounts typically recommended. There have been a few reports of the oil causing allergic skin reactions. If you apply lavender oil and subsequently develop irritation or a rash, stop using it.

While ingesting a few drops of lavender oil is probably harmless, as little as a teaspoon can be toxic, especially to children and the elderly.

Growing Information

Native to the Mediterranean, lavender is a pleasantly aromatic, woody, branching perennial shrub that grows to about 3 feet. Its narrow, fuzzy leaves change color from gray to green as they mature. In summer, lavender produces small blue or purple flowers that develop on spikes 6 to 8 inches long, creating beautiful, aromatic bouquets.

There are more than 25 species of lavender, all of which grow easily in sunny locations. The plants prefer sandy soil but will tolerate a wide range of soil conditions.

If you'd like to grow lavender for medicinal purposes, *Lavandula angustifolia* is considered the best species. Other species presumably have comparable benefits, because the oil they produce is the same or very similar. Consult a nursery for the species that grows best in your area.

The fragrance of lavender remains potent long after the flowers are dried.

Lemon Balm

Family: Labiatae; other members include mints

Genus and species: *Melissa officinalis*

Also known as: Balm, bee balm, melissa, sweet balm, and cure-all

Parts used: Leaves

Bees love lemon balm, which has been a favorite among beekeepers for more than 2,000 years. It's not surprising that its genus name, *Melissa*, is Greek for "bee."

Lemon balm is also a honey of a healer. It calms the stomach, soothes the nerves, promotes restful sleep, and helps treat herpes.

Healing History

The ancient Greek physician Dioscorides applied lemon balm leaves to skin wounds and added the herb to wine to treat a variety of illnesses. The Roman naturalist Pliny recommended lemon balm to stop bleeding.

During the 10th century, Arab doctors recommended lemon balm for nervousness and anxiety. The great 11th-century Arab physician Avicenna wrote, "Balm causeth the mind and heart to become merry."

Medieval Europeans adopted the Arabs' practice of using lemon balm for nervousness and anxiety. Melissa water, or *eau de Melisse*, became so popular as a tranquilizer and sedative that the emperor Charlemagne ordered the plant grown in every medicinal herb garden, or "physic garden," in his realm to guarantee an adequate supply.

During the Middle Ages, European herbalists greatly expanded on lemon balm's earlier uses, prescribing it for just about everything: insomnia, arthritis, headache, toothache, sores, digestive problems, and cramps and other menstrual problems. In fact, they recommended the herb for so many ailments that lemon balm was referred to as cure-all.

In his influential herbal, 17th-century English herbalist Nicholas Culpeper echoed Avicenna, commenting, "[Lemon balm] causeth the mind and heart to become merry, and driveth away all troublesome cares and thoughts arising from melancholy. . . ." Culpeper also recommended lemon balm for "faintings and swoonings . . . to help digestion . . . open obstructions of the brain . . . [and] procure women's courses [menstruation]."

In North America, colonists had surprisingly little regard for the bees' favorite herb. They used lemon balm primarily to relieve menstrual cramps and to induce sweating, a traditional treatment for fever.

America's 19th-century Eclectic physicians, forerunners of today's naturopaths, also had few uses for lemon balm. Despite the herb's long history as a tranquilizer, it was considered only a moderate stimulant.

Contemporary herbalists tout lemon balm's traditional roles as a tranquilizer, digestive aid, and treatment for wounds and viral infections.

Therapeutic Uses

Culpeper was way off-base when he reported that lemon balm "opens obstructions in the brain," but many of the plant's other traditional uses have stood up to scientific scrutiny. Researchers have even determined that lemon balm is a potent antiviral, a benefit that the ancients knew nothing about.

Wounds. Dioscorides was right about at least one of lemon balm's therapeutic properties. The herb contains chemicals called polyphenols that help fight several infection-causing bacteria, among them streptococcus and mycobacteria. Lemon balm also contains eugenol, a natural anesthetic that may help relieve wound pain.

Herpes and other viral infections. Research has shown that lemon balm has antiviral action.

In one German study, 116 people with herpes lesions (cold sores or genital herpes) were given either a medically inactive placebo cream or a cream containing 1 percent lemon balm extract. The participants applied the creams two to four times a day for up to 10 days. By the second day, those using the lemon balm showed greater healing, and by the fifth, their sores were 50 percent more likely to have cleared entirely. The researchers concluded: "Melissa was judged conclusively superior to the placebo by physician and patient alike." To be effective, however, treatment with lemon balm must begin as soon as a sore begins to erupt.

In Germany, where herbal medicine is more mainstream than in the United States, lemon balm extract is an active ingredient in ointments intended for the treatment of cold sores and genital herpes. Experts say that compresses of lemon balm infusion should also help.

Insomnia. Animal studies have found that several compounds in lemon balm—including the oil, which gives the plant its pleasant fragrance—have tranquilizing properties. This supports lemon balm's traditional role as a relaxant.

In Germany, lemon balm is widely used as a tranquilizer and sedative. In one German study, a combination of lemon balm and valerian provided significant relief to 68 people with insomnia. In another study, the same herb combination proved as effective as the pharmaceutical tranquilizer/sedative triazolam (Halcion), but unlike the drug, it caused no morning "hangover."

Commission E, the expert panel that evaluates herbal medicines for the German counterpart of the FDA, approves lemon balm as a treatment for insomnia.

Digestive problems. German researchers have discovered that lemon balm relaxes the smooth muscle tissue of the digestive tract, thus supporting the herb's age-old reputation as a digestive aid. Many other herbs in the mint family, notably peppermint, are also traditional digestive aids. Commission E endorses lemon balm for treating indigestion.

Women's health concerns. Herbs that relax the digestive tract may also calm another smooth muscle, the uterus. This potential effect could explain lemon balm's traditional role in treating menstrual cramps.

Curiously, lemon balm has also been recommended as a uterine stimulant to promote menstruation. No contemporary research clarifies this confusing situation. For this reason, pregnant women should not take the herb.

Intriguing Possibility

Animal studies have found that lemon balm interferes with the activity of thyroid-stimulating hormone, suggesting that it may prove useful as a treatment for an overactive thyroid gland (hyperthyroidism or Grave's disease).

Rx Recommendations

For a relaxing bath, tie a handful of balm into a cloth and run the bath water over it. In addition to feeling the tranquilizing effect, you'll love the lemony aroma.

To treat wounds or herpes sores, make a hot compress using 2 teaspoons of leaves per cup of water. Boil for 10 minutes, strain, and apply with a clean cloth.

To treat a minor cut, crush some fresh balm leaves and apply them directly to the wound.

For a light, lemony-tasting infusion that helps soothe the stomach or promote sleep, use 2 teaspoons of leaves per cup of water. Steep for 10 to 20 minutes, then strain. Drink up to 3 cups a day.

As a homemade tincture, take ½ to 1½ teaspoons up to three times a day.

When using commercial preparations, follow the package directions.

Do not give medicinal infusions or tinctures of lemon balm to children under age 2. For older children and adults over age 65, start with low-strength preparations and increase the strength if necessary.

The Safety Factor

Because lemon balm interferes with thyroid-stimulating hormone, it may aggravate problems associated with an underactive thyroid (hypothyroidism). Although there are no published reports of the herb having this effect, anyone with hypothyroidism should consult a physician before taking lemon balm.

Wise-Use Guidelines

Balm is on the FDA list of herbs generally regarded as safe. The medical literature contains no reports of toxicity. For adults who are not pregnant or nursing and do not have a thyroid condition, balm is considered safe when used in the amounts typically recommended.

You should take medicinal amounts of balm only in consultation with your doctor. If it causes minor discomfort, such as stomach upset or diarrhea, reduce the dosage or stop using it altogether. Let your doctor know if you experience any unpleasant effects or if the symptoms for which you're using the herb do not improve significantly within 2 weeks.

Growing Information

Lemon balm is an erect, branching perennial that grows to 2 feet. It has the mint family's characteristic square stems and small, two-lipped white or yellow flowers, which bloom in bunches throughout the summer. The above-ground parts die back each winter, but the root is perennial.

Lemon balm grows easily from seeds sown in spring or from cuttings or root divisions. Seeds germinate indoors or out and often do best when left uncovered. Simply keep them moist. Germination typically takes 3 to 4 weeks.

Lemon balm likes well-drained soil with a pH near neutral. Thin seedlings to 12-inch spacing. The herb prefers partial shade; it wilts in full sun and loses some aroma.

For medicinal use, the leaves should be harvested before the plant flowers. Cut the entire plant back to a few inches above the ground. Dry the leaves quickly, or they may turn black.

Lemon balm loses much of its fragrance when dried. After drying, powder the leaves, then store them in tightly sealed opaque containers to preserve the volatile oil.

Licorice

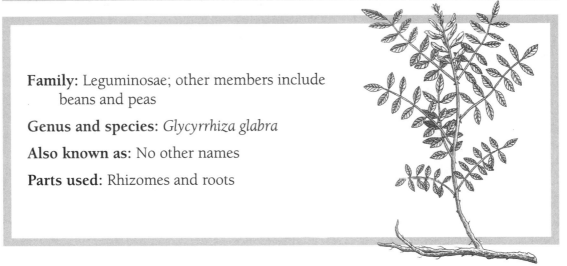

Family: Leguminosae; other members include beans and peas

Genus and species: *Glycyrrhiza glabra*

Also known as: No other names

Parts used: Rhizomes and roots

Licorice is both beneficial and controversial. Advocates point out that the herb has been used around the world for thousands of years to treat coughs, colds, rashes, arthritis, ulcers, hepatitis, cirrhosis, and infections. Critics concede the herb's effectiveness but insist that its "potentially life-threatening side effects" make it too dangerous to use.

In a small number of cases, the concentrated licorice extracts that flavor candies have caused some harm when eaten in enormous amounts. For healthy adults who ingest the herb in moderation, however, licorice's benefits greatly outweigh its risks.

Healing History

Licorice appears prominently in the first great Chinese herbal, the *Pen Tsao Ching* (*Classic of Herbs*), attributed to the mythical emperor-sage Shen Nung around 3000 B.C. According to legend, the emperor tested dozens of herbs on himself and died after taking a bit too much of a poison plant. Since Shen Nung's time, licorice has remained one of China's most popular healing herbs.

Licorice has a long history in Western herbalism as well. Amid the treasures of King Tut's tomb, archeologists found a bundle of licorice sticks.

During the 3rd century B.C., Hippocrates extolled licorice for coughs, asthma, and other respiratory complaints. He called it sweet root—in Greek, *glukos riza*, which evolved into the herb's genus name, *Glycyrrhiza*.

The Romans changed *Glycyrrhiza* to *Liquiritia*, which evolved into "licorice." The noted 1st-century Roman naturalist Pliny recommended the herb as an expectorant and stomach soother. The Greek physician Dioscorides, who served in the Roman army, prescribed licorice juice for colds, sore throats, and chest and gastrointestinal complaints.

India's ancient Ayurvedic physicians recommended licorice as an expectorant, diuretic, and menstruation promoter.

The 12th-century medieval German abbess/herbalist Hildegard of Bingen prescribed licorice for stomach and heart problems. The herb was mentioned frequently in 14th- and 15th-century German and Italian herbals as a cough and respiratory remedy.

The 17th-century English herbalist Nicholas Culpeper described licorice as "a fine medicine . . . for those that have dry cough or hoarseness, wheezing or shortness of breath, phthisis [tuberculosis], heat of urine [burning], and griefs of the breast and lungs."

North American colonists found Native Americans drinking a tea brewed from American licorice as a cough remedy, laxative, earache treatment, and mask for the bitter flavor of other herbs.

America's 19th-century Eclectic physicians, forerunners of today's naturopaths, prescribed licorice for urinary problems, coughs, colds, and other "bronchial and pectoral [chest] affections."

Among American folk herbalists, licorice was considered a treatment for menstrual discomforts. It was included in Lydia E. Pinkham's Vegetable Compound, the popular 19th-century patent medicine for "female hysteria," which was that era's description of menstrual and menopausal complaints.

Many cultures around the world have used licorice to treat a variety of cancers.

In contemporary Chinese medicine, licorice is known as the great harmonizer. Its sweetness masks the bitter taste of many other medicinal herbs. Chinese physicians believe that in their multi-herb formulas, licorice improves the ability of the ingredients to work together. It is found in a variety of formulas, including those for indigestion, asthma, depression, varicose veins, and conditions that cause inflammation.

Contemporary American herbalists recommend licorice for its soothing effects on the respiratory, urinary, and gastrointestinal tracts, especially as a treatment for ulcers. They also follow the Chinese example of using licorice to mask the bitter taste of other healing herbs.

A few herbalists believe that licorice has hormonelike action. They recommend it as a treatment for Addison's disease, a condition in which the adrenal glands produce abnormally low amounts of certain hormones.

Therapeutic Uses

True to its Greek name, sweet root, licorice is 50 times sweeter than sugar. The herb contains a remarkable chemical, called glycyrrhetinic acid (GA), that has a broad range of healing powers. But a bitter battle has erupted over the sweet root's hazards.

Colds, coughs, and sore throats. Several studies support licorice's traditional role as a cough remedy. Glycyrrhetinic acid has some cough-suppressant properties.

In Europe, licorice is quite common in cough and cold formulas. Commission E, the expert panel that evaluates herbal medicines for the German counterpart of the FDA, approves the herb as a cold and cough treatment.

Ulcers. Back in 1946, a Dutch pharmacist noticed that licorice candies and cough remedies were unusually popular with customers who had gastrointestinal ulcers. They told him that licorice provided better, longer-lasting relief than other ulcer medicines. Intrigued, the pharmacist published a report in a Dutch medical journal.

Soon after, the British medical journal *Lancet* and the *Journal of the American Medical Association* published studies showing that concentrated GA extracted from licorice heals ulcers in both animals and people. Unfortunately, it also causes swollen ankles, which is a classic sign of water retention.

Water retention is potentially serious. It can lead to elevated blood pressure, which can be dangerous for women who are pregnant or nursing and for anyone with diabetes, glaucoma, high blood pressure, heart disease, or a history of stroke.

By the late 1970s, mainstream medicine had developed an effective ulcer drug called cimetidine (Tagamet). Several studies compared licorice head-to-head against Tagamet. Overall, while the pharmaceutical was more effective for stomach ulcers, the two treatments were equally effective for duodenal (small intestine) ulcers, with the licorice extract actually providing better protection against recurrences. Water retention related to glycyrrhetinic acid continued to be a problem, however.

Eventually, researchers figured out why GA causes water retention. The chemical acts like the adrenal hormone aldosterone, which is involved in salt and water metabolism. Large amounts of aldosterone can cause a potentially serious condition called pseudoaldosteronism, with symptoms that include water retention as well as headache, lethargy, elevated blood pressure, and possibly heart failure.

Fortunately, scientists also discovered that they could retain licorice's ulcer-healing benefits but eliminate its hormonal side effects by removing 97 percent of its glycyrrhetinic acid. This led to the creation of a new semi-herbal medicine, deglycyrrhizinated licorice (DGL).

European and British journals featured research demonstrating DGL's anti-ulcer effectiveness and lack of serious side effects. In one 12-week study of 874 people with duodenal ulcers, published in the *Irish Medical Journal*, DGL healed ulcers faster than Tagamet.

American scientists, who had dismissed glycyrrhetinic acid as too hazardous, decided to take a second look. In the late 1970s, they conducted several studies, but they unknowingly used improperly prepared DGL. It produced such poor results that the scientists deemed DGL to be totally ineffective against ulcers.

These unfortunate findings crushed any interest in licorice as an ulcer treatment in the United States. As it turned out, the improperly prepared DGL had released very little medicine (in other words, it had poor bioavailability).

In the late 1980s, research revealed that most ulcers are caused by bacteria and can be treated with antibiotics. As a result, DGL is of little use to most American physicians, but it remains a popular ulcer remedy in Europe. Commission E endorses licorice as a treatment for ulcers.

People with ulcers who are interested in incorporating licorice into their treatment regimens should discuss the herb with their physicians.

Arthritis. Licorice has anti-inflammatory and anti-arthritis properties. One study found that GA could be applied like hydrocortisone cream to treat skin inflammations such as eczema. These findings led to several animal studies, which concluded that licorice taken internally has anti-inflammatory, and specifically anti-arthritis, effects.

People with arthritis who want to try licorice should discuss it with their physicians.

Canker sores. Canker sores are painful mouth sores that can last a week before clearing up. In one study, Indian researchers asked 20 people with canker sores to use a DGL mouthwash. Fifteen of them (75 percent) experienced substantial relief after 1 day, with complete healing by the third day.

Herpes. According to a study published in *Microbiology and Immunology*, licorice stimulates cell production of interferon, the body's own antiviral compound. Not surprisingly, other studies have shown that licorice fights the herpes simplex virus, which causes genital herpes and cold sores. Sprinkling some powdered licorice root on sores may speed healing.

Hepatitis. Chinese physicians have used licorice for centuries to treat liver problems. Hepatitis C is a viral infection that can cause liver failure and liver cancer.

Japanese researchers injected 453 people who had hepatitis C with a licorice preparation (100 milliliters a day for 8 weeks, then several times a week for 10 years). Within 15 years, 25 percent of the people in a second group that didn't receive the injections had developed liver cancer. By comparison, only 12 percent of those in the licorice group had gotten cancer.

In a similar study, Indian researchers injected 18 people who had hepatitis with the same licorice preparation (40 milliliters a day for 30 days, then 100 milliliters three times a week for 8 weeks). Among those who didn't re-

ceive injections, the survival rate was 31 percent. Among those treated with licorice, the survival rate jumped to 72 percent.

The injectable licorice preparation used in these studies (Stronger Neo-Minophagen C) is not available in the United States. Nonetheless, the studies provide convincing evidence that licorice is a potent antiviral. The herb has also shown liver-protecting ability in people with cirrhosis as well as some action against influenza viruses and HIV, the virus that causes AIDS.

People who want to take advantage of licorice's possible healing action against liver disease or HIV should discuss the herb with their physicians.

Infections. Many laboratory studies have found that licorice fights disease-causing bacteria (staphylococcus and streptococcus) and the fungus responsible for vaginal yeast infections (*Candida albicans*). Sprinkling some powdered licorice root on clean wounds may help prevent infection.

Menopausal complaints. Lydia Pinkham was on the right track when she included licorice in her Vegetable Compound. In a small pilot study, naturopathic researchers in Portland and Seattle gave 13 women who were experiencing hot flashes either medically inactive placebos or an herbal formula containing equal parts of licorice and four other herbs used to treat menopausal complaints: Chinese angelica, motherwort, burdock, and wild yam root. The women took 1,500-milligram capsules of the formula three times a day.

After 3 months, 6 percent of the women in the placebo group reported significant relief from their hot flashes. Among those using the herb formula, that figure rose to 100 percent.

Intriguing Possibility

Immune stimulation may help explain licorice's anti-tumor activity against cancerous melanomas in experimental animals. It's too early to deem the herb a treatment for such tumors, but that day may come.

Rx Recommendations

To help keep a minor wound from becoming infected, first wash it with soap and water, then sprinkle it with powdered licorice. The herb can also be used in this way on herpes sores, but check with your physician before doing so.

To help soothe a cough or sore throat, add a pinch of sweet-tasting licorice to any herbal beverage tea.

To make a decoction for canker sores, gently boil ½ teaspoon of powdered herb per cup of water for 10 minutes, then strain if you wish. Drink up to 2 cups a day, holding the liquid in your mouth for a while so it washes over the sores.

As a homemade tincture, take ½ to 1 teaspoon up to twice a day.

When using commercial preparations, follow the package directions.

Do not give licorice to children under age 2. For older children and adults over age 65, start with low-strength preparations and increase the strength if necessary.

The Safety Factor

In the United States, medical journals have been slow to pick up on licorice's therapeutic benefits, but they've jumped all over its potential to cause pseudoaldosteronism. The problem is real, and some people should not take the herb. In moderation, however, most people can use it safely.

There have been no reports of licorice sticks or powdered herb causing adverse reactions. According to the few dozen reports that have appeared in the world medical literature, problems have been caused by the highly concentrated licorice extracts used in some candies, laxatives, and tobacco products. The vast majority of these problems have resulted from overindulgence in licorice candies.

The *Journal of the American Medical Association* recounted the case of a man who ate 2 to 4 ounces of real licorice candies every day for 7 years. He developed weakness and hormone disturbances and required hospitalization. Another man ate more than a pound of licorice candy a day for 9 days. He, too, required hospital treatment. And a 15-year-old boy developed severely high blood pressure after eating more than a pound of licorice candy.

Clearly, consuming unusually large amounts of licorice can have adverse effects. For this reason, women who are pregnant or nursing and anyone with a history of diabetes, glaucoma, high blood pressure, stroke, or heart disease should be cautious about using the herb. It may raise blood pressure and cause potentially serious problems.

Healthy adults may take licorice, but they should familiarize themselves with overdose symptoms, which include headache, facial puffiness, ankle swelling, weakness, and lethargy.

Remember, though, that in the United States, most "licorice" candies are made with anise, not licorice. Real licorice is available in specialty shops.

Wise-Use Guidelines

Despite its well-publicized potential hazards, licorice is included in the FDA list of herbs generally regarded as safe. For adults who are not pregnant or nursing; do not have diabetes, glaucoma, high blood pressure, or a history of heart disease or stroke; and are not being treated for adrenal problems, licorice is considered safe when used cautiously for brief periods in the amounts typically recommended.

You should take medicinal amounts of licorice only in consultation with your doctor. If it causes minor discomfort, such as stomach upset or diarrhea, reduce the dosage or stop using it altogether. Let your doctor know if you experience unpleasant effects or if the symptoms for which you're using the herb do not improve significantly within 2 weeks.

Growing Information

Licorice is an erect, hardy perennial that reaches 3 to 7 feet. Small, alternate, inch-long leaflets and ½-inch purple midsummer flowers give the plant a graceful beauty

Mature plants have long taproots that send out creeping horizontal rhizomes (stolons), which are the source of other shoots and more branching roots. This creates a tangled mass of underground growth. Licorice roots have brown bark and sweet, juicy, yellow pulp.

Hard freezes kill licorice. It grows best in warm, sunny climates or in greenhouses in pots 48 inches deep. Greenhouse licorice often requires artificial light.

Licorice is usually propagated from root cuttings containing eyes. Plant them vertically about an inch below the soil surface, with 18-inch spacing. Beds should be rich, well-dug, well-manured, and well-drained. Once established, the herb can become extremely invasive, so be sure to keep it contained.

Licorice requires little care other than weeding. Expect slow growth the first year or two, then harvest rhizomes and roots during the fall of the third or fourth year. The year that you plan to harvest, pinch the flowers back. Flowering drains some of the roots' sweet sap.

Thick roots should be split to dry. Shade-dry the roots for 6 months. Licorice root keeps for a long time. Scientists who analyzed a sample from A.D. 756 found that even after 1,200 years, it still contained active compounds.

Marshmallow

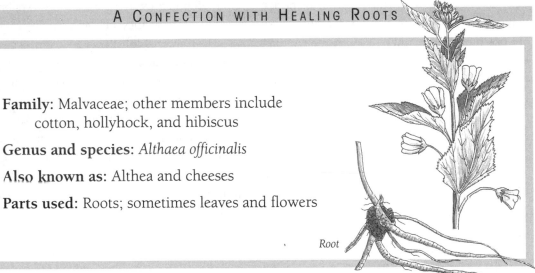

Family: Malvaceae; other members include cotton, hollyhock, and hibiscus

Genus and species: *Althaea officinalis*

Also known as: Althea and cheeses

Parts used: Roots; sometimes leaves and flowers

Root

Yes, marshmallow is the plant that inspired the pillowy white confections toasted over campfires. But today's marshmallows contain none of their namesake herb and bear no resemblance to the marshmallow sweets of old.

It's a shame that so few people know marshmallow as anything other than a candy. The herb has a healing tradition that dates back some 2,500 years.

Healing History

Marshmallow was a food before it became a medicine. The Book of Job (30:4) refers to a plant whose name translates as mallow (or possibly broom) that was eaten during famines. And during the Middle Ages, when crops failed, people boiled marshmallow roots, then fried them with onions in butter. Even today, back-

packing guides suggest the plant for wilderness foragers.

Marshmallow's history as a healing herb goes back to Hippocrates, who prescribed a root decoction to treat bruises and blood loss from wounds. Four hundred years later, the Greek physician Dioscorides recommended marshmallow root poultices for insect bites and stings. He also prescribed a decoction for toothache and vomiting and as an antidote to poisons.

The Romans loved marshmallow. The Roman naturalist Pliny enthused, "Whosoever shall take a spoonful of the mallows shall that day be free from all diseases."

Tenth-century Arab physicians applied marshmallow leaf poultices as a treatment for inflammation. Early European folk healers used marshmallow root both internally and externally to relieve toothache, sore throat, digestive upset, and urinary irritation.

Marshmallow was a special favorite of 17th-century English herbalist Nicholas Culpeper. "You may remember that not long since, there was a raging disease called the bloody flux . . . the college of physicians not knowing what to make of it," he wrote. "My son was taken with [it] and . . . the only thing I gave him was mallows bruised and boiled in milk and drunk. In two days (the blessing of God be upon it), it cured him. And I here, to show my thankfulness to God in communicating it to his creatures, leave it to posterity."

Culpeper recommended marshmallow roots, leaves, and seeds for their soothing action in treating "agues [fever] . . . torments of the belly . . . pleurisy, phthisis [tuberculosis], and other diseases of the chest . . . coughs, hoarseness . . . shortness of breath, wheezing, cramps . . . and swellings in women's breasts . . . and other offensive humors."

Early colonists introduced marshmallow into North America, and by the mid-19th century, it had found its way into the *U.S. Pharmacopoeia*, a standard drug reference. The Eclectic physicians of that time, the forerunners of today's naturopaths, prescribed the herb externally for "wounds, bruises, burns, scalds, and swellings of every kind." They also recommended a root decoction internally for colds, hoarseness, diarrhea, gonorrhea, gastrointestinal problems, and "nearly every affection of the kidney and bladder."

Contemporary herbalists generally limit their recommendations of marshmallow to respiratory and gastrointestinal irritation. Some tout the herb for urinary complaints.

Incidentally, you can thank the French for the spongy confection that bears the herb's name. They made the first candied marshmallow roots centuries ago. They peeled the root bark to expose the white pulp and boiled it to soften it and release its sweetness. Then they added sugar. The result: sweet, white, somewhat spongy sticks that over time evolved into today's campfire treat.

Therapeutic Uses

The spongy material in marshmallow roots is a fiber called mucilage. When mucilage comes in contact with water, it absorbs the liquid, swells, and forms a soothing, protective gel.

Wounds. Applied topically, the mucilage gel from marshmallow helps soothe and protect cuts, scrapes, wounds, and burns.

Respiratory problems. Taken internally, marshmallow helps relieve stomach upset and the respiratory rawness associated with sore throats, coughs, colds, flu, and bronchitis. Commission E, the expert panel that evaluates herbal medicines for the German counterpart of the FDA, approves marshmallow for treating coughs.

Enhanced immunity. In one experiment, marshmallow improved the ability of white blood cells to devour disease microbes, a process called phagocytosis. This suggests that marshmallow's traditional role in treating wounds and gastrointestinal infections may have been therapeutic as well as soothing.

Intriguing Possibility

One animal study has found that marshmallow root reduces levels of blood sugar (glucose), an indication that the herb may have value in managing diabetes.

Rx Recommendations

Prepare a sweet decoction to take advantage of marshmallow's soothing powers and possible infection-fighting abilities. Gently boil ½ to 1 teaspoon of chopped or crushed root per cup of water for 10 to 15 minutes. Drink up to 3 cups a day.

When using commercial preparations, follow the package directions.

For external use, chop the root very fine and add enough water to produce a gooey gel. Apply the gel directly to superficial wounds or sunburn. If you have a serious wound or sunburn, however, see your physician for advice regarding treatment.

You may give low-strength marshmallow decoctions cautiously to children under age 2.

The Safety Factor

The medical literature contains no reports of any harm from marshmallow. For adults who are not pregnant or nursing, the herb is considered safe in the amounts typically recommended.

You should use medicinal amounts of marshmallow only in consultation with your doctor. If it causes minor discomfort, such as stomach upset or diarrhea, reduce the dosage or stop using it altogether. Let your doctor know if you experience any unpleasant effects or if the symptoms for which you're using the herb do not improve significantly within 2 weeks.

Growing Information

You can guess from its name where marshmallow grows: in marshes, bogs, and damp meadows and along stream banks. The plant is a downy, erect, 5-foot perennial with a long taproot. The stems, which die back each autumn, are hairy and branching. The roundish, gray-green leaves, 1 to 3 inches long, are lobed, toothed, and covered with velvety hairs. Pink or white flowers bloom in summer. They are up to 2 inches across and give rise to round fruits called cheeses, which is one of the herb's names.

In moist soil under full sun, marshmallow is a hardy plant that grows easily from seeds, cuttings, or root divisions. Seeds should be planted in spring and root divisions in autumn. Thin them to 2-foot spacing.

Do not harvest roots from plants less than 2 years old. In autumn, when the topgrowth has died back, dig out mature roots and remove the lateral rootlets. Wash, peel, and dry them whole or in slices.

Maté

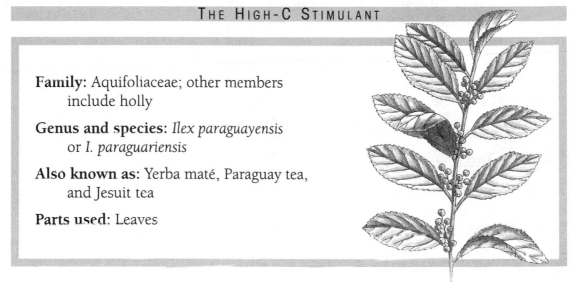

Family: Aquifoliaceae; other members include holly

Genus and species: *Ilex paraguayensis* or *I. paraguariensis*

Also known as: Yerba maté, Paraguay tea, and Jesuit tea

Parts used: Leaves

More than 300 years ago, Jesuit missionaries noticed that South American Indians ate a virtually all-meat diet. In spite of this, however, they didn't develop "sailor's sickness" (scurvy), which decimated European mariners who ate similar diets while at sea.

The Jesuits concluded that the Indians must be protected by the tea they drank out of cups made from calabash gourds. The missionaries dubbed it *maté*, from the Spanish for "gourd." They began cultivating the hollylike shrub and using its leathery leaves to produce the bitter tea.

Maté (pronounced *MAH-tay*), also called yerba maté or Paraguay tea, was introduced into the United States in the 1970s as a non-caffeinated coffee substitute. That claim was in error, because maté does contain caffeine. It also contains a surprisingly large number of nutrients, including vitamin C, several B vitamins, magnesium, calcium, iron, potassium, manganese, and zinc. Because of this, it's much more nutritious than other caffeine-containing herbal beverages (coffee, tea, cola, and cocoa).

Healing History

The Jesuits introduced maté to European colonists. Today, the herb is one of South America's favorite stimulants. In Argentina, Paraguay, and Uruguay, it's considerably more popular than either coffee or tea. More than 200 brands of maté are currently marketed in Argentina alone.

Argentinians consume 11 pounds of maté per capita annually. In Uruguay, that figure is 22 pounds. South American breads often have maté added. The herb is also a key ingredient in a popular South American soft drink.

South Americans consider maté not only a pleasant stimulant but also an appetite suppressant and a diuretic. Although there has been no scientific research to back it up, maté has a longstanding reputation as a digestive aid. Argentinian cowboys (gauchos) sometimes live on just meat and maté, like the Indians of old.

Therapeutic Uses

A 6-ounce cup of maté contains about 50 milligrams of caffeine, about as much as a cup of tea or a can of cola. By comparison, a cup of instant coffee has about 65 milligrams of caffeine; a cup of brewed coffee has 100 to 150 milligrams. (For details on the health benefits of caffeine, see Coffee on page 144.)

Fatigue. Because maté contains only one-third to one-half as much caffeine as a comparable-size cup of brewed coffee, its effects would be only a fraction as intense. On the other hand, it's still a stimulant. Commission E, the expert panel that evaluates herbal medicines for the German counterpart of the FDA, approves maté as a treatment for fatigue.

Colds. The Jesuits were right about maté preventing scurvy. The herb is fairly high in vitamin C, which also helps treat the common cold. Drinking maté when you have a cold gives you an extra dose of C.

Premenstrual syndrome (PMS). Diuretics help relieve the bloated feeling caused by premenstrual fluid retention. Women bothered by PMS might try maté during the uncomfortable days just before their periods.

Rx Recommendations

Maté has a distinctive odor that some people find offensive. Others get used to it and actually come to enjoy it.

For a pleasantly bitter infusion, use 1 teaspoon of dried crushed herb per cup of boiling water and steep for 10 minutes. Add honey and lemon to taste, if you like. Drink up to 3 cups a day.

When using commercial preparations, follow the package directions.

Do not give maté to children under age 2. For older children and adults over age 65, start with low-strength preparations and increase the strength if necessary.

The Safety Factor

Caffeine is classically addictive. Large amounts may cause significant harm. Because, cup for cup, maté contains less caffeine than coffee, however, it should cause fewer problems. (For a more detailed discussion of caffeine's safety, see page 148.)

Maté also contains tannins, which have both pro- and anti-cancer action. A Uruguayan study, published in the *Journal of the National Cancer Institute*, found that heavy maté users have an increased risk of esophageal cancer. The average Uruguayan consumes 22 pounds of the herb a year, so it's anyone's guess how much *heavy* users consume.

This finding appears to have no real significance to Americans who drink only an occasional cup of maté tea. Nevertheless, people who have been diagnosed with esophageal cancer should not use the herb.

Wise-Use Guidelines

For adults who are not pregnant or nursing, are not taking other substances or medications containing caffeine, and do not have esophageal cancer, maté is considered relatively safe in the amounts typically recommended.

You should use medicinal amounts of maté only in consultation with your doctor. If it causes minor discomfort, such as stomach upset or diarrhea, reduce the dosage or stop taking it altogether. Let your doctor know if you experience unpleasant effects or if the symptoms for which you're using the herb do not improve significantly within 2 weeks.

Growing Information

Maté is not cultivated in the United States. In South America, the plant grows wild near streams, but it is also extensively cultivated, especially in Argentina.

Maté is a perennial shrub with spineless, oval, toothed, leathery leaves. Its fruits (berries) are red, black, or yellow and about the size of black peppercorns.

Meadowsweet

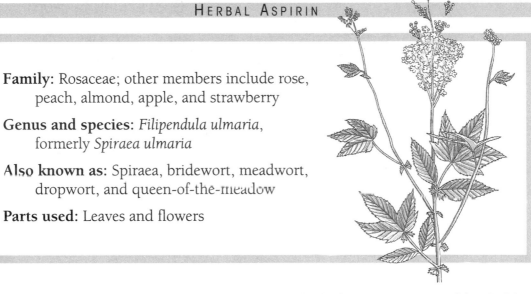

Family: Rosaceae; other members include rose, peach, almond, apple, and strawberry

Genus and species: *Filipendula ulmaria,* formerly *Spiraea ulmaria*

Also known as: Spiraea, bridewort, meadwort, dropwort, and queen-of-the-meadow

Parts used: Leaves and flowers

It's rare to find a medicine cabinet that doesn't contain aspirin. It's even rarer to find anyone who knows that we owe the word *aspirin* to the beautiful, aromatic meadowsweet.

Healing History

During the Middle Ages, meadowsweet's delicate almond fragrance made it a popular air freshener, or "strewing herb." It was scattered around homes to minimize odors at a time when people rarely bathed and when farm animals often shared human living quarters.

Early British herbalist John Gerard wrote of the herb, "The leaves and floures of Meadowsweet farre excelle all other strowing herbs for to decke up houses . . . for the smell thereof delighteth the senses." One fan of meadowsweet as a strewing herb was none other than Queen Elizabeth I, who had the flowers spread around her living quarters.

The herb's sweet aroma and lovely blossoms earned it a place in bridal bouquets, hence its name bridewort (*wort* is Old English for "plant"). Meadowsweet was also used to flavor mead, a fermented beverage made from honey and fruit juices, hence another of its names, meadwort.

Gerard documented meadowsweet's contributions to healing: "The floures boiled in wine and drunke do take away fits of ague [fever]. The distilled water of the floures dropped into the eies taketh away burning and itching thereof and cleareth the sight." Later, herbalists recommended meadowsweet to treat diarrhea, fevers, arthritis, "falling sickness" (epilepsy), and respiratory ailments.

Colonists introduced the herb into the Western Hemisphere. America's 19th-century Eclectic physicians, forerunners of today's naturopaths, considered meadowsweet "an excellent astringent . . . in diarrhea. [It] is less offensive to the stomach than other agents of its kind." They also prescribed it for menstrual cramps and vaginal discharge.

Contemporary herbalists recommend meadowsweet for colds and flu; nausea, heartburn, childhood diarrhea, and other digestive ailments; muscle aches; and congestive heart failure.

From Salicin to Aspirin

In 1839, a German chemist discovered that meadowsweet's flower buds contain salicin, the same chemical that had been isolated from white willow bark 11 years earlier. Salicin has powerful pain-relieving (analgesic), fever-reducing, and anti-inflammatory properties.

Unfortunately, salicin (and its close chemical relatives, notably salicylic acid) can also cause potentially serious side effects, including stomach upset, nausea, diarrhea, bleeding in the stomach, and ringing in the ears (tinnitus). In high doses, it can even cause respiratory paralysis and death.

Chemists began tinkering with salicin and salicylic acid, hoping to preserve the benefits while minimizing the hazards. In 1853, German chemists added a molecular acetyl group to a meadowsweet extract and synthesized acetylsalicylic acid.

"Acetylsalicylic acid" proved to be quite a mouthful, so the scientists who created the compound combined the "a-" from *acetyl* with "-spirin," a variation of meadowsweet's former Latin name, *Spiraea*, to create *aspirin*.

The new compound provided greater relief from fever, pain, and inflammation than either salicin or salicylic acid. Unfortunately, it still had its predecessors' side effects, which disappointed its creators. They published news of aspirin's development in an obscure German medical journal, and the drug was promptly forgotten for almost 50 years.

In the late 1890s, a German chemist, Felix Hoffman, became upset that his father's rheumatoid arthritis medication provided so little relief and so much stomach upset. So Hoffman, who worked at the Fredrich Bayer pharmaceutical company, began combing the journals for leads on a better arthritis treatment. He came across the old report about aspirin and decided to make a batch of the drug himself. As the story goes, he gave some to his father, who pronounced aspirin effective, with fewer side effects than the medications he'd been taking.

At first, Hoffman had a tough time selling aspirin to his superiors at Bayer. Eventually, though, they saw its potential. In 1899, they introduced acetylsalicylic acid in Europe and North America under the brand name Aspirin.

Aspirin quickly became the household drug of choice for relief of pain, fever, and inflammation. Later, in one of the earliest U.S. trademark-protection battles, Bayer lost its trademark to the name Aspirin. The court ruled that the word had passed into general usage. Ever since, the company has promoted its product as Bayer Aspirin.

Therapeutic Uses

While meadowsweet gave us aspirin, the herb can't match all of the pharmaceutical's therapeutic effects. Still, it has some impressive benefits of its own.

Pain, fever, and inflammation. Meadowsweet does not pack aspirin's pain-relieving, fever-reducing, and anti-inflammatory punch.

The herb has a small amount of salicylate, so even strong infusions may not have much effect. Tinctures provide more salicylate and greater relief.

On the other hand, meadowsweet is less likely to produce aspirin's major side effect, stomach upset. In fact, a few laboratory trials have shown that the herb protects experimental animals from aspirin-induced stomach ulcers. This finding supports the Eclectics' observation that meadowsweet is gentle to the stomach. At least one animal study, however, suggests that meadowsweet increases the risk of ulcers when given with drugs that cause them.

If you'd rather take an herbal preparation than a pharmaceutical, especially if aspirin upsets your stomach, you can try meadowsweet for headache, arthritis, menstrual cramps, low-grade fever, and other types of pain and inflammation. The herb may help. And if it's taken in combination with aspirin or another pain reliever, it may let you reduce your dose of the drug.

Colds. Because meadowsweet helps relieve pain and fever, Commission E, the expert panel that evaluates herbal medicines for the German counterpart of the FDA, approves the herb as a treatment for the common cold.

Diarrhea. Meadowsweet contains astringent tannins that can help relieve diarrhea. In addition, a European study found the herb to be effective against *Shigella dysenteriae*, one of the bacteria that cause infectious diarrhea. This finding lends some credence to the herb's traditional use for this condition.

Urinary tract infections. Meadowsweet is active against *Escherichia coli*, the bacteria most likely to cause urinary tract infections.

One report describes the herb as a urinary antiseptic.

Intriguing Possibilities

A great deal of research has shown that low-dose aspirin (one-half to one standard tablet a day) helps prevent the blood clots that trigger heart attack and most strokes. Meadowsweet's effect on heart disease and stroke has not been well-researched, but a few animal studies have determined that the herb has anticoagulant (blood-thinning) properties, so it's likely that it provides similar cardiovascular protection.

Aspirin has also been shown to reduce the risk of digestive tract cancers, notably colon cancer. To date, no studies have linked meadowsweet to reduced risk of these conditions, but again, it seems reasonable to assume that the herb may offer similar benefits.

One study revealed that salicin reduces blood sugar (glucose) levels, suggesting that meadowsweet may be of value in managing diabetes.

Rx Recommendations

To prepare a pleasantly astringent infusion, use 1 to 2 teaspoons of dried, powdered herb per cup of boiling water. Steep for 10 minutes, then strain if you wish. Drink up to 3 cups a day.

As a homemade tincture, take ½ to 1 teaspoon up to three times a day.

When using commercial preparations, follow the package directions.

Do not give meadowsweet to children under age 2 or to children under age 16 who have colds, flu, or chickenpox. For other children and adults over age 65, start with low-strength preparations and increase the strength if necessary.

The Safety Factor

Aspirin is a well-documented asthma trigger. Research has shown that meadowsweet has the same effect. For this reason, people with asthma or any aspirin sensitivity should not take meadowsweet.

In children under age 16 who have fevers from colds, flu, or chickenpox, aspirin is associated with Reye's syndrome, a rare but potentially fatal condition. Meadowsweet has never been linked to Reye's syndrome, but because it's related to aspirin, children who have fevers from those illnesses should not take it.

European animal studies suggest that meadowsweet may stimulate uterine contractions. The herb has no history of use as a menstruation promoter, but because aspirin has been associated with an increased risk of birth defects, women who are pregnant or trying to conceive should not take meadowsweet.

Wise-Use Guidelines

The FDA lists meadowsweet as an herb of undefined safety. For adults who are not pregnant or nursing; do not have ulcers, gastritis, other chronic gastrointestinal conditions, or clotting conditions; and are not taking other medications containing aspirin or salicylates, the herb

is considered safe when used in the amounts typically recommended.

You should take medicinal amounts of meadowsweet only in consultation with your doctor. If it causes minor discomfort, such as stomach upset or ringing in the ears, reduce the dosage or stop using it altogether. Let your doctor know if you experience any unpleasant effects or if the symptoms for which you're using the herb do not improve significantly within 2 weeks.

Growing Information

Meadowsweet is an eye-catching perennial with stems that reach 2 to 6 feet. It has elmlike leaves and large clusters of small, coiled white or pink flowers that bloom throughout summer and have a fragrant, sweet almond aroma. The flower clusters droop, hence the common name dropwort. The plant stands taller and has more striking flowers than most other meadow plants, hence another of its common names, queen-of-the-meadow.

Meadowsweet grows wild from Newfoundland to Ohio in marshes, along stream banks, and in moist forests and meadows. It is best propagated from cuttings of its creeping underground perennial stem (rhizome).

Meadowsweet does best in rich, moist, well-drained soil under partial shade. Harvest the leaves and flowers when the plant is in bloom.

Milk Thistle

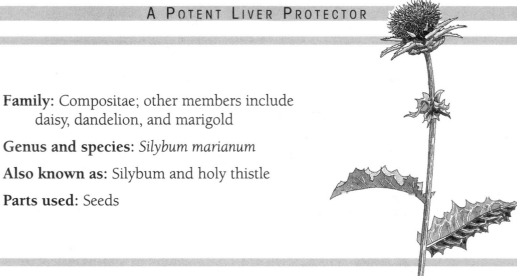

Family: Compositae; other members include daisy, dandelion, and marigold

Genus and species: *Silybum marianum*

Also known as: Silybum and holy thistle

Parts used: Seeds

Milk thistle has a longstanding reputation as a liver protector. Its use as a treatment for liver conditions dates back more than 2,000 years.

Homeopaths use a microdose of the herb to treat liver disorders, gallstones, and varicose veins.

Healing History

While the ancient Greek physician Dioscorides recommended milk thistle seed as a treatment for snakebite, others recognized the herb's potential as a liver tonic. The 1st-century Roman naturalist Pliny wrote that the herb's juice helped "carry off bile." And influential 17th-century British herbalist Nicholas Culpeper endorsed milk thistle as a treatment for jaundice, the yellowing of the skin and eyes caused by liver disease.

America's 19th-century Eclectic physicians, forerunners of today's naturopaths, prescribed milk thistle to treat liver conditions as well as varicose veins, menstrual complaints, and kidney problems.

Therapeutic Uses

In 1968, German researchers isolated three liver-protective compounds from milk thistle seeds: silibinin, silidianin, and silicristin. Collectively, these compounds are known as silymarin.

Silymarin benefits the liver in several ways. It binds tightly to the receptors on liver cell membranes that allow toxins in, thus locking them out. It's a powerful antioxidant, protecting liver cells from the chemical process responsible for a great deal of harm in the body. It spurs the repair of damaged liver cells, and it stimulates the immune system.

Medicine needs a good liver protector. Many conditions attack the liver, notably cirrhosis, mushroom poisoning, and hepatitis A, B, and C. Unfortunately, mainstream medicine doesn't have much to offer people with liver disease.

For hepatitis, doctors advise resting and refraining from behavior that could further damage the liver, such as drinking alcohol or taking drugs. For mushroom poisoning, conventional treatment often fails, with fatal consequences. For cirrhosis, doctors can only offer relief from complications.

Research has shown that milk thistle extract can help treat all of these conditions safely and effectively. In fact, Commission E, the expert panel that evaluates herbal medicines for the German counterpart of the FDA, approves milk thistle extract as a treatment for liver conditions.

Hepatitis. Several European studies have found that compared with hepatitis patients who did not receive silymarin, those who did recovered more quickly. In an Italian study, 20 people with hepatitis were given either medically inactive placebos or silymarin. Those taking the herb showed greater normalization of liver function.

Mushroom poisoning. Amanita mushrooms are called death caps for good reason: They contain a potent liver poison. Every year, the news media issue reports of serious illness and death among people who pick wild mushrooms without knowing how to distinguish the Amanita from edible species.

Without treatment, the death rate from Amanita poisoning is around 50 percent. Standard medical treatment (activated charcoal) saves some lives, but the death rate may still be as high as 40 percent. With silymarin, the odds of survival are much greater.

Silymarin works by blocking the Amanita poison from entering liver cells. In one German study, 60 people were treated with silymarin after accidentally eating death caps, and none died. In another German study, this one involving 205 people with Amanita poisoning, 189 received standard medical care and 16 received silymarin. Of those given standard care, 24 percent died. Of those given silymarin, none died.

In a multicenter European study, researchers looked at 220 cases of Amanita poisoning in which the patients had been treated with silymarin. The death rate was 13 percent, well below the rate associated with conventional medical treatment.

Cirrhosis. Several studies have determined that milk thistle helps stabilize liver function in people with cirrhosis. In one study, 170 people—91 of whom had alcoholic cirrhosis (the others had cirrhosis from other causes)—were given either placebos or 200 milligrams of milk thistle extract three times a day. Four years later, 31 members of the placebo group had died of liver disease. In the milk thistle group, there were only 18 deaths.

For another study, Scandinavian researchers recruited 97 heavy drinkers who had liver damage but not cirrhosis. Forty-seven of the study participants were given silymarin for 4 weeks. Compared with those taking placebos, those taking silymarin showed significant decreases in several liver enzymes that had been abnormally high. The researchers concluded that the people taking silymarin had greater potential for regaining normal liver function.

Drug-induced liver damage. Alcohol is not the only drug that can harm the liver. In large-enough doses, even everyday medications like acetaminophen can do damage.

In one laboratory trial, silymarin protected

the livers of animals that were given large doses of acetaminophen. In other studies, the compound has prevented the liver damage associated with antibiotics, antidepressants, and antipsychotic medications.

Toxin-induced liver damage. Research has shown that silymarin can minimize the damage associated with long-term exposure to several toxic industrial chemicals. In one study, workers with liver damage from the chemicals toluene and xylene took 140 milligrams of silymarin three times a day for a month. The treatment produced substantial reductions in liver enzymes that had been at abnormally high levels.

Intriguing Possibilities

Some research suggests that silymarin lowers cholesterol and may reduce the risk of complications from diabetes.

Rx Recommendations

Silymarin is not very soluble in water, so infusions and decoctions don't supply very high doses of the compound. Neither does wild milk thistle.

German plant scientists have bred a high-silymarin variety of milk thistle that produces a standardized extract. A 200-milligram dose of the extract contains 140 milligrams of silymarin. This dose, taken in tablets or capsules three or four times a day, has become the standard in milk thistle research.

Look for a standardized extract containing 70 percent silymarin and use it according to the package directions.

The Safety Factor

If you have liver disease, talk to your doctor before taking milk thistle. While the herb is generally regarded as safe, there have been a few reports linking it with stomach upset or a laxative effect. Allergic reactions are also possible.

If you suspect that you have mushroom poisoning, seek emergency medical care immediately.

Wise-Use Guidelines

For adults who are not pregnant or nursing, milk thistle is considered safe in the amounts typically recommended.

If the herb causes minor discomfort, such as stomach upset, reduce the dosage or stop taking it altogether. Let your doctor know if you experience any unpleasant effects or if the symptoms for which you're using the herb do not improve significantly within 2 weeks.

Growing Information

Native to Kashmir in India-Pakistan, milk thistle is a weedy plant that now grows throughout the temperate world. It typically reaches 5 to 10 feet and produces large, prickly leaves. When broken, the leaves and stems exude milky sap, hence the name milk thistle. The plant produces reddish purple flowers that are ringed with sharp spines. The flowers resemble miniature artichokes.

Like its close botanical relative, artichoke, milk thistle was once grown in Europe as a vegetable. Backpacking guides still suggest that back-country foragers steam the prickly young leaves and stalks, which taste similar to spinach. Young leaves may also be eaten in salads.

Mistletoe

Family: Loranthaceae; all members are called mistletoe

Genus and species: *Viscum album* (European); *Phoradendron serotinum* or *P. tomentosum* (American)

Also known as: Viscum, herbe de la croix, and lignum crucis

Parts used: Leaves, fruits (berries), and young twigs

Mistletoe is best known for the sprigs under which people kiss at Christmas, a custom with an ironically gruesome origin. As a healing herb, mistletoe is also fraught with irony. One scientific authority calls it "gentle . . . [and] nontoxic." Others call it poisonous and insist that "all parts of the plant should be regarded as toxic."

The fact is, mistletoe's purported toxicity has been overstated. Europeans have used it extensively—and safely—to help treat high blood pressure and cancer.

Healing History

We owe mistletoe's association with kissing to Norse mythology. Balder, god of peace, was slain by an arrow made from mistletoe. When his parents, god-king Odin and goddess-queen Frigga, restored him to life, they gave the plant to the goddess of love and decreed that anyone who passed under it should receive a kiss.

Early Christians believed that mistletoe was a freestanding tree during Jesus' time and that its wood was used to make the cross of the Crucifixion. God punished the plant for its role in the Crucifixion by turning it into a parasite. It was because of this story that mistletoe came to be called *lignum crucis* ("wood of the cross") in Latin and *herbe de la croix* in French.

Hippocrates prescribed mistletoe for disorders of the spleen. Most other ancient physicians, particularly Dioscorides and Galen, advised limiting the herb to external use, foreshadowing the current controversy over its safety.

A French medical text from 1682 recommended mistletoe for "falling sickness" (epilepsy). Some herbals still prescribe it for convulsions (ironically, high doses may cause convulsions).

Seventeenth-century English herbalist Nicholas Culpeper reiterated Hippocrates' recommendation, asserting that mistletoe "doth mollify hardness of the spleen, and helpeth old sores." He also advocated mistletoe for "falling sickness and apoplexy [stroke]," and advised wearing a sprig around the neck to "remedy witchcraft."

In the United States, several Native American tribes used American mistletoe to induce abortion and to stimulate contractions during childbirth.

America's 19th-century Eclectic physicians, forerunners of today's naturopaths, recommended both European and American mistletoe for epilepsy, typhoid fever, and dropsy (congestive heart failure). They also prescribed the herb for "hysterical" (gynecological) complaints, recommending it for relief of menstrual cramps, menstruation promotion, and treatment of postpartum hemorrhage. But the Eclectic text *King's American Dispensatory* (1898) warned that large amounts "possess toxic properties. Vomiting, catharsis, muscular spasms, coma, convulsions, and death have been reported from eating the leaves and berries."

Somewhere along the line, herbalists came to believe that European and American mistletoe had opposite effects. European mistletoe was reputed to reduce blood pressure and soothe the digestive tract, while the American variety was said to raise blood pressure and stimulate uterine and intestinal contractions.

Contemporary herbalists are divided on mistletoe. Some say the two varieties have opposite effects, while others make no distinction between them. Some consider the herb calming, asserting that it reduces blood pressure, quiets the heart, and relaxes the nervous system. Others believe that it raises blood pressure and stimulates uterine contractions. Some describe the plant as poisonous. Others deem it safe.

Koreans use mistletoe tea to treat colds, muscle weakness, and arthritis. Chinese physicians prescribe the dried inner stems as a laxative, digestive aid, sedative, and uterine relaxant during pregnancy.

Therapeutic Uses

Despite the traditional belief that European and American mistletoe have opposite actions, science has determined that the plants contain similar active chemicals and have similar effects. Mistletoe has the ability to slow the pulse, stimulate gastrointestinal and uterine contractions, and lower blood pressure.

Blood pressure regulation. While mistletoe contains substances that both raise and lower blood pressure, those that have a lowering effect predominate.

In Germany, where herbal medicine is considerably more mainstream than in the United States, mistletoe extract is an ingredient in many medications prescribed to reduce blood pressure. German medical herbalist Rudolph Fritz Weiss, M.D., writes, "Anyone who treats hypertension [high blood pressure] will confirm that mistletoe by mouth has definite benefit. . . . For a gentle antihypertensive drug that is well tolerated . . . and nontoxic in the usual dosage . . . mistletoe is the drug of choice."

High blood pressure is a serious condition that requires medical supervision. Use the herb only in consultation with your doctor.

Enhanced immunity. In one experiment, cells damaged by x-ray radiation regenerated more quickly when exposed to a commercial mistletoe extract (the Swiss drug Iscador). Injected preparations of mistletoe improve immune function in people with AIDS.

Cancer. Studies going back 30 years show that when injected, mistletoe preparations enhance immune activity against various types of cancer. In this way, the herb slows and sometimes even reverses tumor growth and extends survival times.

When mistletoe is combined with radiation and chemotherapy, the mainstream treatments are better-tolerated. What's more, in clinical trials involving cancer patients, mistletoe improved general well-being, increased appetite, reduced pain, and normalized sleep. Dr. Weiss writes, "The great advantage offered by mistletoe extracts is that unlike [other chemotherapeutic] drugs, their immunostimulant and tonic effects are nontoxic and well tolerated."

Commission E, the expert panel that evaluates herbal medicines for the German counterpart of the FDA, approves mistletoe as a complementary cancer therapy to be used in combination with mainstream treatments.

In the United States, mistletoe has not been seriously studied as a cancer treatment because of the herb's reputation as a poison. Ironically, many approved cancer drugs are also toxic.

Rx Recommendations

You should take mistletoe only under the close supervision of a physician who has knowledge of herbs.

To treat high blood pressure, Dr. Weiss recommends a tea made from equal parts of mistletoe, hawthorn, and lemon balm. "Infuse 2 teaspoons of the mixture for 5 to 10 minutes," he writes "Take 1 cup in the morning and 1 at night." Other herbalists recommend 1 cup a day of an infusion made with 1 teaspoon of freshly dried plant material steeped in 1 cup of boiling water for 10 minutes.

As a homemade tincture, the recommended dose for blood pressure control is five drops daily.

When using commercial preparations, follow the package directions.

Do not give mistletoe to children. It may also have adverse effects in the elderly.

The Safety Factor

Most authorities on this side of the Atlantic scoff at Dr. Weiss's suggestion that mistletoe is gentle, nontoxic, and well-tolerated. The FDA has deemed the herb unsafe and has not approved any mistletoe preparation as a treatment for any disease. In *Natural Product Medicine*, pharmacognosists Ara Der Marderosian, Ph.D., and Lawrence Liberti speak for most American experts when they write, "Mistletoe's use should be discouraged because of the documented toxicity associated with ingestion of all parts of the plant."

How toxic is it, really? The Eclectics reported coma, convulsions, and death from the ingestion of large doses of mistletoe leaves and berries. Since then, there have been scattered reports of fatalities from consuming the berries or beverages made from them.

On the other hand, a 1986 review of more than 300 cases of mistletoe ingestion, published in *Annals of Emergency Medicine*, found no deaths associated with the herb. A majority of those who consumed the plant—typically its berries—developed no symptoms of poisoning.

In a 1996 review of 11 cases of mistletoe ingestion (amounts up to 20 berries), researchers affiliated with the Kentucky Regional Poison Control Center reported generally minor stomach upset, except in two infants who suffered more severe reactions. There were no deaths. The researchers concluded that ingesting mistletoe causes "infrequent symptoms, and in all but one case would not require direct medical supervision."

Based on these findings, it would appear that mistletoe's reputation for toxicity is undeserved. Nonetheless, keep the herb away from young children.

Mistletoe contains a chemical called tyramine that may stimulate uterine contractions. For this reason, pregnant women should not use the herb, except possibly at term and only under the supervision of a physician to induce labor.

Mistletoe's abortion-inducing dose is close to its fatal dose. It should never be used to terminate pregnancy.

People who are taking MAO inhibitor antidepressants such as isocarboxazid (Marplan), phenelzine sulfate (Nardil), and tranylcypromine (Parnate) should avoid mistletoe. Interaction between the herb and the drugs may cause a serious elevation in blood pressure.

People with heart disease or a history of stroke should not take mistletoe, as the herb may slow the heart rate.

Wise-Use Guidelines

You may use mistletoe cautiously in low doses, but only under the supervision of a medical professional. For adults who are not pregnant, nursing, or taking MAO inhibitors or blood pressure medications, the herb is believed to be relatively safe when taken in small amounts for brief periods.

If mistletoe causes minor discomfort, such as stomach upset or diarrhea, reduce the dosage or stop using it altogether. Let your doctor know if you experience unpleasant effects or if the symptoms for which you're using the herb do not improve significantly within 2 weeks.

If you experience any symptoms of toxicity—nausea, vomiting, diarrhea, headache, decreased heart rate, hallucinations, muscle spasms, or convulsions—seek emergency treatment immediately.

Growing Information

Mistletoe is a parasitic shrub that grows in trees, rooting into their bark. Both European and American mistletoe are branching, woody evergreens that live on a large number of trees. The European herb has thin, leathery, tongue-shaped 2-inch leaves. The American variety also has leathery leaves, but they are broader and up to 3 inches long. Both plants produce small, sticky white berries, which contain single seeds.

Mistletoe is well-adapted to its aerial existence. Its sticky white berries attract birds, which carry them to perches in other trees. The birds eat some but drop others, which stick to the tree bark. Within a few days, the seeds inside newly "planted" mistletoe berries produce tiny roots, which bore their way into the host tree and establish new plants.

Mistletoe is gathered from the wild, not cultivated, although some crafters of mistletoe Christmas products reportedly "plant" the sticky seeds by inserting them into the bark of host trees.

Motherwort

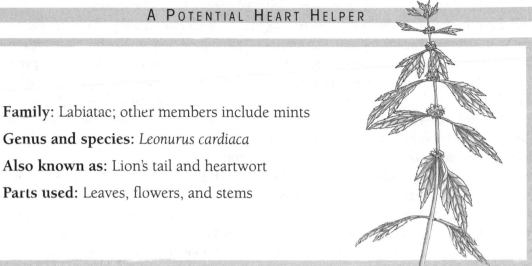

Family: Labiatae; other members include mints

Genus and species: *Leonurus cardiaca*

Also known as: Lion's tail and heartwort

Parts used: Leaves, flowers, and stems

The word *wort* is Old English for "plant," but the name *motherwort* is somewhat misleading. The herb is more likely to prevent motherhood than to promote it.

Also, despite one of the herb's popular names, lion's tail, motherwort won't strengthen the lion-hearted. In fact, it's more apt to turn lions into lambs.

Healing History

The ancient Greeks and Romans used motherwort to treat both physical and emotional problems of the heart—namely, palpitations and depression.

In ancient China, motherwort was reputed to promote longevity. According to legend, a youth who had committed a minor crime was banished from his village to a remote valley with a spring surrounded by motherwort. Supposedly, he lived to be 300.

In Europe, motherwort first gained prominence as a treatment for cattle diseases. Sixteenth-century British herbalist John Gerard called it "a remedy against certain diseases in cattell . . . and for that husbandmen much desire it." Gerard also recommended the herb for "infirmities of the heart."

Seventeenth-century English herbalist Nicholas Culpeper wrote, "There is no better herb to take melancholy vapors from the heart . . . and make a merry, cheerful soul." While Culpeper viewed motherwort primarily as an antidepressant, he also said, "It is . . . of much use in trembling of the heart [palpitations], and faintings, and swoonings, from whence it took the name cardiaca. . . . It took the name motherwort [because] it settles mothers' wombs . . . and is a wonderful help to women in their sore travail [delivery]. . . . It also provoketh women's courses [menstruation]."

As the centuries passed, herbalists used motherwort in contradictory ways, both to relax the uterus during pregnancy and after childbirth and to stimulate menstruation and labor. Eventually, it came to be known as a uterine stimulant.

Colonists introduced motherwort into North America. The 19th-century Eclectic physicians, forerunners of today's naturopaths, recommended the herb as a menstruation promoter and an aid to expelling the afterbirth. They also prescribed it as a tranquilizer for "morbid nervous excitement, and all diseases with restlessness [and] disturbed sleep." The Eclectics did not consider motherwort a heart remedy.

Contemporary herbalists recommend motherwort as a tranquilizer, a women's health tonic, and a remedy for heart palpitations and delayed or suppressed menstruation.

Therapeutic Uses

Until recently, scientists dismissed motherwort as useless. Studies have indicated, however, that the ancients who named the herb cardiaca may have been onto something.

Heart disease. In China, laboratory studies have shown that motherwort helps relax heart cells. Other Chinese research suggests that it helps prevent the blood clots that trigger heart attack. Russian researchers have also found that the herb contains compounds that reduce blood pressure.

These findings are preliminary, but they lend credence to the ancient view that motherwort has a general tonic effect on the heart.

Commission E, the expert panel that evaluates herbal medicines for the German counterpart of the FDA, approves motherwort as a treatment for "nervous cardiac disorders."

In generally healthy adults, occasional heart palpitations are usually no cause for alarm. If the palpitations are frequent and persistent, however, they may be a sign of a heart rhythm disturbance (cardiac arrhythmia), a potentially serious condition that requires professional attention. If you experience frequent palpitations, consult your physician.

If you have high blood pressure or heart disease and would like to incorporate motherwort into your treatment plan, do so only in consultation with your physician.

Insomnia and anxiety. German studies have determined that motherwort has mild sedative action. It may be effective in relieving insomnia and anxiety.

Women's health concerns. Not many tranquilizers are also uterine stimulants, but motherwort contains a compound called leonurine that encourages uterine contractions. This lends support to the herb's traditional role in childbirth and menstruation promotion.

Women who are trying to conceive or are pregnant should not take motherwort, except possibly at term and only under the supervision of a physician to help stimulate labor. For other women, the herb may help induce periods.

Rx Recommendations

To make a possibly tranquilizing, uterine-stimulating, blood-pressure-lowering infusion, use 1 to 2 teaspoons of dried herb per cup of boiling water. Steep for 10 minutes, then strain.

Drink up to 2 cups a day, a tablespoon at a time. Motherwort tastes very bitter; you can add sugar, honey, and lemon, or mix it into an herbal beverage tea to improve the flavor.

As a homemade tincture, take ½ to 1 teaspoon up to twice a day.

When using commercial preparations, follow the package directions.

Do not give motherwort to children under age 2. For older children and adults over age 65, start with low-strength preparations and increase the strength if necessary.

The Safety Factor

Because of motherwort's possible anti-clotting effect, people who are taking anticoagulants (blood thinners)—whether medications (including aspirin), herbs (garlic and willow bark), or supplements (vitamin E)—should not use it. People with clotting disorders should also avoid motherwort.

Some people develop rashes from contact with the plant.

Wise-Use Guidelines

The FDA lists motherwort as an herb of undefined safety. For adults who are not pregnant or nursing, do not have clotting disorders, and are not taking anticoagulant, sedative, or heart or blood pressure medications, motherwort is considered safe when used in the amounts typically recommended.

You should use medicinal amounts of motherwort only in consultation with your doctor. If it causes minor discomforts, such as stomach upset or diarrhea, reduce the dosage or stop using it altogether. Let your doctor know if you experience unpleasant effects or if the symptoms for which you're using the herb do not improve significantly within 2 weeks.

Growing Information

Motherwort's perennial root gives rise to stout, square stems that are tinged with red or violet and grow to 4 feet. The plant's lower leaves are sharply lobed, like maple leaves. Its upper leaves are narrow and toothed. It also produces whorls of small white, pink, or red flowers, which bloom in summer.

This herb grows so easily that it may become a pest. Plant seeds in spring and thin seedlings to 12-inch spacing. Motherwort prefers rich, moist, well-drained soil and full sun, but it tolerates considerably less ideal conditions. Harvest the entire plant after the flowers blossom.

Mullein

Family: Scrophulariaceae; other members
include figwort, foxglove, and eyebright

Genus and species: *Verbascum thapsus*

Also known as: Candlewick plant, torches,
velvet dock, flannel plant, feltwort, Aaron's
rod, shepherd's staff, and lungwort

Parts used: Leaves, flowers, and roots

Mullein (its name rhymes with *sullen*) grows everywhere and is hard to miss. Despite this, however, few who encounter the velvet-leafed weed with its rodlike stem and striking yellow flowers appreciate its place in herbal healing as a treatment for cough.

Healing History

When dried, mullein burns readily. Before the introduction of cotton, mullein's leaves and stems were used by the ancients as candle wicks, earning the herb the name candlewick plant. The dried stems and flowers were dipped in suet to make them burn longer, hence another of the herb's popular names, torches.

Ancient cultures around the world considered mullein a magical protector against witchcraft and evil spirits. Like other herbs used in magic, mullein has a long history as a healer. Its botanical family name, Scrophulariaceae, is derived from *scrofula*, an old term for chronically swollen lymph glands. The condition was later identified as a form of tuberculosis.

The 1st-century Greek physician Dioscorides prescribed a decoction of mullein root in wine as a treatment for "lask and fluxes of the belly" (diarrhea). During the Middle Ages, the French used the herb to treat malandre, an animal disease that causes boils on horses' necks. *Malandre* eventually became *malen* and finally, *mullein*.

Early on, the herb gained a reputation as a respiratory remedy, which endures to this day. In ancient India, Ayurvedic physicians prescribed mullein for cough. Seventeenth-century English herbalist Nicholas Culpeper wrote that gargling a mullein decoction "easeth toothache . . . and old cough." His contemporary, herbalist William Coles, wrote that farmers "give it their cattle against cough."

Colonists introduced mullein into North America, and Native Americans quickly adopted the herb for coughs, bronchitis, and asthma. The accepted way of taking mullein in early America seems ridiculous today: People smoked it.

America's 19th-century Eclectic physicians, forerunners of today's naturopaths, viewed mullein as a diuretic to treat water retention and as a stomach and respiratory soother, with mild pain-relieving and tranquilizing action. The Eclectic text *King's American Dispensatory* (1898) asserted, "Upon the upper portion of the respiratory tract, its influence is pronounced." The Eclectics recommended mullein for colds, coughs, asthma, and tonsillitis, as well as diarrhea, hemorrhoids, and urinary tract infections.

During the late 19th and early 20th centuries, mullein was listed in the *National Formulary,* the pharmacists' reference, as a cough remedy. It was deleted in 1936 for lack of proof of effectiveness. Nonetheless, in his 1986 survey of folk medicine in Indiana, noted herb expert Varro E. Tyler, Ph.D., found mullein "a very popular Hoosier remedy for all types of respiratory complaints."

Contemporary herbalists recommend mullein as an internal treatment for coughs, colds, sore throat, and other respiratory complaints and as an external treatment (in compresses) for hemorrhoids.

Therapeutic Uses

In laboratory studies, at least, mullein inhibits the growth of the bacteria that cause tuberculosis, so perhaps it was of some value against scrofula. Today, the herb is used mostly to soothe minor respiratory irritations.

Coughs and sore throats. Mullein contains a soluble fiber called mucilage that swells and turns into a slippery gel when it absorbs water. This accounts for the herb's soothing action on the throat and skin.

Distinguished German medical herbalist Rudolph Fritz Weiss, M.D., writes that mullein has a "well-founded reputation as a cough remedy." Commission E, the expert panel that evaluates herbal medicines for the German counterpart of the FDA, endorses mullein as a treatment for colds.

Hemorrhoids. Its mucilage is not the only reason that mullein soothes hemorrhoids. The herb also contains astringent tannins, which are widely used to treat hemorrhoids and other skin conditions. One study showed that mullein has anti-inflammatory properties as well.

Diarrhea. The astringent tannins probably account for mullein's traditional role in treating diarrhea.

Intriguing Possibility

In a laboratory study, mullein infusion helped to combat the virus that causes genital herpes and cold sores. If you develop either of these conditions, you might apply a compress made from a strong mullein infusion.

Rx Recommendations

For an infusion that can soothe cough and sore throat and may help relieve diarrhea, use 1 to 2 teaspoons of dried leaves, flowers, or roots per cup of boiling water. Steep for 10 minutes, then strain. Drink up to 3 cups a day.

Mullein has a bitter taste. To improve its flavor, you can add sugar, honey, and lemon to the tea, or mix it into an herbal beverage blend.

To help treat hemorrhoids, apply a compress made with a strong, cool infusion.

As a homemade tincture, take $\frac{1}{2}$ to 1 teaspoon up to three times a day.

When using commercial preparations, follow the package directions.

You may give dilute mullein infusions cautiously to children under age 2 to help soothe coughs.

The Safety Factor

Mullein seeds are toxic and may cause poisoning. There have been no reports of adverse effects from the herb's leaves, flowers, and roots.

Wise-Use Guidelines

The FDA includes mullein in its list of herbs generally regarded as safe. For adults who are not pregnant or nursing, mullein is considered safe when used in the amounts typically recommended.

You should take medicinal amounts of mullein only in consultation with your doctor. If it causes minor discomfort, such as stomach upset or diarrhea, reduce the dosage or stop using it altogether. Let your doctor know if you

experience unpleasant effects or if the symptoms for which you're taking the herb do not improve significantly within 2 weeks.

Growing Information

Mullein is a hardy biennial that grows almost anywhere in temperate climates. During its first year, the plant produces a rosette of 6- to 15-inch leaves that are greenish white, tongue-shaped, and hairy—hence its common names velvet dock, flannel plant, and feltwort. In its second year, mullein sends up a solitary, fibrous stem that reaches 3 to 6 feet, the source of common names such as Aaron's rod and shepherd's staff. In summer, a striking, cylindrical spike of small, dense, yellow, honey-scented flowers develops atop the stem.

Mullein grows easily from seed in light sandy soil under full sun, but it tolerates other conditions. Sow seeds in spring after the danger of frost has passed.

Harvest up to one-third of the leaves during the plant's first year and the rest the following year, before the flowers bloom. Pick the flowers as they open. Harvest the roots in autumn.

Mullein is a prolific self-sower. Many authorities recommend removing the flower heads before the seeds ripen to keep it under control.

Myrrh

Family: Burseraceae; other members include balm of Gilead

Genus and species: *Commiphora abyssinica* or *C. myrrha*

Also known as: Balsamodendron

Part used: Gum-resin from incisions in bark

In the biblical account, Joseph's jealous brothers decided to sell him into slavery. Egypt was the place to sell slaves, but who would take him there? The answer soon appeared on the horizon: "And looking up, they saw a caravan of Ishmaelites coming from Gilead [Jordan], with their camels bearing gum, balm, and myrrh on their way to carry it down to Egypt" (Genesis 37:25). They sold Joseph to the Ishmaelites.

This is just the first of a dozen biblical references to myrrh, the hardened, tear-shaped nuggets of clear or reddish brown aromatic resin that exude from incisions in the bark of a small Middle Eastern tree. Of course, the Bible's best-known mention of myrrh involves the three Magi offering the rare and costly herb to the newborn Jesus (Matthew 2:11).

Healing History

The world's oldest surviving medical text, the *Ebers Papyrus* (1500 B.C.), discusses myrrh. The ancient Egyptians used the herb as an ingredient in embalming mixtures and as a treatment for wounds. From these humble beginnings, myrrh emerged in the Bible as an all-purpose aromatic for perfumes and insect repellents.

The Arabs called the herb *murr*, meaning "bitter." When the ancient Greeks adopted the herb, they attributed its teardrop shape to Myrrha, daughter of the Syrian king Thesis. Myrrha refused to worship Aphrodite, the goddess of love. Angered by this blasphemy, Aphrodite tricked Myrrha into committing incest with her father. When Thesis realized what he had done, he threatened to kill his daughter. To save her, the gods transformed her into a myrrh tree, whose teardrop resin recalls the girl's sorrow.

Hippocrates recommended myrrh to treat mouth sores, and the Greeks also considered the herb an antidote to poisons.

As the centuries passed, myrrh became valued primarily as a mouthwash to treat bleeding gums, mouth ulcers, and sore throats. The 12th-century German abbess/herbalist Hildegard of Bingen prescribed a mixture of powdered myrrh and aloe for dental problems. Later herbalists recommended myrrh as an expectorant for colds and chest congestion.

By the Middle Ages, the belief that myrrh protected against poisons grew to encompass infectious disease. In 1665, when the Black Plague struck London, however, myrrh offered no benefit, and belief in its protective powers faded. Nonetheless, the powdered resin continued to be used to treat sores in the mouth and on the skin.

America's 19th-century Eclectic physicians, forerunners of today's naturopaths, considered myrrh an antiseptic for the external treatment of "indolent sores and gangrenous ulcers." They prescribed the herb internally for colds, laryngitis, asthma, bronchitis, indigestion, gonorrhea, sore throat, dental cavities, and bad breath. The Eclectics also cautioned that large doses of myrrh could have violent laxative action and cause sweating, nausea, vomiting, and accelerated heartbeat.

Contemporary herbalists recommend using powdered myrrh on well-washed wounds as an antiseptic. They also consider a gargle made from the herb to be effective against sore throats, colds, sore teeth and gums, coughs, asthma, and chest congestion.

Therapeutic Uses

Today, myrrh continues to be used for oral hygiene, just as it has been for 1,000 years.

Mouthwash. Myrrh contains tannins, which have an astringent, drawing effect on tissues. Chinese researchers have identified other substances in the herb that fight bacteria, and Indian scientists have discovered that the herb has anti-inflammatory action. All of these factors make myrrh an effective mouthwash.

Myrrh tastes bitter but refreshing. It may help relieve the inflammation and destroy the bacteria involved in gingivitis, the early form of gum disease. Commission E, the expert panel that evaluates herbal medicines for the German counterpart of the FDA, approves myrrh as a treatment for mouth sores.

Toothpaste. Myrrh is a common ingredient in European toothpastes. It's used to help fight the bacteria that cause tooth decay and gum disease. In the United States, some health food stores carry Merfluan, one brand of myrrh toothpaste.

Pain reliever. In an Italian study, treatment with myrrh appeared to raise the pain threshold of laboratory mice. The herb's pain-blocking action would enhance its effectiveness in treating mouth problems.

Intriguing Possibility

Myrrh may help prevent heart disease. Preliminary Indian studies suggest that the herb reduces cholesterol. It may also protect against the blood clots that trigger heart attack.

Rx Recommendations

To prepare a mouthwash, steep 1 teaspoon of powdered herb and 1 teaspoon of powdered boric acid in 1 pint of boiling water. Let stand for 30 minutes, then strain if you wish. Be sure the rinse is cool before using it. Do not swallow it

For an infusion that may help prevent heart disease, use 1 teaspoon of powdered herb per cup of boiling water. Steep for 10 minutes, then strain if you wish. Drink up to 2 cups a day. Myrrh has an unpleasant, bitter taste; to improve its flavor, you can add sugar, honey, and lemon, or mix it into an herbal beverage blend.

As a homemade tincture, take 1/4 to 1 teaspoon up to three times a day.

When using commercial preparations, follow the package directions.

Do not give myrrh to children under age 2. For older children and adults over age 65, start with low-strength preparations and increase the strength if necessary.

The Safety Factor

Myrrh has not been shown to stimulate uterine contractions, but its traditional use as a menstruation promoter should serve as a red flag to pregnant women.

Large doses of the herb may produce a violent laxative action. They could also cause other symptoms described by the Eclectics, including sweating, nausea, vomiting, and rapid heartbeat.

Wise-Use Guidelines

Myrrh appears in the FDA list of herbs generally regarded as safe. For adults who are not pregnant or nursing, myrrh is considered safe when used in the amounts typically recommended.

You should take medicinal amounts of myrrh only in consultation with your doctor. If it causes minor discomfort, such as stomach upset or diarrhea, reduce the dosage or stop using it altogether. Let your doctor know if you experience unpleasant effects or if the symptoms for which you're taking the herb do not improve significantly within 2 weeks. If you have gum or tooth pain or bleeding gums for more than 2 weeks, consult a dentist.

Growing Information

Myrrh is a large shrub or small tree that grows in the Middle East, Ethiopia, and Somalia. Pale yellow oil drips from cuts in its dull gray bark and hardens to form teardrop-shaped nuggets, which are powdered for medicinal purposes.

Nettle

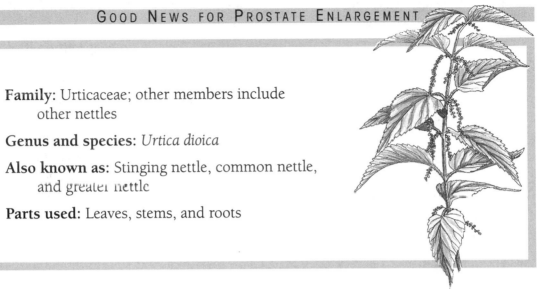

Family: Urticaceae; other members include other nettles

Genus and species: *Urtica dioica*

Also known as: Stinging nettle, common nettle, and greater nettle

Parts used: Leaves, stems, and roots

While everyone agrees that nettle stings hurt, controversy surrounds the herb's use in healing. One modern herbalist calls nettle "one of the most widely applicable plants we have," but many scientists contend that the herb "has no pharmacologic value when administered orally."

Nettle is no wonder herb, but its diuretic action can benefit a number of conditions. And, according to recent research, nettle has potential as a treatment for benign prostate enlargement.

Healing History

Nettle's role in healing dates back to ancient times. Around the 3rd century B.C., Hippocrates' Greek contemporaries prescribed nettle juice externally to treat snakebite and scorpion stings and internally as an antidote to plant poisons such as hemlock and henbane. (Nettle is not an antidote to these poisons.)

When in cold climates, Roman soldiers flailed themselves with nettle branches because the herb's sting warmed their skin. This practice, called urtication, evolved into a treatment for the joint stiffness of arthritis that is still in use today.

Early European herbalists touted nettle tea to combat cough and tuberculosis. Strange as it seems today, they recommended smoking the herb as a treatment for asthma. Herbalists also prescribed nettle to cure scurvy and stop bleeding, particularly nosebleeds.

Somewhere along the way, nettle juice gained a reputation as a hair-growth stimulant. It remained an ingredient in hair-growth nostrums well into the 19th century.

Seventeenth-century English herbalist Nicholas Culpeper endorsed all of the nettle prescriptions that preceded him. He also added one of his own: "The decoction of the leaves in wine is singularly good to provoke women's courses [menstruation]."

Native American women believed that drinking nettle tea during pregnancy strengthened the fetus and eased delivery. They also used the herb to stop uterine bleeding after childbirth, an application that early settlers adopted. Nursing mothers took nettle to increase their milk production.

America's 19th-century Eclectic physicians, forerunners of today's naturopaths, recommended nettle primarily as a diuretic to treat urinary, bladder, and kidney problems. The Eclectic text *King's American Dispensatory* (1898) describes the herb as an excellent styptic (bleeding stopper) and as a treatment for infant diarrhea, hemorrhoids, and eczema.

Contemporary herbalists have adopted many of nettle's traditional uses, notably as a diuretic. Based on recent research, a growing number of herbalists also recommend nettle as a treatment for arthritis and benign prostate enlargement.

Therapeutic Uses

Modern science has validated the Eclectics' claim that nettle is a diuretic. Researchers have also determined that the herb may help relieve arthritis and benign prostate enlargement.

Urinary tract infections. As a diuretic, nettle can help flush the bladder of the bacteria that cause urinary tract infections (UTIs). Commission E, the expert panel that evaluates herbal medicines for the German counterpart of the FDA, approves nettle leaf preparations for the prevention of UTIs and kidney stones.

High blood pressure. Diuretics are often used to treat high blood pressure. In the United States, physicians prescribe pharmaceutical di-

uretics. In Germany, where herbal medicine is more mainstream, doctors may prescribe nettle.

According to noted German medical herbalist Rudolph Fritz Weiss, M.D., "Nettle juice is definitely useful [in] diuretic therapy. It has the advantage of being well tolerated and safe, as distinct from the [pharmaceutical] thiazides."

High blood pressure is a serious condition that requires professional care. If you'd like to include nettle in your overall treatment plan, do so only under the supervision of your physician.

Congestive heart failure. Physicians often prescribe diuretics to combat the fluid accumulation associated with congestive heart failure. This condition demands professional care. If you'd like to include nettle in your overall treatment plan, do so only with the approval and supervision of your physician.

Premenstrual syndrome (PMS). Diuretics help relieve the bloating caused by premenstrual fluid buildup. Women who are bothered by PMS may want to try taking nettle in the days before their periods.

Benign prostate enlargement. Doctors refer to this condition as benign prostatic hypertrophy, or BPH. It affects middle-aged men with symptoms such as decreased urine flow, difficulty starting and finishing urination, and nighttime waking to urinate.

Traditionally, doctors have prescribed diuretics to treat BPH. In 1950, a German researcher tried nettle root, with some success: increased urine volume and fewer nighttime wakings. Most of the studies examining nettle as a treatment for BPH have occurred since the late 1970s.

Nettle works by inhibiting 5-alpha-reductase, an enzyme that plays a key role in the overgrowth of prostate tissue that's characteristic of BPH. To date, researchers have found that nettle root is most effective when it's combined with an extract of the bark of pygeum (*Pygeum africanum*), an African tree.

Treatment with a nettle-pygeum combination is not as well-researched as treatment with another herb, saw palmetto (see page 362), but nettle appears to have a future as a remedy for BPH. Commission E endorses nettle root preparations for mild to moderate BPH.

Hay fever. A study at the National College of Naturopathic Medicine in Portland, Oregon, found that taking two 300-milligram capsules of freeze-dried nettle provides significant relief from hay fever symptoms.

Arthritis. At the University of Frankfurt in Germany, researchers assessed the pain of 40 people with various forms of arthritis, including osteoarthritis, rheumatoid arthritis, and gout. Then they gave 20 of their recruits a standard dose of the prescription arthritis medication diclofenac (Voltaren, 200 milligrams a day). The rest of the volunteers took just 50 milligrams of the drug plus about 2 ounces of stewed nettle leaves. (Cooking removes the nettle hairs and their sting, making the leaves a vegetable similar to spinach.) After 2 weeks, both the drug-only group and the drug-nettle group reported about 70 percent improvement in their pain scores.

Diclofenac is a nonsteroidal anti-inflammatory drug (NSAID). NSAIDs are notorious for causing abdominal distress and gastrointestinal bleeding, which can become serious. Combining diclofenac with nettle provided equivalent pain relief while allowing a substantial decrease in the NSAID dose—which means less risk of NSAID side effects.

Since this study, a new class of arthritis drugs, called COX-2 inhibitors, has been shown to be as effective as NSAIDs but have fewer gastrointestinal side effects. To date, no research has examined the use of nettle in combination with COX-2 inhibitors. It seems reasonable to assume that the herb may increase the effectiveness of these new drugs while minimizing their side effects.

Scurvy. Nettle is a good source of vitamin C. This validates the herb's traditional role in treating scurvy, which is caused by a vitamin C deficiency.

Rx Recommendations

To prepare a pleasant-tasting diuretic infusion, use 1 to 2 teaspoons of dried herb per cup of boiling water. Steep for 10 minutes, then strain. Drink up to 3 cups a day.

As a tincture, use ¼ to 1 teaspoon up to twice a day.

To treat hay fever, look for freeze-dried nettle capsules in health food stores. If you can't find them, try an infusion or a tincture.

For arthritis, harvest nettle leaves (wearing gloves and protective clothing), then steam the leaves until they are wilted. If you don't have access to nettle leaves, try an infusion or a tincture.

To treat BPH, buy a commercial root preparation and follow the package directions.

Do not give nettle to children under age 2. For older children and adults over age 65, start with low-strength preparations and increase the strength if necessary.

The Safety Factor

Nettle's main safety issue is its sting. The hairs that give the herb a downy appearance are actually hollow needles attached to sacs filled with irritant chemicals, notably histamine. Brushing against the plant bends the hairs, squeezing the irritants onto the skin. The pain can last for 12 hours or longer.

Herbal folklore is filled with remedies for nettle stings. One age-old recommendation is to rub the affected area with nettle juice. Rubbing with other herbs—notably peppermint and other plants of the mint family, such as rosemary—also reportedly helps. This makes some sense, since the menthol in peppermint has some anesthetic action.

The most famous remedy for nettle stings is dock, immortalized in this old British rhyme: "Nettle in, dock out / Dock rub nettle out." Nonherbal treatments include washing the affected skin with soap and water, applying topical hydrocortisone cream (such as Cort-Aid), and taking oral antihistamines.

Diuretics deplete the body of potassium, an essential nutrient. If you take nettle frequently, be sure to eat potassium-rich foods such as bananas and fresh vegetables.

Some weight-loss programs tout diuretics to eliminate water weight, but weight-loss experts advise against taking diuretics. Any pounds lost this way almost invariably return. The key to permanent weight control is a low-fat, high-fiber diet and regular, moderate exercise.

Nettle has been shown to stimulate uterine contractions in rabbits. For this reason, and because of its diuretic action, pregnant women should not take the herb internally. Nursing women should also avoid diuretics.

Wise-Use Guidelines

The FDA describes nettle as an herb of undefined safety. For adults who are not pregnant or nursing and are not taking other diuretics, nettle is considered safe when used in the amounts typically recommended.

You should take medicinal amounts of nettle only in consultation with your doctor. If it causes minor discomfort, such as stomach upset or diarrhea, reduce the dosage or stop using it altogether. Let your doctor know if you experience unpleasant effects or if the symptoms for which you're taking the herb do not improve significantly within 2 weeks.

Growing Information

Nettle is only one of 500 species of *Urtica*, a name derived from the Latin *uro*, meaning "to burn." And burn they do. Just be thankful that the Javanese species, *U. urentissima*, doesn't grow in North America. Its burn is said to last a year.

Nettle's erect stem grows from a creeping underground rhizome. It has opposite, serrated, heart-shaped, dark green leaves. It is dioecious, meaning that male and female flowers grow on separate plants. If you harvest nettle, wear heavy gloves, a long-sleeved shirt, and long pants to avoid contact with the hairs and the irritants they transmit.

Nettle grows very easily from seeds or root divisions in just about any soil. Plant seeds in spring. Take root divisions in autumn after the leaves have died back.

Harvest the leaves (wearing gloves and protective clothing) before the plants flower in late spring or early summer. You may boil or steam young leaves like spinach and eat them as a vegetable. Boiling or drying eliminates the sting. The fresh tender shoots do not sting and may be used in salads.

Nettle has a reputation for increasing the aromatic oil content of angelica, marjoram, oregano, peppermint, sage, valerian, and other fragrant herbs. Nettle also reputedly speeds decomposition in compost.

Papaya

Family: Caricaceae; other members include custard apple

Genus and species: *Carica papaya*

Also known as: Pawpaw and melon tree

Parts used: Fruits, leaves, and latex

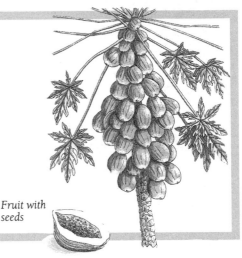

Fruit with seeds

Cookbooks caution that gelatin won't gel if you add pineapple. The same is true if you add papaya, only more so. Both fruits contain digestive enzymes that prevent the proteins in gelatin from solidifying. Those powerful enzymes are key to papaya's therapeutic powers.

Healing History

Centuries ago, the Caribbean Indians noticed that meat wrapped in papaya's broad leaves became more tender. Today, papaya extract is the active ingredient in most commercial meat tenderizers.

The Indians cut incisions into mature but unripe papayas, collected the milky fluid (latex), and applied it to their skin to treat psoriasis, ringworm, wounds, and infections. Caribbean Indian women ate unripe papayas to trigger menstruation, abortion, and labor.

After Europeans introduced papaya into tropical Asia, it quickly became incorporated into local healing practices. Filipinos used a root decoction to treat hemorrhoids. The Javanese believed that eating papaya fruit prevented arthritis. The Japanese used the latex to treat digestive disorders. Throughout Asia, the leaves were applied to wounds, and the latex was dabbed onto the cervix at term to stimulate labor.

Papaya did not play a role in traditional American herbal medicine. Over the past 25 years, however, as tropical fruits have become more widely available in this country, papaya has grown in popularity. The plant's leaves and latex are commonly sold in specialty herb shops.

Contemporary herbalists recommend papaya fruit and leaf infusions to aid digestion, ease stomach upset, and eliminate intestinal worms. They also suggest applying the leaves and latex externally to wounds.

Therapeutic Uses

Papaya fruits, leaves, and latex contain several enzymes that account for the herb's action as a digestive aid and its ability to tenderize—that is, predigest—the protein in meat. The latex contains the most enzymes, followed by the leaves and then the fruits, but even the fruit has enough enzymes to enhance digestion. (Incidentally, one of those enzymes, papain, is the active ingredient in the cleaning solutions developed for soft contact lenses.)

Digestive problems. Of all papaya's enzymes, papain may be the most important. It's similar to the human digestive enzyme pepsin, which helps break down proteins. In fact, papain is sometimes called vegetable pepsin. Papaya's other enzymes include one similar to rennin, which breaks down milk proteins, and one similar to pectase, which helps digest starches.

Ulcers. One laboratory study found that papaya exerts a direct effect on the stomach, helping to prevent ulcers. In the study, two groups of experimental animals were fed large doses of ulcer-inducing aspirin and steroids. Those that were also fed papaya for 6 days prior to receiving the drugs developed significantly fewer ulcers. This finding suggests that papaya may be of particular benefit to people with inflammatory conditions who take aspirin or steroids.

Slipped disks. In 1982, the FDA approved another papaya enzyme, chymopapain, as a treatment for herniated ("slipped") vertebral disks in the back. Injected directly into the affected area, chymopapain helps dissolve cellular debris.

Rx Recommendations

Papaya fruit is soft when ripe, and it tastes similar to cantaloupe. Have some as an appetizer before meals to stimulate digestion.

For a pleasant-tasting infusion to aid digestion, use 1 to 2 teaspoons of dried, powdered leaves per cup of boiling water. Steep for 10 minutes, then strain if you wish. Drink during or after meals, especially those high in protein (red meat and dairy products). Do not boil papaya leaves; boiling deactivates the papain.

When using commercial preparations, follow the package directions.

You may give papaya fruit to children under age 2, but papaya leaf tea should be given cautiously.

The Safety Factor

Pregnant women may eat ripe papaya fruit in moderation but should stay away from papaya latex and medicinal doses of the herb's leaves. Many cultures used papaya as a menstruation promoter and labor inducer. In addition, Indian researchers have found that papain causes birth defects and fetal death in animals.

Some allergic reactions, including asthma,

have been reported with papaya. The latex may cause stomach inflammation (gastritis).

Wise-Use Guidelines

For adults who are not pregnant or nursing, papaya is considered safe in the amounts typically recommended.

You should use medicinal amounts of papaya only in consultation with your doctor. If it causes minor discomfort, such as stomach upset, reduce the dosage or stop using it altogether. Let your doctor know if you experience any unpleasant effects or if the symptoms for which you're using the herb do not improve significantly within 2 weeks.

Growing Information

Native to the Caribbean and now naturalized throughout the tropics, papaya trees can reach 25 feet. The trunk is hollow, with spongy wood and fibrous, light-colored bark that is used to make rope. Its leaves are smooth, hand-shaped (palmate), and large, often 2 feet across.

The fruits are yellow-green, pear-shaped melons with tasty orange-yellow pulp. Papayas sold in the United States are typically about the size of large potatoes, but in the tropics, they grow to the size of large honeydews and can weigh up to 10 pounds. That's where the name melon tree comes from.

Parsley

Family: Umbelliferae; other members include carrot, celery, fennel, dill, and angelica

Genus and species: *Petroselinum crispurn*, *P. hortense*, and *P. sativurn*

Also known as: Rock selinon

Parts used: Leaves, fruits (seeds), and roots

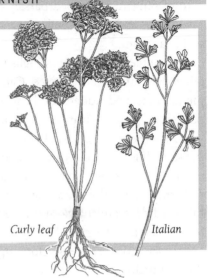

Curly leaf   Italian

ew herbs are more familiar than parsley. Its lacy sprigs typically adorn restaurant plates—and usually remain uneaten. This is unfortunate, for parsley is nutritious and an effective after-dinner breath freshener. It has other benefits, too.

Healing History

Parsley is one of the first herbs to appear in spring. For centuries, it has been used in the Seder, the ritual Jewish Passover meal, as a symbol of new beginnings.

The ancient Greeks had a different view of the herb. In Greek mythology, parsley sprang from the blood of Opheltes, infant son of King Lycurgus of Nemea, who was killed by a serpent while his nanny directed some thirsty soldiers to a spring. For centuries, Greek soldiers believed that any contact with parsley before battle signaled impending death.

Because of its association with death, parsley was planted on Greek graves. Ironically, this custom gradually changed public perception of the herb. To honor the memory of important figures, the Greeks held athletic contests and crowned the winners with parsley wreaths. Over the course of a few centuries, the herb came to symbolize strength.

The shadow of bad luck clung to the herb well into the Middle Ages, however. Some Europeans considered parsley a "devil's herb," sure to bring disaster upon those who grew it—unless they planted it on Good Friday.

Parsley was not widely used in ancient medicine, but the Roman physician Galen prescribed it for "falling sickness" (epilepsy) and as a diuretic for water retention. The Romans also munched sprigs to freshen their breath—the beginnings of the parsley garnish on restaurant plates today.

Medieval German abbess/herbalist Hildegard of Bingen prescribed parsley compresses for arthritis and parsley boiled in wine for chest and heart pain.

Seventeenth-century English herbalist Nicholas Culpeper reiterated Galen's recommendations and added to them, prescribing parsley to "provoke urine and women's courses [menstruation] . . . to expel wind . . . to break the stone [kidney stones] and ease the pains and torments thereof . . . and against cough." Culpeper also endorsed parsley compresses for inflamed eyes and black-and-blue marks and suggested that the herb be "fried with butter and applied to [the] breasts" for nipple soreness due to nursing.

Over the centuries, herbalists recommended topical applications of parsley to treat insect bites, wounds, and lice and internal doses to treat dysentery, gallstones, and some tumors.

From the 1850s through 1926, parsley was recognized by the *U.S. Pharmacopoeia*, a standard drug reference, as a laxative, a diuretic for kidney problems and the fluid accumulation of congestive heart failure, and a substitute for quinine in treating malaria.

America's 19th-century Eclectic physicians, forerunners of today's naturopaths, echoed the *Pharmacopoeia*. Their main text, *King's American Dispensatory* (1898), chronicled the isolation of a chemical called apiol from parsley oil. It recommended apiol as a treatment for "menstrual derangements," although it also noted that high doses could cause "intoxication, giddiness, flashes of light, vertigo, and ringing in the ears [tinnitus]."

During the early 20th century, large doses of apiol were used to induce abortion, despite its considerable toxicity.

Contemporary herbalists recommend parsley in cooking as a rich source of vitamins A and C, plus calcium and iron. They suggest the fresh herb as a breath freshener and an infusion or a tincture as a diuretic, digestive aid, and gas expeller.

Therapeutic Uses

Parsley roots, leaves, and fruits (seeds) all contain the plant's volatile oil, but the highest concentrations are in the seeds.

Parsley oil contains the chemicals apiol and myristicin, two significant diuretics that are also uterine stimulants and mild laxatives. Commission E, the expert panel that evaluates herbal medicines for the German counterpart of the FDA, approves parsley as a diuretic.

High blood pressure. Physicians often prescribe diuretics to treat high blood pressure. A study published in the *American Journal of Chinese Medicine* suggests that parsley's diuretic action can also help control the condition. In Germany, where herbal medicine is more mainstream than in the United States, parsley seed tea is often prescribed for high blood pressure.

High blood pressure is a serious health problem that requires professional care. If you'd like to include parsley in your overall treatment plan, do so only with the approval of your physician.

Congestive heart failure. Physicians often prescribe diuretics to combat the fluid accumulation associated with congestive heart failure. This condition demands professional care, so if you'd like to include parsley in your overall treatment plan, do so only with the approval and supervision of your physician.

Bad breath. Parsley has one of the highest levels of chlorophyll of any herb. Chlorophyll is the active ingredient in many breath fresheners, such as Clorets. This supports the herb's use as a breath freshener, a practice that dates back to Roman times.

Women's health concerns. Both apiol and myristicin are uterine stimulants. In Russia, a preparation called Supetin, which contains 85 percent parsley juice, is used to induce uterine contractions during labor.

Pregnant women may eat culinary amounts of parsley, but they should not take medicinal preparations, except possibly at term and under the supervision of a physician, to help induce labor. Other women might try parsley tea to bring on their periods.

As a diuretic, parsley may help relieve the bloated feeling caused by premenstrual fluid buildup. Women who are bothered by premenstrual syndrome may want to try some parsley in the days leading up to their periods.

Allergies. A study published in the *Journal of Allergy and Clinical Immunology* found that parsley inhibits the secretion of histamine, a compound that's produced by the body and is responsible for triggering allergy symptoms. Parsley's apparent antihistamine action may help people with hay fever or hives.

Fever. Parsley has never been proven effective against malaria, so the *Pharmacopoeia* was incorrect on that score. But apiol has some fever-reducing (antipyretic) properties. While you shouldn't count on parsley to take the place of aspirin, ibuprofen, or acetaminophen, you may want to try it in addition to mainstream medications.

Intriguing Possibility

Parsley contains psoralen, a chemical that's best known for causing sun sensitivity. But psoralen shows promise in the treatment of one form of cancer, cutaneous T-cell lymphoma. Although it's premature to recommend parsley as a cancer therapy, testing the herb for this purpose is certainly warranted.

Rx Recommendations

To freshen breath, chewing on a few sprigs of fresh parsley is usually sufficient.

For a pleasant-tasting infusion that may help treat high blood pressure, congestive heart failure, allergies, or fever or induce labor, use 2 teaspoons of dried leaves or root or 1 teaspoon of crushed seeds per cup of boiling water. Steep for 10 minutes, then strain. Drink up to 3 cups a day.

As a homemade tincture, take ½ to 1 teaspoon up to three times a day.

When using commercial preparations, follow the package directions.

Do not give medicinal doses of parsley to children under age 2. For older children and adults over age 65, start with low-strength preparations and increase the strength if necessary.

The Safety Factor

Diuretics deplete the body of potassium, an essential nutrient. If you frequently take medicinal preparations of parsley, be sure to eat potassium-rich foods such as bananas and fresh vegetables.

Although some weight-loss programs tout diuretics to eliminate water weight, weight-management experts discourage the use of diuretics for this purpose. Any pounds taken off with diuretics almost invariably return. The key to permanent weight control is a low-fat, high-fiber diet and regular aerobic exercise.

Pregnant and nursing women should avoid all diuretics, including parsley.

The psoralen in parsley has been known to cause skin rashes in agricultural workers who harvest large quantities. People with sensitive skin should be aware of this possible side effect.

The Eclectics were right about large doses of parsley oil causing headache, nausea, vertigo, giddiness, hives, and liver and kidney damage. Nevertheless, the medical literature contains no reports of problems from the herb itself, even when used in medicinal quantities.

Wise-Use Guidelines

For adults who are not pregnant, nursing, or taking diuretic medications, parsley is safe in the amounts typically recommended.

If parsley causes any discomfort, reduce the dosage or stop taking it altogether. Let your doctor know if you experience any unpleasant effects or if the symptoms for which you are using the herb do not improve significantly within 2 weeks.

Growing Information

Parsley is a small, bright green biennial that reaches 12 inches the first year and up to 3 feet the second year, when it flowers. The plant has a thick, carrotlike taproot and juicy stems terminating in feathery, deeply divided, curly or flat leaves, depending on the variety. Its tiny yellow-green flowers develop on the umbrella-like canopy (umbels) characteristic of the Umbelliferae family.

Although it's a biennial, parsley should be cultivated as an annual. The seeds are slow to germinate, often requiring up to 6 weeks. Sow them any time from early spring to autumn. Parsley can be sown indoors and transplanted, but most authorities recommend outdoor planting with ¼ inch of soil cover.

Parsley grows best in moist, sandy, well-drained loam with a neutral pH. Thin seedlings to 8-inch spacing. Late-season planting is fine. Even as a seedling, the herb usually survives one or two frosts.

You may harvest the leaves once the plants have reached about 8 inches. Harvest the fruits when they appear full-size and gray brown. Dig the roots during the autumn of the first year or the spring of the second.

Caution: Unless you are an experienced field botanist, do not pick wild parsley. It closely resembles three potentially lethal plants: water hemlock, poison parsley (also known as poison hemlock), and fool's parsley (dog parsley or small hemlock).

Passionflower

Family: Passifloraceae; other members include granadilla, sweet calabash, and Jamaican honeysuckle

Genus and species: *Passiflora incarnata*

Also known as: Maypop, apricot vine, and water lemon

Parts used: Leaves

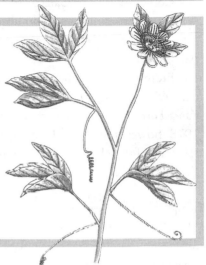

In the 1560s, 20 years after Francisco Pizarro brutally suppressed the Incas' last rebellion and forced their conversion to Christianity, Dr. Nicolas Monardes of Seville apparently developed a guilty conscience for the carnage his countrymen had wrought. An avid botanist, he searched among the plants sent back from the New World for some sign of divine approval of the Spanish conquest. He found it in a vine that had large, beautiful blossoms with parts that seemed to evoke the Passion of the Crucifixion.

To Dr. Monardes, the plant's three styles represented the three nails of the cross. Its ovary looked like a hammer. Its corona evoked the crown of thorns, and its 10 petals suggested the 10 true apostles (the original 12 minus Judas, the betrayer, and Peter, who denied Christ). Dr. Monardes christened the vine passionflower.

Healing History

The Incas brewed a tonic tea from passionflower. The herb's pleasant taste and its Christian symbolism quickly turned its leaves into a popular item in Europe, where it was used as a tranquilizer and mild sedative.

When colonists settled the American Gulf Coast, they found that the area's Native Americans used a tea made from their local passionflower to calm nervousness and applied the herb's crushed leaves as poultices on cuts and bruises.

Southerners adopted passionflower as both an ornamental and a medicinal vine. It remained a folk remedy until 1839, when two Gulf Coast Eclectic physicians touted it in the *New Orleans Medical Journal* as a non-narcotic sedative and digestive aid.

The Eclectics, forerunners of today's naturopaths, adopted passionflower as "an important remedy" for insomnia, restlessness, menstrual discomforts, diarrhea, epilepsy, and whooping cough. They also prescribed juice from the leaves externally for burns, scalds, wounds, and toothache.

Contemporary herbalists recommend passionflower primarily as a tranquilizer and sedative. They also consider it a digestive aid and pain reliever.

From 1916 to 1936, passionflower was recognized as a tranquilizer and sedative in the *National Formulary*, the pharmacists' reference. In 1978, however, the FDA banned the herb from sleep aids for lack of proven effectiveness.

Therapeutic Uses

The FDA had a reasonable argument for banning passionflower before it had been extensively studied. Unfortunately, the agency has not kept up with more recent research findings.

Stress, anxiety, and insomnia. Passionflower contains compounds that are indeed tranquilizing (maltol, flavonoids, and passiflorine, which is chemically similar to morphine). It also has substances that are potentially stimulating (harmala compounds). Various researchers have concluded that the herb has complex activity in the central nervous system, with an overall mild tranquilizing-sedative effect despite the presence of stimulants.

The herb is clearly sedative in animals, and that effect has been confirmed by research in humans. French researchers gave 91 people with anxiety problems either medically inactive placebos or an herbal preparation containing passionflower and several other herbs (including hawthorn and valerian). After 28 days, those taking the herb formula reported significantly greater anxiety relief.

In Europe, passionflower is an ingredient in many tranquilizing and sedative preparations. It's non-narcotic, so there's no need for a prescription, and there's no possibility of addiction. Commission E, the expert panel that evaluates herbal medicines for the German counterpart of the FDA, approves passionflower for nervousness and restlessness.

Digestive problems. Passionflower relaxes the smooth muscle lining the digestive tract, which means that it is an antispasmodic. This property lends credence to the herb's traditional role as a digestive aid.

Women's health concerns. Antispasmodics relax not only the digestive tract but also other smooth muscles, such as the uterus. This supports passionflower's traditional use as a remedy for menstrual discomforts.

Wounds. One study suggests that passionflower helps relieve pain, while two others show that it kills many disease-causing molds, fungi, and bacteria. These findings support the Native American and Eclectic use of passionflower as a wound treatment.

Intriguing Possibilities

In animal studies, the harmala compounds in passionflower dilate (open) the coronary arteries. Blocked coronary arteries result in heart attack, so the herb may help prevent heart disease.

Of course, heart disease is a serious condition requiring professional care. If you'd like to incorporate passionflower into your overall treatment plan, consult your physician.

Rx Recommendations

For first-aid in the garden, crush a few passionflower leaves and flowers into minor cuts until you can wash and bandage them.

For a pleasant-tasting infusion that may help you relax, calm down, or fall asleep, use 1 teaspoon of dried leaves per cup of boiling water. Steep for 10 to 15 minutes, then strain. For insomnia, drink a cup of tea before bed. For other conditions, drink up to 3 cups a day.

As a homemade tincture, take ¼ to 1 teaspoon up to three times a day.

When using commercial preparations, follow the label directions.

Do not give passionflower to children under age 2. For older children and adults over age 65, start with low-strength preparations and increase the strength if necessary.

The Safety Factor

While most sources attest to passionflower's safety, one report cites liver damage in a small group of people who drank large amounts of passionflower tea for long periods. Don't consume more than the recommended amounts. People with liver disease should probably not use the herb.

The harmala compounds in passionflower are uterine stimulants. Whole passionflower has not been associated with miscarriage, but pregnant women would be prudent to stay away from an herb with such complex effects on the central nervous system.

Some sources warn that passionflower contains cyanide, a potent poison. This is a botanical error. Ornamental blue passionflower, *Passiflora caerulea*, contains the poison. The healing herb, *P. incarnata*, does not. When buying passionflower, check the label to be sure that the product is *P. incarnata*.

Wise-Use Guidelines

For adults who are not pregnant, nursing, or taking other tranquilizers or sedatives, passionflower is considered safe in the amounts typically recommended.

You should use medicinal amounts of passionflower only in consultation with your doctor. If it causes minor discomfort, such as stomach upset or diarrhea, reduce the dosage or stop using it altogether. Let your doctor know if you experience unpleasant effects or if the symptoms for which you're using the herb do not improve significantly within 2 weeks.

Growing Information

Passionflower has a perennial root with fast-growing, climbing, annual tendrils that may reach 30 feet. The leaves are dull green, 4 to 6 inches long, and deeply divided into three to five lobes with serrated edges. Its sweet-scented white flowers are 3 inches across and tinged with purple. They bloom in May, hence the name maypops, and produce egg-size yellow or orange edible fruits, the source of the names apricot vine and water lemon.

Passionflower grows easily from seeds, cuttings, or root runners divided in autumn. It prefers rich, slightly acidic, well-watered, well-drained loam in locations that have plenty of light but are shaded from strong, direct summer sun.

The perennial root is hardy but may not survive temperatures below −15°F. The vine tendrils need something to climb, such as a fence or trellis.

Harvest the leaves around the time the flowers bloom. When the plant is generously watered, the fruits are edible and sweet.

Pennyroyal

A GOOD HERB WITH A BAD REPUTATION

Family: Labiatae; other members include mints

Genus and species: *Mentha pulegium* (European); *Hedeoma pulegioides* (American)

Also known as: Pulegium, hedeoma, fleabane, tickweed, mosquito plant, and squawmint

Parts used: Leaves and flowers

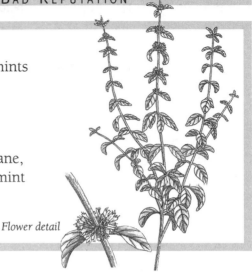

Flower detail

ew healing herbs have a reputation as bad—or as undeserved—as pennyroyal's. Critics charge that ingesting even small amounts can be fatal.

It is true that as little as 2 tablespoons of pennyroyal *oil* can cause death. But the dried herb is not dangerous. Pennyroyal's highly aromatic leaves and flowers are a safe decongestant, cough remedy, and digestive aid.

Healing History

Pennyroyal became popular during the 1st century A.D. after the Roman naturalist Pliny noted that the aromatic plant repelled fleas (hence its common name, fleabane). When crushed and rubbed on the skin or strewn, pennyroyal repels other insects as well, so it's also called tickweed and mosquito plant.

Pliny also touted pennyroyal as a cough remedy and digestive aid. He recommended hanging the plant in sickrooms in the belief that its fragrance promoted healing. The Greek physician Dioscorides seconded Pliny's recommendations, adding that pennyroyal stimulates menstruation and helps expel the afterbirth.

During the early Middle Ages, pennyroyal was recommended for truly bizarre purposes. Physician-philosopher St. Albertus Magnus wrote that by covering drowning bees in the herb's warm ashes, "they shall recover their lyfe after a space of one houre." It remains unclear why anyone would want to revive drowning bees.

In the 16th century, British herbalist John Gerard touted pennyroyal's ancient use as an expectorant: "Penny-royale taken with honey cleanseth the lungs and cleareth the breast from all gross and thick humors."

Seventeenth-century English herbalist Nicholas Culpeper recommended the herb for many other conditions: "Drunk with wine, it is of singular service to those stung or bit by any venomous beast . . . applied to the nostrils with vinegar, it is very reviving [for] fainting . . . being dried and burnt, it strengtheneth the gums, and is helpful for those troubled with the gout . . . being applied as a plaster, it taketh away carbuncles [boils]."

Early American colonists introduced European pennyroyal (*Mentha pulegium*) into North America. They found, however, that Native Americans were already using the American herb (*Hedeoma pulegioides*) for similar purposes—externally to dress wounds and repel insects and internally to treat colds, flu, coughs, and congestion and to stimulate menstruation and abortion. Folk healers also recommended aromatic pennyroyal garlands for headache and dizziness.

During the early 19th century, Thomsonian herbalists packed pennyroyal leaves into the nostrils to treat nosebleeds. After the Civil War, Eclectic physicians, forerunners of today's naturopaths, adopted pennyroyal as a stimulant, fever treatment, digestive aid, and menstruation promoter. Their text *King's American Dispensatory* (1898) described the herb as "an excellent remedy for the common cold" and recommended it for arthritis, whooping cough (pertussis), "colic in children . . . and hysteria" (menstrual discomforts).

Around 1887, the Eclectics began using pennyroyal oil, which they considered more convenient than the raw herb. They also recognized its potential hazards. *King's Dispensatory* mentioned a case of pennyroyal poisoning caused by ingesting just 1 tablespoon.

From 1831 to 1916, pennyroyal was listed in the *U.S. Pharmacopoeia*, a standard drug reference, as a stimulant, digestive aid, and menstruation promoter. From 1916 to 1931, pennyroyal oil was listed as an intestinal irritant and abortion inducer.

Contemporary herbalists advise against taking pennyroyal oil because of its toxicity, but they recommend using the herb externally as an insect repellent and treatment for cuts and burns. They also suggest taking the herb (not the oil) internally for colds, coughs, upset stomach, flatulence, anxiety, and menstruation promotion.

Therapeutic Uses

Pennyroyal oil contains pulegone, a compound that accounts for its actions as an insect repellent, menstruation promoter, and abortion inducer.

Insect repellent. Pliny was right: Pennyroyal oil helps repel flies, gnats, mosquitoes, fleas, and ticks. It is the active ingredient in most natural insect repellents. If you buy an herbal flea collar for your dog or cat, it's likely to contain pennyroyal oil.

Congestion and coughs. Because pennyroyal is one of the most aromatic mints, the strong aroma of a pennyroyal infusion can serve as a decongestant and possible expectorant.

Digestive problems. Pennyroyal contains compounds similar to the stomach-soothing menthol in its botanical relative, peppermint. While pennyroyal's stomach-settling action is not as strong as peppermint's, the herb is still an effective digestive aid.

Rx Recommendations

To repel insects, rub fresh, crushed plant material over your body, or mix pennyroyal tincture into a skin cream and apply.

To make an herbal flea collar, try hanging a pennyroyal garland or a bag of the herb from a regular collar. Do not apply pennyroyal oil to your pet's fur or skin. The animal may get a toxic dose from licking itself.

For an infusion to help treat coughs, congestion, or stomach upset, use 1 to 2 teaspoons of dried herb per cup of boiling water. Steep for 10 to 15 minutes, then strain. Drink up to 2 cups a day. Its aroma resembles spearmint's, but it's sharper and not quite as inviting. The taste is warm and pleasant, initially bitter with a cool finish.

As a homemade tincture, use ¼ to ½ teaspoon up to twice a day.

When using commercial preparations, follow the package directions.

Do not give pennyroyal to children under age 2. For older children and adults over age 65, start with low-strength preparations and increase the strength if necessary.

The Safety Factor

Ever since pennyroyal's abortion-inducing oil was first distilled more than 100 years ago, the herb has been notorious because the oil is so toxic. Pulegone does indeed stimulate uterine contractions. Unfortunately, the dose necessary for abortion is quite close to the lethal dose, a fact that many women learned the hard way. As little as ½ teaspoon of pennyroyal oil can cause convulsions. Doses not much larger can be fatal.

The British medical journal *Lancet* cited a case of abortion-related pennyroyal oil poisoning as early as 1897. Since then, many similar reports have appeared in the medical literature. According to one such report in the *Journal of the American Medical Association*, a pregnant 18-year-old woman died within 2 hours after taking 2 tablespoons of the oil, despite emergency treatment.

Clearly, women wishing to terminate pregnancy should not use pennyroyal oil. In fact, no one should.

Although small amounts of pennyroyal oil can be fatal, the oil is a superconcentrated extract of the herb. Drinking a few cups of pennyroyal infusion poses no hazard. University of Illinois pharmacognosist Norman Farnsworth, Ph.D., estimates that it would take 75 gallons of strong pennyroyal infusion to approach the potential toxicity of a fatal dose of pennyroyal oil.

Wise-Use Guidelines

For adults who are not pregnant or nursing, pennyroyal herb—again, not the oil—is considered safe in the amounts typically recommended.

You should use medicinal amounts of pennyroyal only in consultation with your doctor. If it causes minor discomfort, such as stomach upset or diarrhea, reduce the dosage or stop using it altogether. Let your doctor know if you experience unpleasant effects or if the symptoms for which you're using the herb do not improve significantly within 2 weeks.

Growing Information

Despite their botanical differences, both European and American pennyroyal yield similar oils and are used interchangeably.

The European herb is a perennial that spreads by underground runners. Its square stems grow to about 12 inches, and its opposite, oval leaves are smooth or slightly hairy. Tight whorls of small lilac flowers appear in mid-summer. European pennyroyal may be propagated from root runner divisions in early spring or fall or by rooting stem cuttings during summer.

American pennyroyal is an annual with square stems that reach 15 inches. Its leaves resemble those of the European variety, but its summer-blooming flowers tend to be smaller and more bluish. It must be grown from seeds sown in spring or fall. Cover them with ¼ inch of soil. Thin seedlings to about 5-inch spacing.

Both types do best in rich, well-watered, sandy, slightly acidic loam under full sun, although the European herb tolerates partial shade. It also needs room to spread. Its runners emerge after it flowers.

Harvest the leaves and flowers of both plants when they are in full bloom. In the fall, cut them back to a few inches above the ground and hang the herb to dry.

Peppermint and Spearmint

Family: Labiatae; other members include balm, basil, catnip, horehound, marjoram, and pennyroyal

Genus and species: *Mentha piperita* (peppermint); *M. spicata, M. viridis, M. aquatica, M. cardiaca* (spearmint)

Also known as: No other names, but there are hundreds of varieties of mint

Parts used: Leaves and flowers

Peppermint   *Spearmint*

Have you ever had an after-dinner mint? Those familiar candies evolved from the ancient custom of concluding feasts with a sprig of mint to soothe the stomach. Modern research has shown the wisdom of this age-old practice and has verified other therapeutic uses of peppermint and spearmint.

Both mints are popular in herbal medicine, and both have similar effects. But of the two, peppermint is much tastier. It's more potent, too.

Spearmint was the original medicinal mint. Peppermint appeared later, a natural hybrid of spearmint species. Authorities aren't exactly sure which species combined to form the spicier mint or when it actually appeared. All of the mints were considered one plant, called mint, until 1696. That's when British botanist John Ray differentiated them.

Healing History

Mint was mentioned as a stomach soother in the *Ebers Papyrus*, the world's oldest surviving medical text. From Egypt, mint spread to Palestine, where it was accepted as payment for taxes. In Luke (11:39), Jesus scolds the Pharisees, "You pay tithes of mint and rue . . . but have no care for justice and the love of God."

From the Holy Land, mint spread to Greece and entered Greek mythology. It seems that Pluto, god of the dead, fell in love with the beautiful nymph Minthe. Pluto's goddess-wife, Persephone, became jealous and changed Minthe into mint. Pluto could not bring Minthe back to life, but he gave her plant form a fragrant aroma. *Minthe* evolved into the mints' genus name, *Mentha*.

Greek and Roman homemakers added

mint to milk to prevent spoilage and served the herb after meals as a digestive aid. The Roman naturalist Pliny wrote that mint "reanimates the spirit" and recommended hanging it in sickrooms to assist convalescence. The Greek physician Dioscorides considered mint "heating" and therefore a promoter of lust. Other Greek and Roman herbalists prescribed mint for everything from hiccups to leprosy.

Chinese and Ayurvedic physicians have used mint for centuries as a tonic and digestive aid and as a treatment for colds, coughs, and fevers.

Twelfth-century German abbess/herbalist Hildegard of Bingen recommended mint for digestion and gout.

Seventeenth-century English herbalist Nicholas Culpeper wrote, "[Mint] is very profitable to the stomach . . . especial to dissolve wind [and] help the colic. . . . It is good to repress the milk in women's breasts . . . and a very powerful medicine to stay women's courses [stop menstrual flow]. It helpeth the biting of a mad dog . . . and is good to wash the heads of young children against all manner of breaking out, sores, and scabs. . . ."

Culpeper disagreed with Dioscorides on mint and sex, however. Instead of calling it a lust promoter, Culpeper considered it "an especial remedy for venereal [sexual] dreams and pollutions in the night [nocturnal emissions], being applied outwardly to the testicles."

Shortly after Culpeper's time, peppermint and spearmint were differentiated. Herbalists decided that the former was the better digestive aid, cough remedy, and treatment for colds and fever.

Early colonists found Native Americans using the American mints to treat coughs, chest congestion, and pneumonia. The colonists introduced peppermint and spearmint, and the plants quickly went wild.

By the late 19th century, the Eclectic physicians, forerunners of today's naturopaths, prescribed peppermint for headache, coughs, bronchitis, stomach distress, and hysteria (menstrual discomforts). They also added it to laxatives to minimize intestinal cramping and disguise their unpleasant taste.

The Eclectics also valued spearmint but considered it "somewhat inferior to peppermint" except for its superior ability to treat fever.

Chemists distilled menthol from peppermint oil in the early 1880s. The Eclectic text *King's American Dispensatory* (1898) touted menthol's "active germicidal properties," and its "considerable anesthetic power" when applied to wounds, burns, scalds, insect bites and stings, eczema, hives, and toothache. The Eclectics also used menthol vapors in inhalants and chest rubs to relieve asthma, hay fever, and morning sickness.

Contemporary herbalists recommend peppermint externally for itching and inflammations and internally as a digestive aid and treatment for menstrual cramps, motion sickness, morning sickness, colds, cough, flu, congestion, headache, heartburn, fever, and insomnia. Some herbalists consider peppermint and spearmint interchangeable, but most believe peppermint to be more potent. As they do with so many other aromatic herbs, herbalists also recommend these herbs for relaxing herbal baths.

Therapeutic Uses

Both spearmint and peppermint owe their value in healing to their aromatic oils. Peppermint oil is mostly menthol. Spearmint oil contains a similar compound, carvone. These chemicals have similar properties, but as the herbalists of old believed, menthol is the more potent and is the one more widely used in herbal medicine.

Digestive problems. Thumbs-up for the after-dinner mint. Menthol and carvone soothe the smooth muscle lining the digestive tract, preventing muscle spasms, which means that they are antispasmodics.

In Germany, where herbal medicine is more mainstream than in the United States, an over-the-counter digestive capsule called Enteroplant has two active ingredients: peppermint oil (90 milligrams) and caraway oil (50 milligrams). German researchers gave 45 people with chronic indigestion either placebos or Enteroplant at doses of one capsule three times a day with meals. After 4 weeks, those taking the placebos reported no change in abdominal distress. In comparison, 94.5 percent of the peppermint-caraway group reported significant improvement, with 63 percent declaring themselves free from pain.

In a separate German study, another herbal digestive aid—this one containing peppermint, caraway, fennel, and wormwood—produced similar relief from indigestion in only 2 weeks. It's no wonder that Commission E, the expert panel that evaluates herbal medicines for the German counterpart of the FDA, endorses peppermint for indigestion and abdominal distress.

Other German and Russian research suggests that peppermint may help to prevent stomach ulcers and stimulate bile secretion.

Irritable bowel syndrome. Also known as spastic colon and functional bowel disorder, irritable bowel syndrome causes a variety of symptoms: abdominal cramps, bloating, flatulence, diarrhea or constipation, and possibly heartburn and queasiness.

British researchers analyzed five studies involving the treatment of irritable bowel syndrome with peppermint oil. The three that showed benefit all used enteric-coated peppermint oil capsules (0.2 to 0.4 milliliter three times a day) that delivered the oil to the colon. The two that showed no effect used uncoated peppermint oil capsules that allowed the oil to be absorbed before it reached the colon.

Pain. The Eclectics were on the right track about menthol's "considerable anesthetic power." It's an ingredient in many over-the-counter pain-relieving skin creams, including Absorbine and Bengay. It is also added to throat lozenges such as Cepacol. It's also an ingredient in many ointments marketed to soothe insect bites and stings as well as rashes caused by poison ivy, poison oak, and sumac.

Commission E approves peppermint oil as a treatment for muscle aches.

Congestion. Menthol vapors do indeed help relieve nasal, sinus, and chest congestion. Menthol is an ingredient in Afrin Nasal Spray, Mentholatum, and Vicks VapoRub.

Peppermint is an FDA-approved remedy for the common cold, primarily because of its decongestant action. Commission E also approves peppermint as a cold remedy.

Coughs. Several studies show that in addition to its decongestant action, menthol is an effective cough suppressant. Researchers in

England had 20 volunteers inhale citric acid, which triggers coughing. Five minutes beforehand, the participants received either one of two medically inactive placebos or menthol. For the people treated with menthol, coughing was significantly reduced. Menthol is an ingredient in Hall's, Luden's, Ricola, Robitussin, and Vicks Cough Drops.

Infections. The Eclectics may have been onto something when they described menthol as being actively germicidal. In laboratory studies, peppermint oil kills several types of bacteria and the herpes simplex virus, which causes cold sores and genital herpes. These findings seem to validate peppermint's traditional roles in treating wounds and bronchitis.

Headaches. In two very similar studies, German researchers gave people who had tension headaches either placebos or different combinations of peppermint and eucalyptus oils. Participants rubbed the preparations on their foreheads and temples. The herb treatments produced greater relief. The formula that was mostly eucalyptus oil provided the most muscle relaxation, while the one that was mostly peppermint oil yielded the greatest pain relief. The researchers suggest trying an herbal treatment instead of or in addition to over-the-counter pain relievers.

Women's health concerns. Antispasmodics soothe not only the smooth muscle lining the digestive tract but also other smooth muscles, such as the uterus. Several herbals recommend peppermint as a treatment for morning sickness. The *Toxicology of Botanical Medicines,* however, suggests that medicinal concentrations of peppermint may promote menstruation.

Pregnant women who want to try peppermint for morning sickness should stick with dilute, beverage-tea concentrations rather than more potent medicinal infusions. Women with a history of miscarriage should not use this herb while pregnant. Other women may try peppermint to bring on their periods.

Rx Recommendations

For an anesthetic to treat wounds, burns, scalds, and herpes sores, apply a few drops of peppermint oil directly to the affected area.

For a decongestant, cough-suppressant, or digestive infusion, use 1 to 2 teaspoons of dried peppermint or spearmint per cup of boiling water, steep for 10 minutes, and strain. Drink up to 3 cups a day. Peppermint has a sharper taste than spearmint, and it cools the mouth.

As a homemade tincture, take ¼ to 1 teaspoon up to three times a day.

When using commercial preparations, follow the package directions.

For an herbal bath, fill a cloth bag with a few handfuls of dried or fresh herb and let the water run over it.

You may give dilute peppermint or spearmint preparations cautiously to children under age 2, but youngsters may find the taste too pungent and may gag.

The Safety Factor

As dried plant material, neither peppermint nor spearmint has been reported to cause problems, except for skin irritation in sensitive individuals.

Do not ingest pure menthol. As little as a teaspoon (about 2 grams) can be fatal.

Since pure peppermint oil has also been found to produce toxic effects, such as heart rhythm disturbances (cardiac arrhythmias), do not ingest peppermint oil, either.

Wise-Use Guidelines

Peppermint and spearmint are included in the FDA list of herbs generally regarded as safe. For adults who are not pregnant or nursing, the herbs are considered safe when used in the amounts typically recommended.

You should take medicinal amounts of peppermint and spearmint only in consultation with your doctor. If either causes minor discomfort, such as stomach upset or diarrhea, reduce the dosage or stop using it altogether. Let your doctor know if you experience unpleasant effects or if the symptoms for which you're taking the herb do not improve significantly within 2 weeks.

Growing Information

Spearmint is a perennial that reaches 2 feet and spreads by underground root runners. It has the mint family's characteristic square stems with wrinkled, lance-shaped, serrated, 2-inch leaves, and flower spikes with whorls of small white, pink, or lilac flowers that bloom in midsummer.

Peppermint looks like spearmint, except that it grows somewhat taller, spreads by surface runners, has stems with a purplish cast, and has longer, less wrinkled leaves.

Mints crossbreed so easily that it's often impossible to tell what's sprouting from seeds. The best way to propagate true peppermint or spearmint is to use root cuttings. Any piece of root with a joint or node can produce a plant. Contain your mint bed or plant in containers. In rich, moist, well-drained soil, under full sun or partial shade, spreading mints may become pests.

Frequent cutting encourages bushiness. You may harvest leaves as they mature. Cut the entire plant back to within a few inches of the ground when the first flowers appear. Most species become woody after a few years, so dig them out and plant new root cuttings.

Psyllium

Family: Plantaginaceae; other members include about 250 *Plantago* species, including rib grass

Genus and species: *Plantago psyllium*

Also known as: Fleaseed, plantago, and plantain

Parts used: Seeds

Mention psyllium (pronounced *SILLY-um*), and most people say, "Huh?" Mention the brand-name laxative Metamucil instead, and everyone says, "Oh, yes."

The fact is, except for a little sweetening, coloring, and flavoring, Metamucil is psyllium, the seeds of a hardy plant distributed around the world. Psyllium is among the safest, gentlest laxatives, an attribute that earned it a place in herbal healing centuries ago.

In addition, modern research shows that psyllium seed has a remarkable ability to reduce cholesterol. This makes the herb beneficial in preventing heart disease and many strokes.

Healing History

Psyllium is often called plantain, but it should not be confused with the other plantain (*Muca paradisiaca*), a palmlike tree that produces fruits similar to bananas.

For centuries, traditional Chinese and Ayurvedic physicians have used the seeds and leaves of several Asian *Plantago* species to treat diarrhea, hemorrhoids, constipation, urinary problems, and, more recently, high blood pressure.

Psyllium entered European folk medicine in the 16th century as a remedy for diarrhea and constipation. Seventeenth-century English herbalist Nicholas Culpeper recommended the seeds for inflammation, gout, hemorrhoids, and sore nipples (mastitis) in nursing mothers.

European physicians eventually adopted psyllium, but it was not widely used on this side of the Atlantic until after World War I.

Therapeutic Uses

Up to 30 percent of psyllium's seed coat is a soluble fiber called mucilage. When exposed to water, psyllium seeds swell to more than 10 times their original size and become gelatinous. The herb's mucilage accounts for its medicinal action.

Diarrhea. Psyllium absorbs excess fluid in the intestinal tract and helps restore normal bulk to stool. Commission E, the expert panel that evaluates herbal medicines for the German counterpart of the FDA, approves psyllium for the treatment of uncomplicated diarrhea.

Constipation. Israeli researchers gave 35 people with chronic constipation either medically inactive placebos or laxatives containing psyllium and aloe. After 2 weeks, those taking the placebos showed no improvement. Those taking the psyllium-aloe combination reported softer stools, more frequent bowel movements, and less use of pharmaceutical laxatives.

Psyllium's bulk-forming action increases stool volume. Larger stools press on the colon wall, triggering the wavelike contractions (peristalsis) that we recognize as "the urge." As stool gains bulk, it also becomes softer and easier to pass.

In general, Americans eat a low-fiber diet, with fewer fruits, vegetables, beans, and whole grains than experts recommend. This results in hard, dense stools that are difficult and painful to pass. Psyllium's fiber content and water-absorbing action can compensate to some extent for a deficiency of dietary fiber.

Today, psyllium is one of North America's most popular bulk-forming laxatives. It's the active ingredient in Metamucil, Fiberall, Hydrocil, Konsyl, Modane, and Serutan and one of the active ingredients in Innerclean and Perdiem. Commission E endorses psyllium as a treatment for constipation and irritable bowel syndrome, which may involve either constipation or diarrhea.

Hemorrhoids. Because psyllium softens stool, it can bring some relief from the pain and bleeding of hemorrhoids, according to a report in *Diseases of the Colon and Rectum.* This supports Culpeper's recommendation. Commission E approves psyllium as a hemorrhoid treatment.

High cholesterol. Oat bran has garnered much of the publicity, but the fact is, any dietary fiber helps pull cholesterol out of the bloodstream so it doesn't wind up narrowing artery walls and increasing the risk of heart disease and stroke. Many studies show that as dietary fiber increases, the risk of elevated cholesterol decreases. As a form of fiber, psyllium reduces cholesterol.

A study published in *Archives of Internal Medicine* showed that a teaspoon of psyllium three times a day for 8 weeks produced significant decreases in participants' blood cholesterol levels. The researchers concluded that many people with moderately elevated cholesterol may be able to bring it down to healthy levels with psyllium alone, without cholesterol-lowering medication.

A similar study published in the *Journal of the American Medical Association* found that psyllium could reduce total cholesterol by about 5 percent in 12 weeks. Heart disease experts say that for every 1 percent decrease in total cholesterol, heart attack risk drops 2 percent, so this 5 percent cholesterol reduction meant a 10 percent decrease in heart attack risk.

In another study, Mexican researchers placed 125 people with diabetes—all at high risk for heart attack—on a low-fat diet. In addition, the participants were given either placebos or psyllium (about 2 teaspoons three times a day). After 3 months, those taking psyllium had significantly lower cholesterol levels.

In all of these trials, psyllium treatment caused no side effects, making it safer than some prescription drugs prescribed to reduce cholesterol. If you would like to include psyllium in a cholesterol reduction program, consult your physician.

In 1997, the FDA hopped on the psyllium bandwagon. Any food that contains at least 1.7 grams of psyllium can make a label claim that it helps prevent heart disease. Kellogg's Bran Buds cereal contains the requisite amount of psyllium, and other cereals are expected to add the herb. Check the labels to find out which have added it.

Intriguing Possibilities

One study showed that psyllium protects laboratory animals from intestinal damage associated with toxic food additives. The psyllium increased the bulk of the animals' stools, so the toxic chemicals had less direct contact with sensitive intestinal tissues and less opportunity to cause harm. Researchers believe that the same mechanism is the reason that a high-fiber diet is associated with reduced risk of colorectal cancer.

To date, no studies have found that psyllium helps prevent colon cancer, the leading cause of cancer deaths among nonsmokers.

Even so, the American Cancer Society recommends a diet high in fiber such as psyllium to possibly help reduce the risk of colon cancer.

Like other dietary fibers, psyllium reduces blood sugar (glucose) levels in laboratory animals, suggesting a possible role in diabetes management for humans.

Rx Recommendations

Most studies show that a teaspoon or two of psyllium three times a day, along with plenty of water or fruit juice, usually produces significant relief from constipation. Psyllium is odorless and almost tasteless, but it has a gritty texture that some people find unpleasant. If you take a commercial preparation, follow the label directions.

Do not give psyllium to children under age 2. If your infant or child appears constipated, consult a physician.

The Safety Factor

As a laxative and cholesterol cutter, psyllium does not work by itself. It swells only in the presence of fluid. If you take psyllium but don't drink enough water or juice with it, you could end up like the man whose intestine became completely blocked by a large psyllium plug. He required abdominal surgery. Drink at least one tall glass of water or juice every time you take psyllium.

Inhaling dust from psyllium seeds may trigger an allergic reaction. As a result, someone who is sensitive to psyllium could later experience allergy symptoms from ingesting it. Severe allergic reactions are extremely rare, but if you have breathing difficulties after ingesting psyllium, seek emergency help immediately.

Psyllium has no history as a menstruation promoter, but other *Plantago* species do. Although constipation is a common complaint during pregnancy, pregnant women should avoid laxatives, including psyllium, and control constipation by eating high-fiber foods such as fruits, vegetables, beans, and whole-grain bread products.

Wise-Use Guidelines

You should use medicinal amounts of psyllium only in consultation with your doctor. If it causes minor discomforts, such as stomach upset or diarrhea, reduce the dosage or stop using it altogether. Let your doctor know if you experience unpleasant effects or if the symptoms for which you're using the herb do not improve significantly within 2 weeks.

Growing Information

Psyllium is an annual that reaches 18 inches and produces inconspicuous white flowers in summer that soon give way to small brown seed pods.

Most of the psyllium used in this country is imported from France. Although available from specialty seed houses, psyllium is not usually grown as a garden herb. It looks like a weed, and if the seed pods are not harvested before they break open, the wind scatters the seeds. This can be a major problem when you consider that each pod contains up to 15,000 seeds and that the plant grows aggressively.

Raspberry

Family: Rosaceae; other members include rose, peach, almond, apple, and strawberry

Genus and species: *Rubus idaeus* and *R. strigosus*

Also known as: Hindberry and bramble

Parts used: Leaves and fruits

For more than 2,000 years, raspberry was considered a minor healer, a footnote under blackberry. Since the 1940s, however, it has emerged from blackberry's shadow and virtually replaced it in herbal medicine—all because it has become *the* herb for pregnant women. The latest research also shows that raspberry fruits are very high in antioxidants, the nutrients that help prevent many degenerative diseases.

Healing History

The ancient Greeks, Chinese, Ayurvedics, and Native Americans hardly distinguished raspberry from blackberry. They used the leaves of the two bushes interchangeably, externally to treat wounds and in tea to treat diarrhea.

Seventeenth-century English herbalist Nicholas Culpeper recommended raspberry as "very binding" (astringent) and good for "fevers, ulcers, putrid sores of the mouth and secret parts [genitals] . . . spitting blood [tuberculosis] . . . piles [hemorrhoids], stones of the kidney . . . and too much flowing of women's courses [heavy menstrual flow]."

America's 19th-century Eclectic physicians, forerunners of today's naturopaths, continued the long tradition of considering raspberry a footnote under blackberry. The Eclectic text *King's American Dispensatory* (1898) recommended blackberry as being "of much service in dysentery . . . pleasant to the taste, mitigating suffering, and ultimately effecting a cure." Then it noted that raspberry helped, too.

Contemporary herbalists recommend raspberry to relieve diarrhea and to end nausea and vomiting, especially the morning sickness of pregnancy. One herbalist goes so far as to call raspberry a "panacea during pregnancy . . . allaying morning sickness, preventing miscarriage, [and] erasing labor pains." The berries are also increasingly touted for their antioxidant content.

Therapeutic Uses

Raspberry won't erase labor pains, and it's no panacea during pregnancy. But science has shown it to be of some value for pregnant women.

Pregnancy complaints. In 1941, raspberry came into its own when an animal study published in the British medical journal *Lancet* showed that the herb contains a "uterine relaxant principle." Over the next 30 years, several other studies confirmed this finding. Today, physicians in England and Europe prescribe a number of raspberry preparations for morning sickness, uterine irritability, and threatened miscarriage. The herb is also included in many herbal pregnancy blends sold in the United States.

Diarrhea. Raspberry leaves contain tannins, which are astringent. This helps explain the traditional use of raspberry leaf tea as a diarrhea remedy.

General disease prevention. Raspberries owe their red color to high levels of anthocyanosides, compounds that are potent antioxidants. Antioxidants help prevent and reverse the harm to cells caused by highly reactive oxygen molecules called free radicals. Scientists now agree that free radical damage (oxidative damage) is the underlying cause of heart disease, many cancers, and other degenerative illnesses.

Antioxidants—among them, vitamins C and E, the mineral selenium, and anthocyano-sides—are found in plant foods. Researchers at the Jean Mayer USDA Human Nutrition Research Center on Aging at Tufts University in Boston analyzed the antioxidant content of dozens of common plant foods. Those richest in antioxidants turned out to be the dark-colored fruits and berries that contain generous amounts of anthocyanosides, including raspberries and blackberries.

Cataracts. Cataracts are a major cause of vision impairment and blindness among older Americans. They occur when oxidative damage to the normally clear lens of the eye leads to the development of cloudy spots.

For reasons that remain unclear, anthocyanosides have unusually powerful effects on the eyes. In one Italian study, 50 people with early-stage cataracts were given extracts of bilberry, a fruit similar to raspberry, in combination with another antioxidant, vitamin E, three times a day. The treatment stopped cataract progression in 97 percent of the study participants.

Raspberries and bilberries contain comparable amounts of anthocyanosides, so presumably, the berries have similar effects.

Macular degeneration. The nerve-rich retina at the back of the eye plays a key role in vision. Macular degeneration involves deterioration of the macula, the most sensitive part of the retina—the part responsible for seeing fine detail and what's directly in front of you.

In a European study, 31 people with various types of retinal eye problems, including macular degeneration, were given bilberry extract. Those with macular degeneration experienced significant vision improvement.

Again, raspberries presumably produce similar benefits.

Diabetic retinopathy. Diabetes damages all of the blood vessels in the body, including the tiny capillaries in the eye that nourish the retina. When these capillaries are weakened, they leak blood into the eye, causing the blurred vision of retinopathy.

Bilberry's powerful antioxidants help strengthen retinal blood vessels, reducing that blood leakage. In the European macular degeneration study mentioned above, people with diabetic retinopathy showed significant improvement when treated with bilberry. Raspberries probably produce similar benefits.

Intriguing Possibilities

One animal study has found that raspberry helps reduce blood sugar (glucose) levels, suggesting the herb's possible value in diabetes management.

Rx Recommendations

For a treat rich in antioxidants, enjoy raspberries. Whether fresh, frozen, canned, or in preserves, they supply generous amounts of anthocyanosides.

For a pleasantly astringent, sweet infusion to treat diarrhea or the discomforts of pregnancy, use 1 to 2 teaspoons of dried herb per cup of boiling water. Steep for 10 to 15 minutes and strain. Drink as needed.

As a homemade tincture, take ½ to 1 teaspoon up to three times a day.

When using commercial preparations, follow the package directions.

You may use cool, dilute raspberry tea cautiously to treat infant diarrhea in consultation with the child's physician.

The Safety Factor

Standard medical advice warns pregnant women against taking any drugs during pregnancy because of the possibility of harming the fetus. Raspberry used medicinally is an exception to this rule, although you should use it only in consultation with a prenatal care provider.

Raspberry has been widely recommended as a uterine relaxant for decades, and there are no reports in the medical literature of any problems with it. Women with a history of miscarriage may find it especially valuable. On the other hand, prudence dictates using the lowest effective dose. Start with a weak infusion and increase the concentration if necessary.

Tannins have both pro- and anti-cancer action. People with a history of cancer who want to use raspberry should consult their physicians.

Wise-Use Guidelines

For adults, raspberry is safe in the amounts typically recommended.

You should use medicinal amounts of raspberry only in consultation with your doctor. If it causes minor discomfort, such as stomach upset or diarrhea, reduce the dosage or stop using it altogether. Let your doctor know if you experience unpleasant effects or if the symptoms for which you're using the herb do not improve significantly within 2 weeks.

Growing Information

Raspberry's perennial invasive roots produce a dense, spreading mass of thorny biennial stems that can grow to 10 feet. The bush has serrated, lance-shaped leaves; small white summer-blooming flowers; and hanging clusters of tart red berries that become very sweet as they ripen.

Raspberry bushes grow so vigorously and invasively that they quickly become impenetrable pests. Rooting them out is quite difficult.

Even when cleared, stray root fragments send up new shoots. Be sure that your raspberries are well-contained.

Plant ½-inch root cuttings in a few inches of soil. Raspberry grows best under full sun in loose, rich, well-drained soil amended with manure or compost.

You can harvest the leaves at any time. Mature fruits appear in summer. For ease of harvesting the berries, train the branches along supports, and prune mercilessly.

Red Clover

Family: Leguminosae; other members include beans and peas

Genus and species: *Trifolium pratense*

Also known as: Trifolium, purple clover, sweet clover, and cow clover

Parts used: Flowers

Red clover is one of the world's oldest agricultural crops, cultivated as forage since prehistoric times. The small, ball-shaped flowers of the three-leafed herb have been used for almost as long in herbal healing.

Red clover's century-old role as a cancer treatment remains extremely controversial. Increasingly, however, the herb is finding a place on the herbal medicine shelf as a remedy for menopausal discomforts, despite a lack of research support.

Healing History

Because of its importance in early agriculture, red clover has a long history as a religious symbol. The ancient Greeks and Romans and the Celts of pre-Christian Ireland all revered it. Early Christians linked the plant to the Trinity, and some say red clover is the model for Ireland's symbol, the shamrock. It was also the model for the suit of clubs in playing cards.

During the Middle Ages, red clover was considered a charm against witchcraft. A more potent protector was the rare four-leaf clover, which represented the cross and the four aspects of happiness: health, wealth, fame, and a faithful lover. Modern children still search for four-leaf clovers.

Traditional Chinese physicians have long used red clover blossoms as an expectorant. Russian folk healers recommended the herb for asthma. Other cultures have used it externally in salves for skin sores and eye problems and internally as a diuretic to treat water retention and as a sedative, anti-inflammatory, cough medicine, and cancer treatment.

America's 19th-century Eclectic physicians, forerunners of today's naturopaths, were great promoters of red clover. Their text *King's American Dispensatory* (1898) deemed the herb "one of the few remedies which favorably influences pertussis [whooping cough] . . . possess[ing] a peculiar soothing property." The Eclectics recommended red clover for coughs bronchitis, and tuberculosis. But they waxed truly enthusiastic about the herb as a cancer treatment: "It unquestionably retards the growth of carcinomata."

During the late 19th and early 20th centuries, red clover was the major ingredient in many patent medicines known as Trifolium Compounds. The most popular, produced by the William S. Merrell Chemical Company of Cincinnati, was a combination of red clover and several other herbs. Manufacturers claimed that Trifolium Compounds were tonics and treatments for skin diseases, syphilis, and scrofula (tuberculosis of the lymph nodes).

In 1912, the American Medical Association's Council on Pharmacy and Chemistry attacked Trifolium Compounds, saying, "We have no information to indicate they possess medicinal properties." Nonetheless, red clover remained in the National Formulary, the pharmacists' reference, as a treatment for skin diseases until 1946.

Red clover was also one of the herbs in ex–coal miner Harry Hoxsey's controversial alternative cancer treatment (see page 32).

Contemporary herbalists recommend red clover externally as a treatment for eczema and psoriasis and internally to aid digestion, ease the discomforts of menopause, and relieve coughs, bronchitis, and whooping cough. Some continue to recommend it for cancer.

Therapeutic Uses

Red clover doesn't get much respect among many herbal experts. The FDA says, "There is not sufficient reason to suspect it of any medicinal value."

Cancer. Researchers from the National Cancer Institute (NCI) felt compelled to investigate the anti-tumor properties of red clover after their own Jonathan Hartwell, Ph.D., published a monograph in the *Journal of Natural Products* in which he pointed out that 33 different cultures around the world had used red clover to treat cancer. Sure enough, NCI researchers have confirmed that red clover contains four anti-tumor compounds, including daidzein and genistein, which are also isoflavone plant estrogens (phytoestrogens).

In addition, red clover contains significant amounts of tocopherol, a form of vitamin E. This vitamin is a potent antioxidant that helps prevent cancer and heart disease.

Red clover is no substitute for mainstream cancer treatment, but for those with cancers not aggravated by estrogen (non-estrogen-dependent tumors), red clover may hold some promise. Ask your physician about using it in addition to your regular treatment.

Menopausal complaints. The isoflavone phytoestrogens in red clover are similar to those found in some other plants, notably soybean (page 377). Consumption of soy foods and soy isoflavone supplements has been shown to reduce the hot flashes associated with menopause. Similar isoflavones are included in an Australian red clover supplement, Promensil, now available in the United States.

Unfortunately for Promensil, two 1999 studies pitting the product against medically inactive placebos—one study that involved 37 postmenopausal women and the other 51 women—showed no difference in the ability to reduce hot flashes. At this point, the research does not support red clover as a treatment for the discomforts of menopause.

On the other hand, a study of 27 postmenopausal women by Australian researchers showed that Promensil (40 milligrams a day) improves arterial elasticity 23 percent. This suggests that red clover may help prevent heart disease, the leading cause of death in postmenopausal women.

Intriguing Possibility

One laboratory study found red clover to be effective against several kinds of bacteria, including the type that causes tuberculosis. This finding lends some credence to the Eclectics' use of the herb in treating TB.

Rx Recommendations

For a pleasantly sweet infusion, use 1 to 3 teaspoons of dried flowers per cup of boiling water. Steep for 10 to 15 minutes, then strain. Drink up to 3 cups a day.

As a homemade tincture, use ½ to 1½ teaspoons up to three times a day.

When using commercial preparations, follow the package directions.

Do not give medicinal red clover preparations to children under age 2. For older children and adults over age 65, start with low-strength preparations and increase the strength if necessary.

The Safety Factor

The medical literature contains no reports of harm from red clover. The herb's phytoestrogen content suggests, however, that some people should exercise caution in taking it.

Estrogens are used to treat some prostate cancers but may accelerate the growth of estrogen-dependent breast and gynecological tumors. Estrogen also increases the risk of blood clots (thromboembolisms) and inflammation of blood vessels (thrombophlebitis). People who have a history of any of these disorders or of heart disease or stroke should use red clover cautiously, if at all.

Likewise, women on estrogen-based birth control pills should consult their physicians before using the herb.

Wise-Use Guidelines

The FDA includes red clover in its list of herbs generally regarded as safe. For adults who are not pregnant or nursing and do not have estrogen-dependent cancers or a history of thromboembolism or thrombophlebitis, red clover is considered safe when used in the amounts typically recommended.

You should take medicinal amounts of red clover only in consultation with your doctor. If it causes minor discomfort, such as stomach upset or diarrhea, reduce the dosage or stop using it altogether. Let your doctor know if you experience any unpleasant effects or if the symptoms for which you're taking the herb do not improve significantly within 2 weeks.

Growing Information

Red clover is a three-leafed perennial that grows to 2 feet. Its fragrant, edible, red or purple, ball-shaped flowers are composed of many tiny florets.

Because it's a legume, red clover adds nitrogen to the soil, and its deep roots help break up compacted soil. Plant seeds in spring or fall. In sunny conditions, this herb thrives in a variety of moist, well-drained soils but does not grow well in sand or gravel. Harvest the flowers when the tops are in full bloom.

Red Pepper

MEDICINALLY, IT'S HOT!

Family: Solanaceae; other members include potato, tomato, eggplant, tobacco, and nightshade

Genus and species: *Capsicum annuum* and *C. frutescens* (green and red bell pepper, paprika, and pimiento are all milder varieties of *C. annuum*)

Also known as: Hot, African, Tabasco, Guinea, and bird pepper; Louisiana long (and short) pepper, cayenne chili pepper, and capsicum

Parts used: Fruits

The fiery taste and bright crimson color of red pepper make it one of the world's most noticeable and popular spices. Recently, the herb has become as hot in healing as it is on the tongue. Extracts of red pepper are remarkably effective in relieving certain types of severe, chronic pain. The herb can also help prevent and treat ulcers.

Red pepper has been discovered at Central American archeological sites dating to 7000 B.C. The herb has been a culinary staple in Asia since ancient times. It was unknown in Europe, however, until Columbus returned with it from his first voyage to the New World.

You may hear red pepper referred to as cayenne, a name that comes from the Caribbean Indian word *kian*. Today, Cayenne is the capital of French Guiana. Ironically, only a tiny fraction of the U.S. red pepper supply comes from South America or the Caribbean. Most comes from India and Africa. Tabasco (Louisiana pepper) grows along the Gulf Coast of the United States.

Because so little of the herb comes from around Cayenne, the American Spice Trade Association considers the name cayenne a misnomer and says that it is properly called red pepper.

Healing History

Seventeenth-century English herbalist Nicholas Culpeper wrote that immoderate use of red pepper "inflames the mouth and throat so extremely it is hard to endure," and warned that the herb "might prove dangerous to life." But he believed that sparing amounts were of "considerable service" to "help digestion, provoke urine, relieve toothache, preserve the teeth from rottenness, comfort a cold stomach, expel the stone from the kidney, and take away dimness of sight."

Culpeper urged women to mix red pepper, gentian, and bay laurel oil in cotton and insert it vaginally to "bring down the courses" (menstruation). He warned, though, that "if [it] be put into the womb after delivery, it will make [the woman] barren forever."

During the 18th century, red pepper was mixed with snuff to boost the inhaled tobacco's kick. Herbalist Phillip Miller warned against this, saying that the combination caused "such violent fits of sneezing as to break the blood vessels in the head."

In India, the East Indies, Africa, Mexico, and the Caribbean, red pepper enjoys a long history as a digestive aid. This use never caught on among Europeans, who have traditionally believed that hot spices cause stomach ulcers.

The first North American to advocate red pepper in healing was Samuel Thomson, creator of Thomsonian herbal medicine, which enjoyed considerable popularity before the Civil War. Thomson believed most disease was caused by cold and cured by heat, so he prescribed "warming" herbs, red pepper among them.

After the Civil War, America's Eclectic physicians, forerunners of today's naturopaths, called red pepper capsicum and recommended it externally for arthritis and muscle soreness and internally as a digestive stimulant and treatment for colds, coughs, fever, diarrhea, constipation, nausea, and toothache. The Eclectics also advised placing red pepper in socks to warm cold feet, a use echoed in some herbals today.

The Eclectics considered red pepper invaluable in the treatment of delirium tremens, the combination of hallucinations and violent tremors common among advanced alcoholics: "Capsicum is the very best agent that can be used in delirium tremens. It enables the stomach to take and retain food. The best form is in a tea or strong beef soup. There is no danger of overdose as a [large] quantity may be swallowed with evident pleasure and without ill results."

American folk healers have also recommended dusting children's hands with powdered red pepper to stop thumb sucking and nail biting.

An estimated 25 percent of the world's population uses red pepper daily as a culinary spice. Some 2.5 million acres are planted with the herb.

Contemporary herbalists prescribe capsules of cayenne powder for colds and gastrointestinal and bowel problems, and as a digestive aid. They also recommend cayenne plasters for arthritis and muscle soreness.

Therapeutic Uses

Red pepper owes its heat and its value in herbal healing to one compound found in its fruit—capsaicin. Research supports the herb's traditional uses as a digestive aid and pain reliever.

Digestive problems. Red pepper assists digestion in two ways. First, it stimulates the flow of saliva and stomach secretions. Saliva contains enzymes that initiate the breakdown of carbohydrate, while stomach secretions (gastric juices) contain acids and enzymes that break down food even further. Second, red pepper prevents the growth of *Helicobacter pylori*, the bacteria that cause ulcers.

In cultures with bland cuisines, such as the traditional American meat-and-potatoes fare, people often believe that highly spiced foods damage the stomach and contribute to ulcers. This is not the case. In a study published in the *Journal of the American Medical Association*, researchers used tiny video cameras to examine volunteers' stomach linings after both bland meals and meals liberally spiced with jalapeño peppers. The researchers found no difference in stomach condition, concluding, "Ingestion of highly spiced meals by normal individuals is not associated with [gastrointestinal] damage."

Diarrhea. In addition to its action against *H. pylori*, red pepper helps combat other bacteria. This seems to validate traditional claims that the herb helps treat infectious diarrhea.

Chronic pain. For centuries, herbalists have recommended rubbing red pepper into the skin to treat muscle and joint pain. Medically, this is known as applying a counterirritant. The body can pay attention to only so many pain signals at once. The minor superficial pain caused by counterirritants reduces the nervous system's ability to alert the brain to deeper, more severe pain.

More recently, red pepper has been shown to possess direct pain-relieving properties for certain kinds of chronic pain. For reasons that are still not completely understood, capsaicin interferes with the action of substance P, the chemical in the peripheral nerves that sends pain messages to the brain. Since the mid-1980s, dozens of studies have found capsaicin to be remarkably effective at relieving many types of pain.

The FDA has approved capsaicin for use in many over-the-counter pain-relieving creams, including Arthricare, Capzasin, Dencorub, Icy Hot Arthritis Therapy, Pain-X, and Zostrix.

Osteoarthritis. This is the most common type of arthritis. It causes joint pain and stiffness for more than 16 million Americans, most of them older adults.

At the Veterans Affairs Hospital in Miami, researchers had 113 people with osteoarthritis apply either a medically inactive placebo ointment or one containing capsaicin to their stiff, painful joints four times a day. After 12 weeks, those using the capsaicin ointment reported significantly greater relief.

At Rush-Presbyterian–St. Luke's Medical Center in Chicago, a similar 9-week study of 59 people with osteoarthritis produced similar results. In this trial, the participants rubbed their painful joints with capsaicin cream just twice a day.

Fibromyalgia. Fibromyalgia causes muscle pain and tenderness. At the Medical College of Wisconsin in Milwaukee, 45 people with fibromyalgia rubbed their painful or tender spots four times a day with either a placebo ointment or capsaicin ointment. After a month, those using the capsaicin reported significantly less pain and tenderness.

Psoriasis. In some cases, the red, scaly patches caused by psoriasis become very itchy (pruritic). At the University of Michigan, 197 people with pruritic psoriasis treated their skin patches with either a placebo cream or capsaicin. After 6 weeks, those who applied the capsaicin reported significantly greater relief.

Shingles. Capsaicin ointment is the most effective treatment yet for the severe chronic pain associated with shingles, or herpes zoster. Shingles is an adult disease caused by the same virus that produces chickenpox in children. The virus remains dormant in the body until later in life when, for unknown reasons, it reappears in some people as shingles, causing a rash on one side of the body that progresses from red bumps to blisters to crusty pox resembling chickenpox.

In healthy adults, shingles clears up by itself within 3 weeks. But some people—typically the elderly or those with other illnesses, particularly Hodgkin's disease—develop severe, chronic pain, a condition that doctors call postherpetic neuralgia. Now, thanks to capsaicin, they don't have to suffer as much.

Diabetic neuropathy. A common complication of diabetes, diabetic neuropathy causes pain in the arms, hands, legs, feet, and possibly elsewhere. Researchers at several medical centers around the United States instructed people with diabetic neuropathy to rub either a placebo cream or a capsaicin ointment on the painful parts of their bodies four times a day. After 8 weeks, the capsaisin group reported significantly less pain, improved sleep, and greater ability to walk, work, and participate in recreational activities.

Cluster headaches. Capsaicin helps relieve cluster headaches, which cause extremely severe pain on one side of the head. At the University of Florence in Italy, researchers had 16 people with cluster headaches apply a capsaicin preparation inside their nostrils on the affected side for several days. Eleven of the participants (69 percent) experienced complete relief.

In another study, people with cluster headaches rubbed a capsaicin preparation inside their nostrils and the outside of their noses. Within 5 days, 75 percent reported less pain and fewer headaches. They also reported burning nostrils and runny noses, but these side effects subsided within a week.

Self-defense. Capsaicin is the active ingredient in many self-defense sprays, aptly known as pepper sprays. When directed into an attacker's eyes, pepper spray causes pain and temporary blindness that lasts up to 30 minutes, but does not do permanent eye damage.

Intriguing Possibility

Red pepper may help cut cholesterol and prevent heart disease, according to Indian and U.S. researchers. While it is too early to recommend red pepper for these conditions, the common kitchen spice may someday play a role in heart health.

Rx Recommendations

Season food with red pepper to taste, but err on the side of caution. A little too much can set your mouth afire. If your mouth begins to burn uncomfortably, the best treatment is milk. Casein, a protein in milk, pulls capsaicin off the tastebuds.

For an infusion to aid digestion and help prevent or treat ulcers, use ¼ to ½ teaspoon per cup of boiling water. Drink it after meals.

For external application to help treat pain, mix ¼ to ½ teaspoon into a cup of warm vegetable oil and rub it on the affected area.

When using a commercial capsaicin ointment, follow the label directions.

Do not give red pepper to children under age 2. For older children, start with a small amount and use more if necessary. People over age 65 often experience a loss of sensitivity in their tastebuds and skin nerves, so they may require more red pepper than younger adults.

The Safety Factor

Chopping red peppers may burn the fingertips, a condition dubbed Hunan hand because it was first identified in a man who was preparing a Hunan Chinese recipe that called for chopping many of the fiery fruits. He wound up in an emergency room with severe hand pain.

Red pepper does not wash off the hands easily (vinegar removes it best). Even with careful washing, the pungent herb may remain on the fingertips for hours and cause severe pain if contaminated fingers touch the eyes. Consider wearing rubber gloves when handling red peppers.

One French study shows that red pepper boosts resistance to infection. Some bacteria-fighting spices can be sprinkled on cuts to help prevent infection, but don't do this with red pepper. It burns terribly.

Red pepper has not been linked to menstruation promotion since the 17th century, but some research suggests that the herb's stems and leaves, not the more typically used powdered fruits, stimulate uterine contractions in animals. Women who are pregnant or trying to conceive should stick with products made from the powdered fruits.

Wise-Use Guidelines

Red pepper is on the FDA list of herbs generally regarded as safe. For adults who are not nursing, red pepper is considered safe when used in the amounts typically recommended.

You should use medicinal amounts of red pepper only in consultation with your doctor. If it causes minor discomfort, such as stomach upset, diarrhea, or burning during bowel movements, reduce the dosage or stop using it altogether. Let your doctor know if you experience unpleasant effects or if the symptoms for which you're taking the herb do not improve significantly within 2 weeks.

Growing Information

Red pepper is a shrubby, tropical perennial with shiny, pendulous, leathery fruits. It grows best in tropical or subtropical areas but also prospers in south-facing windows and greenhouses. The fruits' boxy shape is the source of the plant's genus name, *Capsicum*, from the Latin *capsa*, meaning "box."

In southern states, seeds may be sown after the danger of frost has passed. Farther north, sow seeds indoors in flats 8 weeks before the final frost date, then transplant. Space seedlings 12 inches apart.

Red pepper prefers rich, well-watered, sandy soil and full sun, but it tolerates some shade. When harvesting the ripened fruit, be careful not to break the stems, or the peppers may spoil. To dry red peppers, hang them in a warm, dry place. Drying takes several weeks.

Rhubarb

Family: Polygonaceae; other members include buckwheat

Genus and species: *Rheum officinale* and *R. palmatum* (garden rhubarb, *R. rhaponticurn*, has similar but less powerful action)

Also known as: Rheum, or Chinese, Himalayan, Turkish, or medicinal rhubarb

Parts used: Roots

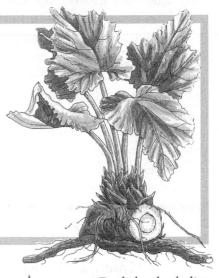

Rhubarb is an odd plant. Its roots are medicinal. Its stems make tasty pies. And its leaves are poisonous.

Healing History

Chinese physicians have used rhubarb root since ancient times. They prescribed it externally as a treatment for cuts and burns and internally in small amounts for dysentery. They also discovered that large amounts have powerful laxative action and promote menstruation. In the 13th century, China traveler Marco Polo mentioned rhubarb as a medicinal plant in his journal.

Over the centuries, the Indians, Russians, and Europeans adopted rhubarb as a healing herb and discovered that their own native species have similar, though less powerful, effects.

Seventeenth-century English herbalist Nicholas Culpeper endorsed rhubarb's laxative action: "This herb purges downward." He also recommended it externally as "a most effectual remedy to heal scabs and running sores." In addition, Culpeper claimed that rhubarb "heals jaundice . . . provokes urine . . . is very effectual for reins [gonorrhea] . . . and helps gout, sciatica . . . toothache . . . the stone [kidney stones] . . . and dimness of sight."

Later herbalists repudiated most of Culpeper's recommendations. They returned to prescribing small doses of rhubarb root for diarrhea and larger doses as a laxative.

America's 19th-century Eclectic physicians, forerunners of today's naturopaths, used rhubarb primarily to treat diarrhea and dysentery. The Eclectic text *King's American Dispensatory* (1898) noted rhubarb's effectiveness for constipation but said "it sometimes produces griping [cramping]." The Eclectics also considered the herb helpful in treating "hepatic derangement" (liver problems) and delirium tremens.

Bacterial dysentery was a common—and often fatal—disease in British East Africa between World Wars I and II. In 1921, Nairobi-based physician R. W. Burkitt wrote in the British medical journal *Lancet* that he'd treated it with rhubarb almost exclusively for 3 years: "I know of no remedy in medicine which has such a magical effect. No one who has ever used rhubarb would dream of using anything else . . . in this dreadful tropical scourge."

Contemporary herbalists are divided on rhubarb. Some recommend low doses for diarrhea and large doses for constipation. Others simply recommend it as a laxative.

Therapeutic Uses

The ancient Chinese appear to have been right about rhubarb's dual effects.

Diarrhea. Studies show that small amounts of rhubarb help relieve diarrhea.

Constipation. Large amounts of rhubarb have powerful laxative action. The herb contains anthraquinones, compounds similar to those found in other laxative herbs such as buckthorn, cascara sagrada, and senna.

Anthraquinone laxatives should be used only as a last resort to treat constipation. First, eat more fresh fruits and vegetables, drink plenty of water, and get more exercise. If that doesn't work, try a bulk-forming laxative such as psyllium (see page 325). If you still need help, try cascara sagrada (see page 110), generally regarded as the gentlest anthraquinone. Finally, if you're still having difficulty, try rhubarb, buckthorn (see page 102), or senna

(see page 368) in consultation with your physician.

Commission E, the expert panel that evaluates herbal medicines for the German counterpart of the FDA, approves rhubarb root as a laxative.

Women's health concerns. Some animal studies suggest that rhubarb stimulates uterine contractions, lending some credence to the herb's use in China as a menstruation promoter. Women who are pregnant or trying to conceive should avoid rhubarb. Other women might try it to begin their periods.

Intriguing Possibility

Chinese researchers have reported that rhubarb root helps prevent the progression of kidney failure.

Rx Recommendations

For diarrhea, make a decoction by gently boiling 1/2 teaspoon of powdered root per cup of water for 10 minutes, then strain if you wish. Take 1 tablespoon at a time periodically, up to 1 cup a day. Rhubarb tastes bitter and unpleasant.

For constipation, make a decoction by boiling 1 to 2 teaspoons of powdered root per cup of water for 10 minutes, then strain if you wish. Take 1 tablespoon at a time, up to 1 cup a day.

If you're using a homemade tincture, take 1/4 teaspoon daily for diarrhea and 1/2 to 1 teaspoon daily for constipation.

When using commercial preparations, follow the package directions.

Do not give rhubarb to children under age 2. For older children and adults over age 65, start with low-strength preparations and increase the strength if necessary.

The Safety Factor

Because of rhubarb's powerful action, laxative amounts should not be used by people with chronic intestinal problems such as ulcers or colitis.

Pregnant and nursing women should not use anthraquinone laxatives.

Do not use laxative amounts of rhubarb for more than 2 weeks. Over time, it causes lazy bowel syndrome, an inability to have bowel movements without chemical stimulation.

Rhubarb stems are used in pie fillings, but the plant's leaf blades contain oxalic acid, which is poisonous. Ingesting the leaves can cause burning in the mouth and throat, nausea, vomiting, weakness, and other symptoms. Deaths have occurred.

Rhubarb may color the urine bright yellow or red, which is harmless.

Wise-Use Guidelines

For adults who are not pregnant or nursing, do not have a gastrointestinal condition, and are not taking other laxatives, rhubarb is considered safe when used in the amounts typically recommended for brief periods.

You should take medicinal amounts of rhubarb only in consultation with your doctor. If it causes minor discomfort, such as stomach upset or diarrhea, reduce the dosage or stop using it altogether. Let your doctor know if you experience unpleasant effects or if the symptoms for which you're using the herb do not improve significantly within 2 weeks.

Growing Information

Medicinal rhubarb is a large, leafy perennial that reaches 10 feet. Its root is thick and branching, brown on the outside and yellow inside. Its round, hollow stems are jointed and terminate in branching spikes of numerous small flowers. The medicinal species are not garden herbs.

Garden rhubarb reaches only 3 feet. It has thick roots—reddish outside and yellow inside—and purple stems. Garden rhubarb is considered less potent in herbal healing. If you use it medicinally, start with the amounts recommended above, but be prepared to adjust them upward.

Garden rhubarb requires a dormant period in winter and does not do well in the South, where winters are warm. Sow seeds or root cuttings 4 feet apart in late spring in deeply dug, well-watered beds under full sun or partial shade. Add compost and mulch in winter. Harvest stems for pies the second year and roots the fourth.

Rose

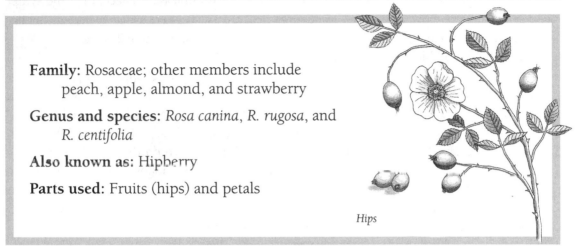

Family: Rosaceae; other members include peach, apple, almond, and strawberry

Genus and species: *Rosa canina*, *R. rugosa*, and *R. centifolia*

Also known as: Hipberry

Parts used: Fruits (hips) and petals

Hips

Prized since the dawn of history, the rose is the queen of flowers. In herbal healing, however, this plant becomes noteworthy only after the velvety petals have fallen away, revealing the cherry-size fruits, or hips.

Rose hips contain vitamin C, but authorities disagree on how much. Some herbalists call rose hips one of the best natural sources of vitamin C. Scientific sources scoff at this claim, asserting that it would take more than a dozen cups of rose hip tea to help treat colds and flu.

While herbalists have generally overstated the herb's vitamin C content, it may still be of some benefit for colds and flu.

Healing History

Roses were a favorite of the ancient Egyptians, who used the fragrant petals as air fresheners and rose water as perfume. During the 1st cen-

tury A.D., when Marc Antony wooed Cleopatra, legend has it that the Egyptian queen ordered the floors of her palace covered knee deep in rose petals.

In Greece, Hippocrates recommended rose flowers mixed with oil for diseases of the uterus. India's traditional Ayurvedic physicians have long considered rose petals cooling and astringent, leading to their application as poultices to treat skin wounds and inflammations. The Ayurvedics also used rose petals and rose water as laxatives.

Western herbalists mirrored the Ayurvedic uses of the herb. The 12th-century German abbess/herbalist Hildegard of Bingen recommended rose hip tea as the initial treatment for just about every illness.

Seventeenth-century English herbalist Nicholas Culpeper called the herb "binding and restringent [astringent]." He wrote that it "strengthens the stomach, prevents vomiting, stops tickling coughs . . . [is] good against all kinds of fluxes [diarrhea] . . . [and is] of great service in consumptions [tuberculosis]."

As the centuries passed, European herbalists recommended dried rose petal tea for headache, dizziness, mouth sores, and menstrual cramps.

Americans have always loved roses. The flowers were among the first planted around the White House, which now boasts an enormous rose garden. American herbalists considered the rose only a minor healing herb, however. The 19th-century Eclectic physicians, forerunners of today's naturopaths, did not use rose petals at all. They beat the hips into a pulp and used it as a base for making pills that contained other medicines.

Roses almost disappeared from early 20th-century herbals. Then came the discovery of vitamin C in the 1930s and the finding that rose hips may contain appreciable amounts.

Contemporary herbalists are almost unanimous in their praise of rose hips as a source of vitamin C. One best-selling herbal claims, "Rose hips are rich in vitamin C, richer by far ounce for ounce than oranges. Some people say we should make rose hip tea a part of our daily diet."

Because of rose hips' vitamin C content, herbalists tout them for colds and flu. Some also recommend the herb as a mild laxative.

Therapeutic Uses

There's nothing wrong with making rose hips a part of your daily diet, but don't count on them—or the prepackaged teas containing them—to supply all the vitamin C you need.

This is especially true if you're using the vitamin to treat the common cold and flu.

While rose hips contain a significant amount of vitamin C, the drying process destroys from 45 to 90 percent of it, and infusions extract only about 40 percent of what's left. That still leaves a fair amount of vitamin C, but it's considerably less than most herbals promise.

Many companies that manufacture vitamin C supplements claim that their products are made from rose hips. In fact, none is made exclusively from rose hips. In commercial "rose hip" vitamin C preparations, the hips are combined with ascorbic acid from other sources.

Colds and flu. The weight of the scientific evidence shows that vitamin C doesn't help prevent colds. Once you've caught one, though, the nutrient helps reduce the severity and duration of your illness, provided that you take at least 2,000 milligrams a day from the moment the first symptoms appear until you feel that you're over the cold.

It's not easy to obtain 2,000 milligrams of vitamin C exclusively from rose hips, but there's no harm in combining the herb with other sources.

Another argument in favor of rose hip infusion is that hot liquids help relieve the sore throat, nasal congestion, and cough associated with colds. They also warm the throat, which helps impair viral replication (cold viruses reproduce best at around 95°F).

Mouth sores. Commission E, the expert panel that evaluates herbal medicines for the German counterpart of the FDA, approves rose petal infusion for one of its many traditional uses: treating sores in the mouth, such as canker sores.

Rx Recommendations

For a pleasant-tasting, mildly astringent infusion that may help treat colds, flu, and mouth sores, use 2 to 3 teaspoons of dried chopped hips or dried powdered petals per cup of boiling water. Steep for 10 minutes and strain if you wish. Drink as needed.

As a homemade tincture, use ½ to 1 teaspoon as needed.

When using commercial preparations, follow the package directions.

You may give dilute rose infusions to children under age 2.

The Safety Factor

High doses of vitamin C cause diarrhea in some people. If you develop diarrhea, reduce your intake of the nutrient.

High doses of vitamin C may also strain the kidneys. This is not a problem for people with healthy kidneys, but those with kidney disease should consult their physicians before using large amounts of rose hips.

Wise-Use Guidelines

Rose hips appear in the FDA list of herbs generally regarded as safe. For adults who do not have kidney disease, rose hips are safe when used in the amounts typically recommended.

Consult a physician if cold or flu symptoms do not improve significantly within 2 weeks, if you develop a fever toward the end of a cold or flu, or if a cold- or flu-related cough brings up brown or red phlegm.

Growing Information

Roses have been bred for every climate. "Old roses" are generally more fragrant than newer hybrids, but they have less showy, faster-wilting flowers. Consult a nursery for the variety best suited to your conditions and desires. Enjoy the flowers, then, when the petals fall, harvest and dry the hips.

Rosemary

Family: Labiatae; other members include mints

Genus and species: *Rosmarinus officinalis*

Also known as: Rosemarine and incensier (French)

Parts used: Leaves

Thousands of years before refrigeration, ancient people noticed that wrapping meats in crushed rosemary leaves preserved them and imparted a fresh fragrance and pleasing flavor. To this day, the herb remains a favorite in meat dishes.

Rosemary's ability to preserve meats also led to the belief that it helped preserve memory. Greek students wore rosemary garlands to assist their powers of recall. As the centuries passed, the herb was incorporated into wedding ceremonies as a symbol of spousal fidelity and into funerals to help survivors to remember the dead. In *Hamlet*, Ophelia gives Hamlet a sprig, saying, "There's rosemary . . . for remembrance."

Healing History

The ancients used rosemary as they used all aromatic, preservative herbs—for head, respiratory, and gastrointestinal problems. Traditional Chinese physicians mixed it with ginger as a treatment for headache, indigestion, insomnia, and malaria.

During the Middle Ages, rosemary's association with weddings evolved into its use as a love charm. If a young person tapped another with a rosemary twig containing an open blossom, the couple would supposedly fall in love.

Placed under a pillow, the aromatic herb was believed to repel bad dreams. Planted around a home, it was reputed to ward off witches. By the 16th century, this practice became a bone of contention in England, where it was believed to signify a household where the woman ruled. Men were known to rip out rosemary plants as evidence that they, not their wives, ruled the roost.

In 1235, Queen Elizabeth of Hungary became paralyzed. According to legend, a hermit soaked a pound of rosemary in a gallon of wine for several days, then rubbed it on her limbs, curing her. Rosemary-wine combinations became known as Queen of Hungary's Water and were used externally for centuries for gout, dandruff, baldness prevention, and skin problems. As the centuries passed, pennyroyal and marjoram were incorporated into what became known as Hungary Water.

The French hung rosemary around sickrooms and in hospitals as a kind of healing incense, calling it *incensier*. As recently as World War II, French nurses burned a mixture of rosemary leaves and juniper berries in hospital rooms as an antiseptic.

Colonists brought rosemary to North America. An early medical guide, *The American New Dispensatory*, recommended the herb's leaves and flowers and Hungary Water for use "in nervous and menstrual affections, for strokes, paralysis, and dizziness."

Oddly, those great proponents of botanical medicine, the Eclectics, forerunners of today's naturopaths, had little use for rosemary. Their text *King's American Dispensatory* (1898) noted its use as a digestive aid and menstruation promoter but declared that it was "seldom used except as a perfume."

Contemporary herbalists say that rosemary stimulates the circulatory, digestive, and nervous systems. They recommend it as a treatment for headache, indigestion, and depression and as a gargle for bad breath. They also advocate its external use for muscle aches and in baths for relaxation.

Central American folk healers use rosemary oil as an insect repellent and menstruation promoter.

Therapeutic Uses

Rosemary may not guarantee A's on exams, marital fidelity, or vivid memories of the dear departed—but the ancients were right about the herb's ability to preserve meats.

Food poisoning. Meats spoil in part because their fats oxidize and turn rancid. Rosemary and its oil contain compounds that are potent antioxidants. In fact, rosemary's preservative power compares favorably with the commercial food preservatives BHA and BHT.

Rosemary's preservative action may help prevent food poisoning on your next picnic. Mix the crushed leaves generously into hamburger meat and tuna, pasta, and potato salads.

Infections. The same compounds that retard spoilage also inhibit the action of many microorganisms that can cause infection. For minor cuts in the garden, press some fresh, crushed rosemary leaves into the wound on the way to wash and bandage it.

Digestive problems. Like most culinary herbs, rosemary may help relax the smooth muscle lining the digestive tract, an action that makes it an antispasmodic. The ancients appear to have been on the right track when they used it as a digestive aid. Commission E, the expert panel that evaluates herbal medicines for the German counterpart of the FDA, approves rosemary as a treatment for indigestion.

Congestion. Like other aromatic herbs, rosemary may help relieve nasal and chest congestion caused by colds, flu, and allergies.

Women's health concerns. Antispasmodics soothe not only the digestive tract but other smooth muscles as well, such as the uterus. As an antispasmodic, rosemary should theoretically calm the uterus, but Italian researchers have discovered that it does exactly the opposite.

Pregnant women should steer clear of medicinal preparations of rosemary. Other women might try the herb to bring on their periods.

Intriguing Possibility

Antioxidants help prevent cancer. The high levels in rosemary led researchers at Pennsylvania State University to add powdered leaves to the food of some laboratory animals. Then all the animals were injected with chemicals known to cause cancer. Compared with the animals that ate plain food, those that consumed rosemary enjoyed significant protection from cancer.

Rx Recommendations

For a pleasantly aromatic infusion to settle the stomach or clear a stuffy nose, use 1 teaspoon of crushed herb per cup of boiling water. Steep for 10 to 15 minutes, then strain. Drink up to 3 cups a day.

As a homemade tincture, use ¼ to ½ teaspoon up to three times a day.

When using commercial preparations, follow the package directions.

You may give dilute rosemary preparations to children under age 2.

The Safety Factor

In culinary amounts, rosemary poses no hazards, but even small amounts of rosemary oil may cause stomach, kidney, and intestinal irritation. Larger doses may cause poisoning. Do not ingest more than a drop or two of concentrated rosemary oil.

Wise-Use Guidelines

Rosemary is included in the FDA list of herbs generally regarded as safe. For adults who are not pregnant or nursing, rosemary is safe when used in the amounts typically recommended.

You should take medicinal amounts of rosemary only in consultation with your doctor. If it causes minor discomfort, such as stomach upset or diarrhea, reduce the dosage or stop using it altogether. Let your doctor know if you experience unpleasant effects or if the symptoms for which you're taking the herb do not improve significantly within 2 weeks.

Growing Information

Rosemary is a woody, pine-scented, evergreen perennial with needlelike leaves. It reaches 3 feet in the United States and produces small, pale blue flowers in summer. Creeping rosemary (*Rosmarinus prostratus*) is widely used in the western United States as a groundcover and cascade over garden walls.

Rosemary can be grown from seeds, but germination can be a problem and seedlings are slow to develop, which is why most herb growers prefer to start with cuttings. If you sow seeds, plant them in the spring, 6 inches apart. Plant cuttings in sandy soil, leaving only one-third of each twig showing.

Rosemary prefers light, sandy, well-drained soil and full sun. Overwatering may cause root rot. It usually survives frigid winter temperatures without special care. If you live where temperatures dip below zero, mulch plants each autumn or grow the herb in pots, bring them indoors each winter, and keep them in a south-facing window.

Cut twigs and strip the leaves any time after the plants have become established.

Sage

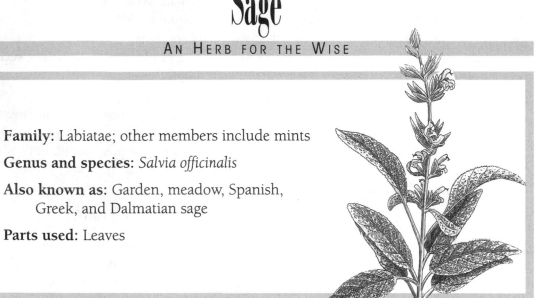

Family: Labiatae; other members include mints

Genus and species: *Salvia officinalis*

Also known as: Garden, meadow, Spanish, Greek, and Dalmatian sage

Parts used: Leaves

Close your eyes and imagine Thanksgiving turkey stuffing. Smell that warm, rich aroma? Chances are, it comes from sage.

Thousands of years before the Pilgrims stuffed the first Thanksgiving turkey, people all over the world were celebrating the healing powers of this aromatic herb. The genus name for sage, *Salvia*, comes from the Latin word meaning "to heal."

Down through history, sage has been used to treat so many maladies that it gained a reputation as a panacea, prompting herb expert Varro E. Tyler, Ph.D., to write, "If one consults enough herbals . . . every sickness known to humanity will be listed as being cured by sage." Sage is no cure-all, but research shows that this herb has some value as an antiperspirant, preservative, wound treatment, and digestive aid.

Healing History

The ancient Greeks and Romans first used sage as a meat preservative. They also believed that like another powerful preservative, rosemary, it could enhance memory.

Sage gained a much broader medicinal reputation, however. The Roman naturalist Pliny prescribed it for snakebite, epilepsy, intestinal worms, chest ailments, and menstruation promotion. The Greek physician Dioscorides considered it a diuretic and menstruation promoter and recommended sage leaves as bandages for wounds.

Around the 10th century, Arab physicians believed that sage extended life to the point of immortality. After the Crusades, this belief showed up in Europe, where students at the medieval world's most prestigious medical school in Salerno, Italy, recited, "Why should a man die who grows sage in his garden?" The same thought evolved into a medieval English proverb: "He that would live foraye [forever] / Must eat sage in May."

The French called the herb *toute bonne*, meaning "all's well," and had their own adage: "Sage helps the nerves, and by its powerful might / Palsy is cured and fever put to flight." Charlemagne ordered sage grown in the medicinal herb gardens on his imperial farms.

"The Knight's Tale" in Chaucer's *Canterbury Tales* echoed the ancient use of sage as a treatment for wounds: "To use on . . . wounds and broken arms . . . sage they drank . . ."

Around the year 1000, an Icelandic herbal recommended sage for bladder infections and kidney stones. The 12th-century German abbess/herbalist Hildegard of Bingen prescribed sage for headache, and gastrointestinal and respiratory ailments, from the common cold to tuberculosis.

During the 16th century, Dutch explorers introduced sage to the Chinese, who prized the herb so highly that they gladly traded 3 pounds of their own tea for each pound of the new European healer. Chinese physicians used sage to treat insomnia, depression, gastrointestinal distress, mental illness, menstrual complaints, and nipple inflammation (mastitis) in nursing mothers.

India's traditional Ayurvedic physicians used Indian sage similarly. They also prescribed it for hemorrhoids, gonorrhea, vaginitis, and eye disorders.

Sixteenth-century British herbalist John Gerard called sage "singularly good for the head and brain. It quickeneth the senses and memory, strengtheneth the sinews, restoreth health to those that have palsy, and taketh away shaky trembling of the members."

In the 17th century, English herbalist Nicholas Culpeper seconded Gerard, and recommended sage "boiled in water or wine to wash sore mouths and throats, cankers, or the secret parts [genitals] of man or woman."

Colonists introduced sage into North America, where it was widely used by folk healers to treat insomnia, epilepsy, measles, seasickness, and intestinal worms.

America's 19th-century Eclectic physicians, forerunners of today's naturopaths, used sage primarily to treat fever. They also prescribed sage poultices for arthritis and the tea as "a valuable anaphrodisiac [sexual depressant] to check excessive venereal desires . . . used in connection with moral . . . and other aids, if necessary."

As late as the 1920s, U.S. medical texts recommended sage tea as a gargle for sore throat and sage leaf poultices for sprains and swellings.

Modern herbalists recommend sage as an external treatment for wounds and insect bites; as a gargle for bleeding gums, sore throat, laryngitis, and tonsillitis; and as an infusion to reduce perspiration, terminate milk production, and relieve dizziness, depression, menstrual irregularity, and intestinal upsets.

Therapeutic Uses

The name *toute bonne* overstates sage's healing potential a bit, but the herb does contain an aromatic oil with some therapeutic value. The oil has one unique property that sets sage apart from all other healing herbs: It reduces perspiration.

Excessive perspiration. Several studies show that sage cuts perspiration by as much as 50 percent, with the maximum effect occurring 2 hours after ingestion. This effect helps explain how sage developed a reputation for treating fever, which causes profuse sweating, and for drying up mothers' milk.

Today, a sage-based antiperspirant (Salysat) is marketed in Germany. In addition, Commission E, the expert panel that evaluates herbal medicines for the German counterpart of the FDA, approves sage infusion as a treatment for "excessive perspiration."

Wounds. In laboratory studies, sage is active against several infection-causing bacteria. This finding lends some credence to the herb's age-old use in treating wounds. Modern physicians would not recommend bandaging wounds with sage leaves as Dioscorides did, but you can use fresh leaves as garden first-aid for minor wounds.

Food poisoning. Meats spoil in part because their fats turn rancid (oxidize). Like rosemary, sage contains powerful antioxidants, which slow spoilage. The antioxidants are comparable to the commercial preservatives BHA and BHT, supporting sage's traditional use as a preservative.

Sage's preservative action may help prevent food poisoning on your next picnic. Mix it generously into hamburger meat and tuna, pasta, and potato salads.

Digestive problems. Like most culinary spices, sage helps relax the smooth muscle lining the digestive tract, an action that makes it an antispasmodic. This property lends support to the herb's traditional role in relieving gastrointestinal complaints. Commission E approves sage as a treatment for indigestion.

Sore throats. Sage contains astringent tannins, which account for its traditional use in treating canker sores, bleeding gums, and sore throat. In Germany, where herbal healing is more mainstream than in the United States, physicians recommend a hot sage gargle for sore throat and tonsillitis.

Women's health concerns. As an antispasmodic, sage should theoretically calm the uterus. Some studies suggest, however, that sage oil may stimulate it instead, possibly explaining its traditional role in menstruation promotion. Pregnant women should not take medicinal doses of sage, but other women might try it to bring on their periods.

Intriguing Possibility

One German study has found that sage reduces blood sugar (glucose) levels in people with diabetes who drink the infusion on an empty stomach. Diabetes is a serious condition requiring professional care. If you'd like to include sage in your overall management plan, discuss it with your physician.

Rx Recommendations

For garden first-aid, crush some fresh leaves into a cut or scrape until you can thoroughly wash and bandage it.

For an infusion to settle the stomach or possibly to help manage diabetes, use 1 to 2 teaspoons of dried leaves per cup of boiling water. Steep for 10 minutes, then strain. Drink up to 3 cups a day. The infusion may also be used as a gargle. Sage tastes warm, pleasantly aromatic, and somewhat pungent.

As a homemade tincture, take ½ to 1 teaspoon up to three times a day. This may help reduce wetness if you perspire a lot.

When using commercial preparations, follow the package directions.

Do not give medicinal doses of sage to children under age 2. For older children and adults over age 65, start with low-strength preparations and increase the strength if necessary.

The Safety Factor

The medical literature contains a few reports of inflammation of the lips and lining of the mouth associated with ingestion of sage tea.

Sage contains relatively high levels of a toxic chemical called thujone. In large amounts, thujone causes a variety of symptoms that culminate in convulsions. The heat used in preparing a sage infusion eliminates much of the chemical, so the risk from consuming recommended amounts of an infusion is negligible.

Concentrated sage oil is toxic and should not be ingested.

Wise-Use Guidelines

Sage appears in the FDA list of herbs generally regarded as safe. For adults who are not pregnant or nursing, sage is considered safe when used in the amounts typically recommended.

You should take medicinal amounts of sage only in consultation with your doctor. If it causes minor discomforts, such as lip or mouth inflammation, reduce the dosage or stop using it altogether. Let your doctor know if you experience any unpleasant effects or if the symptoms for which you're taking the herb do not improve significantly within 2 weeks.

Growing Information

Sage is a perennial, branching, evergreen shrub that reaches about 3 feet. It has square, woolly, woody stems near its base, which become herbaceous toward the top. Its 2-inch leaves are oval, velvety, and gray green, with long stalks. Depending on the species, sage's small, summer-blooming flowers are pink, white, blue, or purple.

Sage is not related to the West's sagebrush, which was so named because of its vaguely sagelike aroma.

Sage may be propagated from seeds or cuttings. Germination takes a few weeks. Sow seeds ½ inch deep in spring. It takes about 2 years to grow good-size plants from seeds, which is why many authorities recommend planting 4-inch cuttings taken in the fall for use the following spring.

Sage grows well in almost any soil, but it requires good drainage and full sun. Water well until the plants have become established, after which they require less water. Sage should be replaced every 3 or 4 years because the plants become woody and less productive. If your winter temperatures fall below zero, mulch your sage in fall.

Harvest leaves before the flower buds open by cutting the plant back to 4 inches above ground. Discard the stems and leaf stalks. Dry the herb, then store it in airtight containers.

St. John's Wort

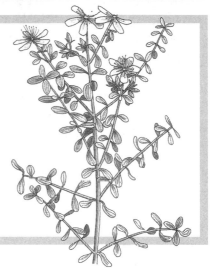

Family: Hypericaceae; other members include rose of Sharon

Genus and species: *Hypericum perforatum*

Also known as: Hypericum

Parts used: Leaves and flowers

St. John's wort has been used in herbal healing for more than 2,000 years, most notably as a treatment for wounds. Today, the herb is more popular than ever—in fact, it's one of the nation's top-selling herbal medicines. That's because in the 1980s, scientists discovered that St. John's wort is as potent an antidepressant as pharmaceutical medications.

Before the herb became known as an antidepressant, its annual sales worldwide totaled around $10 million. Now they top $550 million.

Healing History

The word *wort* is Old English for "plant." The leaves and flowers of St. John's wort contain special glands that release a red oil when pinched. Early Christians named the plant in honor of John the Baptist, because they believed it released its blood-red oil on August 29, the anniversary of the saint's beheading.

In the 1st century, the Roman naturalist Pliny prescribed St. John's wort steeped in wine as a cure for the bites of poisonous snakes. The Greek physician Dioscorides recommended it externally for burns and internally as a diuretic, menstruation promoter, and treatment for sciatica and recurring fevers (malaria).

The Greeks and Romans also believed that St. John's wort protected against witches' spells. Christians adopted this pagan belief, burning the herb in bonfires on St. John's Eve, June 23, to purify the air, drive away evil spirits, and ensure healthy crops. This poem from around 1400 summed up the popular view.

St. John's wort doth charm all witches away
If gathered at midnight on the saint's holy
day.

*Any devils and witches have no power to
    harm
Those that gather the plant for a charm.
Rub the lintels with that red juicy flower;
No thunder nor tempest will then have the
    power
To hurt or hinder your house; and bind
Round your neck a charm of a similar kind.*

Under the Doctrine of Signatures, the medieval belief that herbs' physical appearance revealed their healing value, red plants were believed to be good treatments for bleeding wounds. "The juicy red flower" of St. John's wort was no exception. In the 16th century, herbalist John Gerard recommended it as a "most precious remedy for deepe wounds," and wrote that the herb "provoketh urine and is right good against stone in the bladder."

In 1618, the first *London Pharmacopoeia* advised chopping St. John's wort flowers, immersing them in oil, and placing the mixture in the sun for 3 weeks. The resulting tincture was a standard treatment for wounds and bruises for several hundred years.

Seventeenth-century English herbalist Nicholas Culpeper called St. John's wort "a singular wound herb, boiled in wine and drank, it healeth inward hurts or bruises; made into an ointment, it opens obstructions, dissolves swellings, and closes up the lips of wounds. . . . [It] helpeth all manner of vomiting and spitting blood [tuberculosis]."

Early colonists introduced St. John's wort into North America, but they found Native Americans using the American form of the herb in much same way Europeans used the Old World plant—as a tonic and treatment for diarrhea, fever, snakebite, wounds, and skin problems.

Nineteenth-century botanical medicine authority Charles Millspaugh, M.D., touted St. John's wort's value as a wound treatment during the Civil War: "Lacerations of parts rich in nerves yield nicely to this drug." Dr. Millspaugh railed against the orthodox physicians of his day ("regulars"), who dismissed the herb as obsolete, saying, "Any homeopathic physician of at least 3 months practice can attest to its merits."

Throughout the 19th century, homeopathy was as popular as orthodox medicine. Homeopaths prescribed St. John's wort for a variety of ailments, including wounds, asthma, bites, sciatica, diarrhea, hemorrhoids, and certain forms of paralysis. Contemporary homeopaths continue this tradition.

America's 19th-century Eclectic physicians, forerunners of today's naturopaths, also considered St. John's wort an effective wound healer and tetanus preventive. They advocated the whole herb as a treatment for "hysteria" (menstrual discomforts) because of its "undoubted power over the nervous system and spinal cord."

Contemporary herbalists generally recommend St. John's wort only as an antidepressant, but for this indication they are enthusiastic. Some also suggest it for treating viral illnesses, notably HIV and herpes.

Therapeutic Uses

Unlike many other herbs, St. John's wort has been extensively researched. It contains hypericin, the source of its antidepressant action. It also contains antiviral compounds and immune-boosting chemicals known as flavonoids, which explain its action against viral, bacterial, and fungal infections.

Depression. In the early 1980s, German researchers discovered that hypericin interferes with the activity of a compound in the body known as monoamine oxidase (MAO). MAO inhibitors are an important class of antidepressant drugs. In small pilot studies in Germany, people with mild to moderate depression obtained significant relief after taking St. John's wort, including mood elevation, improved self-esteem, greater interest in life, increased appetite, and more normal sleep patterns.

Herbalists began recommending the herb for depression, but it did not rocket to prominence until 1996. That year, German researchers published a meta-analysis of human studies (clinical trials) in the prestigious *British Medical Journal*. (Meta-analysis is a statistical technique that allows the results of small studies to be combined as if they'd all been part of one large study. In medical research, one large study is more compelling than several small ones.)

The meta-analysis included 23 trials (13 testing St. John's wort against medically inactive placebos) involving 1,757 adults with mild to moderate depression. Combining the results of the trials, the researchers found that 22 percent of the people who took placebos experienced significant mood elevation. Among those who took St. John's wort, 55 percent reported similar results.

Since then, many more studies have shown that St. John's wort is an effective antidepressant. In 1999, researchers at the University of Hawaii School of Medicine performed another meta-analysis of six rigorously scientific trials that had been conducted since the earlier report. Again, St. John's wort provided significant benefit.

How beneficial is the herb? The University of Hawaii research team concluded that it's as effective as one standard class of pharmaceutical antidepressants, the tricyclics.

German researchers then compared St. John's wort to fluoxetine (Prozac), the best known of today's most popular class of pharmaceutical antidepressants, the selective serotonin reuptake inhibitors (SSRIs). Half of the 161 study participants, all of whom had mild to moderate depression, were given 20 milligrams of Prozac a day. The rest received 400 milligrams of St. John's wort twice a day. After 6 weeks, the two treatments produced comparable results—72 percent of those taking Prozac and 71 percent of those taking St. John's wort experienced significant mood elevation. The herb produced somewhat fewer side effects.

St. John's wort is generally recommended for mild to moderate depression, but at least one study suggests that it also helps relieve severe depression. In addition, the herb is beneficial for seasonal affective disorder (SAD), the winter depression caused by short day length and lack of exposure to sunlight.

British researchers gave 301 people with SAD either standard light therapy (exposure to ultrabright light) or light therapy plus St. John's wort. Both treatments produced significant mood elevation. While the light-plus-herb treatment was slightly more beneficial, the difference between that approach and light therapy by itself was not statistically significant. Those who also took the herb reported much more restful and refreshing sleep.

Initially, hypericin was dubbed an antidepressant because it appeared to be an MAO inhibitor. People who take pharmaceutical MAO inhibitors must refrain from eating a large number of foods to avoid unpleasant side effects. Many people taking St. John's wort did not observe these food restrictions but did not develop MAO side effects. German researchers have discovered why: Although hypericin resembles an MAO inhibitor, it is more complicated chemically and more similar to an SSRI, meaning no food restrictions are necessary.

As with pharmaceutical antidepressants, however, St. John's wort requires some patience. According to German medical herbalist Rudolph Fritz Weiss, M.D., the benefit "does not develop quickly . . . [and may take as long as] 2 or 3 months."

Commission E, the expert panel that evaluates herbal medicines for the German counterpart of the FDA, approves St. John's wort as a treatment for depression. According to a 1996 report in the *New York Times*, in Germany, St. John's wort outsells Prozac four to one.

Infections. Hypericin is active against a broad range of viral infections, including influenza, herpes, polio, hepatitis C, and HIV, the virus that causes AIDS. It also helps combat several types of bacteria.

Hypericin's "dramatic" activity against HIV, discovered in 1988 by researchers at New York University and the Weizmann Institute in Israel, sent many people with AIDS rushing to health food stores to stock up on St. John's wort. Some have reported benefits from taking the herb, including increased immune function.

At this time, a hypericin-based AIDS drug is in clinical trials. Enthusiasm for hypericin has waned, however, since the introduction in the late 1990s of the powerful AIDS drugs known as protease inhibitors. Ironically, people who take protease inhibitors should not use St. John's wort because the herb interferes with the action of these drugs.

Wounds. Several studies support St. John's wort's traditional use as a treatment for wounds. Hypericin and other antibiotic and anti-inflammatory compounds in the herb's red oil help prevent infection and speed healing.

One German study showed that compared with conventional treatment, a St. John's wort ointment substantially cut the healing time of burns and caused less scarring. (This product is not available in the United States.) Commission E approves topical application of St. John's wort preparations for the treatment of minor wounds and burns.

Rx Recommendations

To treat depression, buy a standardized extract and use it according to the label directions, in consultation with a physician.

To heal wounds, apply crushed leaves and flowers to the affected area after you have cleaned it with soap and water. Or you can apply a tincture.

For treatment of AIDS, consult a physician.

Do not give St. John's wort to children under age 2. For older children and adults over age 65, start with low-strength preparations and increase the strength if necessary.

The Safety Factor

In livestock fed large amounts of St. John's wort, the hypericin concentrates near the skin and causes sun sensitivity (photosensitization) and blistering sunburn. Laboratory animals injected with large doses of hypericin have died after exposure to sunlight.

As a result of these findings, in 1977, the FDA declared St. John's wort unsafe. The agency presumed that humans would develop the same reactions, but time has proven the FDA's concerns to be unfounded.

Millions of people use St. John's wort to treat depression, but the medical literature contains very few reports of photosensitization and none of serious sun-related harm. On the other hand, if you have fair, sensitive skin or have become photosensitive when using other medications, take extra precautions when out in the sun.

AIDS patients report that the herb is relatively nontoxic, but some have experienced sun sensitivity, drowsiness, nausea, and diarrhea.

St. John's wort oil may irritate sensitive skin.

Do not take St. John's wort in combination with any other antidepressant medication without first consulting your physician. Likewise, don't take the herb if you have HIV and are already taking any of the protease inhibitor medications. It impedes the action of those drugs.

Also, do not take St. John's wort if you are taking cyclosporine to control organ transplant rejection. The herb may interfere with the drug.

Wise-Use Guidelines

For adults who are not pregnant or nursing and are not taking antidepressants, protease in-hibitors, or cyclosporine, St. John's wort is considered safe in the amounts typically recommended.

You should use medicinal amounts of St. John's wort only in consultation with your doctor. If you notice any unusual symptoms, reduce the dosage or stop using it altogether. If the symptoms persist, consult your physician promptly.

Growing Information

St. John's wort is a woody, invasively spreading perennial that reaches 2 feet and has an aroma reminiscent of turpentine. Its leaves are dotted with glands that produce red oil. Its striking star-shaped flowers bloom bright yellow in summer. They also contain the leaf oil and turn red when pinched.

The herb is best propagated from root divisions in spring or fall. It grows in almost any well-drained soil under full sun or partial shade. Contain the herb to control its spread.

Although it is a perennial, St. John's wort is not particularly long-lived. Replant it every few years. Harvest the leaves and flowers as the plants bloom. Dry them and store in airtight containers.

Sarsaparilla

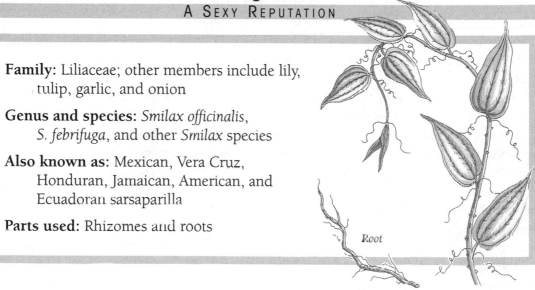

Family: Liliaceae; other members include lily, tulip, garlic, and onion

Genus and species: *Smilax officinalis*, *S. febrifuga*, and other *Smilax* species

Also known as: Mexican, Vera Cruz, Honduran, Jamaican, American, and Ecuadoran sarsaparilla

Parts used: Rhizomes and roots

Root

In old Western movies, the cowboy who didn't want whiskey told the saloon keeper, "Give me a sarsaparilla." Chances are the bartender gave him a bottle of Ayer's Sarsaparilla, a popular beverage back in the days before modern soft drinks.

Cowboys who ordered sarsaparilla usually had more than refreshment in mind. The herb was among the most widely used 19th-century treatments for syphilis, and the men often ordered it after visiting the local brothel.

Scientists say sarsaparilla has no effect against syphilis, but modern studies suggest this herb does have some intriguing benefits.

Healing History

The ancient Greeks and Romans considered European sarsaparilla an antidote to poisons. But the herb was not popular in herbal healing until the 16th century, when Spanish explorers dis-covered the Caribbean species, a prickly (*zarza*) vine (*parra*) that was small (*illa*). That description became our word *sarsaparilla*.

Caribbean Indians and Native Americans used sarsaparilla to treat skin conditions and urinary complaints. They also viewed the herb as a tonic for preserving youth and vigor, both physically and sexually.

In 1494, an epidemic of unusually virulent syphilis swept Europe, killing thousands, rather like the AIDS epidemic today. Europeans considered the disease an import from the New World, and they looked to herbs from across the Atlantic to treat it. They focused on sarsaparilla.

The conquistadors began shipping Mexican sarsaparilla back to Spain around 1530, and by 1600, it was widely used throughout Europe as a strengthening tonic and treatment for syphilis. Sarsaparilla and syphilis have been entwined ever since.

Sarsaparilla enjoyed a meteoric rise in popularity. Seventeenth-century English herbalist Nicholas Culpeper called it the treatment of choice for "the French disease," the British term for syphilis. Echoing the ancients, he wrote, "If the juice of the berries be given to a new-born child, it shall never be hurt by poison." Culpeper also recommended sarsaparilla for eye problems, head colds, gas pains, pimples, and "all manner of aches in the sinews or joints."

By 1800, many physicians denounced sarsaparilla as completely ineffective against syphilis, but their words fell on deaf ears. Mid-19th-century trade records indicate that Britain imported upward of 150,000 pounds a year, much of it for the treatment of syphilis.

In 19th-century America, sexually transmitted diseases were never mentioned in polite conversation. Nonetheless, syphilis was quite prevalent, and physicians experimented with many herbs and patent medicines to treat it. These remedies were known euphemistically as blood purifiers. One of the most popular was Ayer's Sarsaparilla, marketed for blood purification and "disorders of the liver, stomach, and kidneys, as well as tuberculosis, tumors, rheumatism, female weakness, sterility, and pimples."

Sarsaparilla was listed as a syphilis treatment in the *U.S. Pharmacopoeia*, a standard drug reference, from 1820 to 1882. After the Civil War, the anti-sarsaparilla bandwagon gained momentum, and by the late 19th century, most physicians dismissed it as worthless.

Therapeutic Uses

Sarsaparilla may be a minor medicinal herb, but it's not worthless. Research shows that it has some benefits, although not as a treatment for syphilis.

Sarsaparilla contains saponins, compounds that have diuretic action. This property may explain the herb's long association with the genitals. In addition, the herb binds certain toxins produced by bacteria (endotoxins) and speeds their elimination, which makes it a blood purifier, although not in the historical sense. Sarsaparilla also has anti-inflammatory action.

High blood pressure. Physicians often prescribe diuretics for high blood pressure. Since high blood pressure is a serious condition that requires professional care, if you'd like to include sarsaparilla in your overall treatment plan, you should do so only with the approval and supervision of your physician.

Diuretics deplete the body of potassium, an essential nutrient. If you use sarsaparilla frequently, be sure to eat potassium-rich foods such as bananas and fresh vegetables.

Congestive heart failure. Physicians often prescribe diuretics to combat the fluid accumulation associated with congestive heart failure. This condition requires professional care. If you'd like to include sarsaparilla in your overall treatment plan, discuss it with your physician.

Women's health concerns. Pregnant and nursing women should not use diuretics. As a diuretic, though, sarsaparilla may provide some relief for women bothered by premenstrual fluid retention.

Intriguing Possibilities

Preliminary studies from around the world suggest that sarsaparilla helps treat psoriasis and leprosy. Some animal studies indicate that the herb may have liver-protective effects.

While Western investigators insist that sarsaparilla is useless against syphilis, there are unconfirmed reports from China that suggest it may help. Perhaps the Chinese are wrong—or perhaps 19th-century physicians were right when they observed that sarsaparilla takes a long time to show benefit. The question deserves investigation because syphilis has been on the upswing in the United States in recent years.

Medicinal Myths

Sarsaparilla contains a compound, sarsapogenin, that can be chemically converted to the male sex hormone testosterone. Some writers have claimed that sarsaparilla contains testosterone. It does not, and ingesting the herb does not raise testosterone levels.

Sarsaparilla has also enjoyed some popularity among bodybuilders who believe that the herb contains anabolic steroids, chemical relatives of testosterone that are taken, against medical advice, to increase muscle mass. For the record, sarsaparilla contains no anabolic steroids.

Rx Recommendations

For a diuretic decoction, use 1 to 2 teaspoons of powdered root per cup of water. Bring to a boil, simmer for 10 to 15 minutes, then strain if you wish. Drink up to 3 cups a day. Sarsaparilla tastes initially sweetish, then unpleasant.

As a homemade tincture, take ¼ to ½ teaspoon up to three times a day.

When using commercial preparations, follow the package directions.

Do not give sarsaparilla to children under age 2. For older children and adults over age 65, start with low-strength preparations and increase the strength if necessary.

The Safety Factor

No significant side effects from using sarsaparilla have ever been reported.

Some weight-loss programs tout diuretics to eliminate water weight, but weight-loss experts advise against taking diuretics. Any pounds lost with help from diuretics almost invariably return. The key to permanent weight control is a low-fat, high-fiber diet and regular aerobic exercise.

Ingesting large amounts of sarsaparilla's saponins may cause a burning sensation in the mouth and throat as well as stomach and intestinal irritation.

Wise-Use Guidelines

Sarsaparilla appears in the FDA list of herbs generally regarded as safe. For adults who are not pregnant or nursing, sarsaparilla is considered safe when used in the amounts typically recommended.

You should take medicinal amounts of sarsaparilla only in consultation with your doctor. If it causes minor discomfort, such as burning in the mouth or stomach upset, reduce the dosage or stop using it altogether. Let your doctor know if you experience unpleasant effects or if the symptoms for which you're taking the herb do not improve significantly within 2 weeks.

Growing Information

Sarsaparilla is not a garden herb in the United States. It's a perennial, climbing, woody, prickly-stemmed vine with pointed, generally oval-shaped leaves. Its small flowers are dioecious (male and female on different plants), and green, yellow, or bronze. The medicinal parts, the rhizome and long, slender roots, are underground.

Saw Palmetto

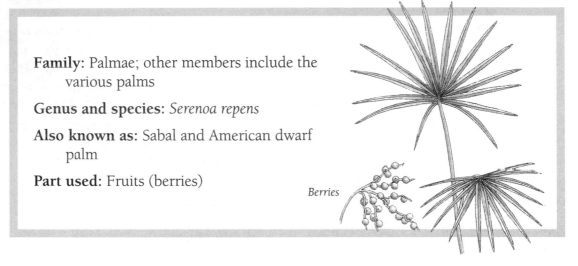

Family: Palmae; other members include the various palms

Genus and species: *Serenoa repens*

Also known as: Sabal and American dwarf palm

Part used: Fruits (berries)

Berries

Saw palmetto is a small palm tree native to Florida and the Gulf Coast that produces a brownish berry. Centuries ago, Native Americans discovered that the berry has diuretic action and began using it to treat urinary problems. Today, saw palmetto is the premier herbal treatment for benign prostate enlargement.

Healing History

Native Americans had many uses for the saw palmetto. They harvested the plant's leaves for mattress stuffing and thatched roofing and to weave into hats and baskets.

White settlers adopted the plant, and during the 19th century, physicians throughout the South recommended berry preparations to treat coughs and bronchitis.

Saw palmetto was used primarily, however, as an aphrodisiac, to enlarge women's breasts, and to treat benign prostate enlargement in men. *King's American Dispensatory* (1898), the standard text for Eclectic physicians, who were forerunners of today's naturopaths, had this to say about the herb: "Long continued use is said to slowly and surely cause the mammary glands to enlarge. Paradoxically, it also reduces hypertrophy [enlargement] of the prostate. [Saw palmetto] has been lauded as 'the old man's friend,' giving relief to the many annoyances commonly attributed to the enlarged prostate. It is reputed to strengthen the sexual appetite and restore sexual activity after exhaustive excesses."

By the early 20th century, as herbal medicine fell from favor among mainstream American doctors, saw palmetto was abandoned. Fortunately, European researchers remained interested in the plant. During the 1960s, they discovered that the Eclectics were right: Saw palmetto fruits contain fatty acids called sitosterols that help counteract prostate enlargement.

Therapeutic Uses

Saw palmetto is no aphrodisiac, nor does it enlarge the breasts. But since the early 1990s, the herb's berry extract has become a widely accepted treatment for benign prostate enlargement (known medically as benign prostatic hypertrophy, or BPH).

Benign prostate enlargement. After age 40, men's levels of testosterone decline, while levels of other hormones, notably prolactin, increase. This results in an elevation of the male sex hormone dihydrotestosterone, which is responsible for the overgrowth of prostate tissue that is characteristic of BPH.

An enzyme, 5-alpha-reductase, converts testosterone to dihydrotestosterone. Pharmaceutical BPH treatments work by interfering with the action of 5-alpha-reductase. Saw palmetto has the same biochemical action, thanks to its sitosterol compounds.

Many studies have shown that saw palmetto shrinks enlarged prostates and relieves BPH symptoms: the need to urinate immediately (urgency), difficulty getting started (hesitancy), decreased flow, difficulty finishing (dribbling), and perhaps most annoying, the need to get up at night to urinate (nocturia).

One of the most impressive studies, conducted at 87 urology clinics in nine European countries, compared a standard European saw palmetto extract (Permixon, a French preparation) to the pharmaceutical 5-alpha-reductase inhibitor finasteride (Proscar). The researchers gave the 1,098 study participants either the herb (160 milligrams twice a day) or a standard dose of the drug (5 milligrams a day).

After 26 weeks, both treatments showed about equal effectiveness. Proscar decreased BPH symptoms by 39 percent, compared with 37 percent for saw palmetto. Urine flow improved by 30 percent in the men taking the drug, compared with 25 percent in those taking the herb. But saw palmetto caused fewer side effects—namely, erection problems and loss of libido.

In another study, Belgian researchers measured prostate size, urine flow rate, and quality of life in 505 men with BPH. Then they gave the men saw palmetto extract. Six weeks later, the men's prostates were smaller, their urine flowed more freely, and they reported significantly improved quality of life. After 90 days on the herb, 88 percent of the men deemed the treatment effective.

In a third study, a team of German researchers gave saw palmetto to 320 men with BPH. Six months later, their urine flow had increased significantly. Three-quarters reported less need to get up at night, and half reported less frequent daytime urination. These improvements were maintained for 3 years.

Commission E, the expert panel that evaluates herbal medicines for the German counterpart of the FDA, approves saw palmetto as a treatment for BPH. In the United States, prescription medications are generally used to treat BPH, but in Europe, saw palmetto is more popular.

Note: Neither saw palmetto nor pharmaceutical treatments cure BPH. They reduce prostate size and relieve symptoms. Continued enlargement may get the better of either herbal or pharmaceutical treatment, and surgery may become necessary.

Intriguing Possiblity

Chinese physicians prescribe an herbal formula whose main ingredient is saw palmetto as a treatment for prostate cancer. At the University of California, San Francisco, Medical Center, researchers gave the Chinese formula to 61 men with advanced prostate cancer whose tumors no longer responded to mainstream medication. Levels of prostate-specific antigen, a standard indicator of tumor activity, declined by at least 50 percent in three-quarters of the men. It's too early to call saw palmetto a treatment for prostate cancer, but that day may come.

Rx Recommendations

Studies showing that saw palmetto reduces the symptoms of prostate enlargement have used 320 milligrams of a standardized extract a day, split into two or three doses. Unfortunately, however, the more doses per day, the less likely people are to take their medicine as they should.

Researchers in Brussels, Belgium, conducted a 1-year study of 132 men with enlarged prostates to compare two different saw palmetto regimens: the standard two doses (160 milligrams each) daily versus one large dose (320 milligrams) a day. The single large dose produced the same symptom improvement as the two smaller doses.

To use saw palmetto, look for a standardized extract and take 320 milligrams a day, as either one or two doses.

The Safety Factor

If saw palmetto produces any side effects, they're mild—stomach upset and headache. Allergic reactions are also possible in some people.

Because saw palmetto has hormonal action, men with hormone disorders should consult a physician before taking it.

If you are already using another BPH medication, do not take saw palmetto without consulting your physician.

If you are having trouble urinating or if you pass blood in your urine, talk to your doctor.

Growing Information

When early explorers sailed along the coast of the United States from the Carolinas to Texas, they saw small palm trees that they called scrub palms, now known as saw palmettos. Saw palmetto grows easily to about 10 feet in sandy soil, and it is used as an ornamental in the Southeast. The plant produces edible brown-black fruits (berries), an extract of which is the herbal medicine.

Scullcap

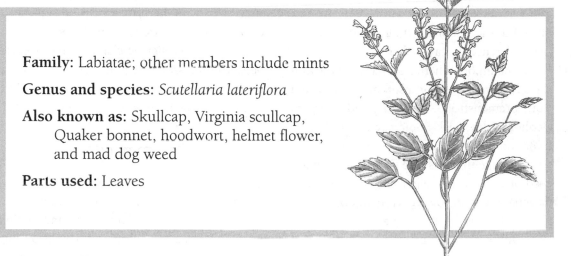

Family: Labiatae; other members include mints

Genus and species: *Scutellaria lateriflora*

Also known as: Skullcap, Virginia scullcap, Quaker bonnet, hoodwort, helmet flower, and mad dog weed

Parts used: Leaves

For an herb reputed to have calming effects, scullcap has caused considerable controversy. One respected herbalist calls the blue-flowered North American native "perhaps the most widely relevant tranquilizer" in medicine. On the other hand, skeptics dismiss it as "nearly worthless and essentially inactive."

The truth is, scullcap's traditional use as a tranquilizer appears to have scientific support.

Healing History

For centuries, Chinese physicians have used Asian scullcap (*Scutellaria baicalensis*) as a tranquilizer-sedative and a treatment for convulsions.

Writing in 1892, medical herbalist Charles F. Millspaugh, M.D., recounted the herb's odd story: "The first introduction of this plant into medicine was the experiments of Dr. Vandesveer [of Roysfield, New Jersey], in 1772,

who claimed it curative and prophylactic [preventive] in hydrophobia [rabies], his reported cases being 1,400. This seems a large number to fall to one physician. His son after him claimed to cure 40 cases more in 3 years. [But] its worthiness was greatly doubted, and the plant much railed against. Many regulars [orthodox physicians] and empirics [folk herbalists] used the remedy with success, while many others wrote essays against it. . . . The plant has also proved itself a useful nervine [tranquilizer], antispasmodic [digestive aid], and tonic in wakefulness, convulsions, and delirium tremens."

America's 19th-century Eclectic physicians, forerunners of today's naturopaths, recommended scullcap primarily as a tranquilizer-sedative for insomnia and nervousness and as a treatment for "intermittent fever" (malaria), convulsions, and the delirium tremens of advanced alcoholism.

Nineteenth-century patent medicine makers used scullcap extensively in tonics for "female weakness" (menstrual discomforts).

Scullcap entered the *U.S. Pharmacopoeia*, a standard drug reference, as a tranquilizer in 1863. It remained there until 1916, when it moved to the *National Formulary*, the pharmacists' reference. It stayed there until 1947.

Contemporary herbalists recommend scullcap as a tranquilizer for insomnia, nervous tension, premenstrual syndrome, and drug and alcohol withdrawal. Some say the herb treats fever and convulsions.

Asian scullcap is one of the most widely used plants in Chinese herbal medicine. Practitioners prescribe it for viral infections (including flu and hepatitis), bacterial infections, fever, and high blood pressure.

Therapeutic Uses

American scientists are almost unanimous in their condemnation of scullcap. They've never gotten over those old, mistaken claims that it treats rabies. They should.

Insomnia and anxiety. European and Russian studies have lent support to scullcap's traditional role as a tranquilizer. European medical experts now accept its potential usefulness as a tranquilizer and sedative. The herb is an ingredient in many European over-the-counter sleep preparations.

Intriguing Possibilities

Japanese researchers have discovered that the Asian species of scullcap has anti-inflammatory properties.

Two other Japanese studies, both involving animals, have shown that scullcap increases levels of "good" cholesterol (high-density lipoprotein, or HDL). As HDL levels increase, the risk of heart attack decreases. These findings suggest that the herb may help prevent heart disease and some strokes in humans.

Chinese physicians claim to have treated hepatitis successfully with the herb. It's too early to tout scullcap for this potentially serious liver disease, but the herb deserves further research.

Rx Recommendations

For a tranquilizing infusion, use 1 to 2 teaspoons of dried herb per cup of boiling water. Steep for 10 to 15 minutes, then strain. Drink up to 3 cups a day. Scullcap tastes bitter; adding honey, sugar, and lemon or mixing it with an herbal beverage blend will improve the flavor.

When using commercial preparations, follow the package directions.

Do not give scullcap to children under age 2. For older children and adults over age 65, start with low-strength preparations and increase the strength if necessary.

The Safety Factor

There are no reports of toxicity from scullcap infusions, but large amounts of tincture can cause confusion, giddiness, twitching, and possibly convulsions.

The FDA lists scullcap as an herb of undefined safety. For adults who are not pregnant or nursing and are not taking other tranquilizers or sedatives, scullcap is considered safe when used in the amounts typically recommended.

You should take medicinal amounts of scullcap only in consultation with your doctor. If it causes minor discomfort, such as stomach upset or diarrhea, reduce the dosage or stop using it altogether. Let your doctor know if you experience unpleasant effects or if the symptoms for which you're taking the herb do not improve significantly within 2 weeks.

Growing Information

Many scullcap species grow in Europe, but the American herb is the one used in herbal healing. It's sometimes called Virginia scullcap, but it grows all over the United States and southern Canada.

The plant is a 2-foot, slender, branching, square-stemmed perennial with opposite, serrated leaves. The flowers have two lips. The upper lip includes an elongated caplike appendage, which is the source of most of the herb's popular names.

Scullcap may be propagated from seeds or root divisions planted in early spring. Thin seedlings to 6-inch spacing. It grows in any well-drained soil under full sun and requires little care. Although it is a perennial, scullcap rarely lives longer than 3 years.

Harvest the leaves in midsummer.

Senna

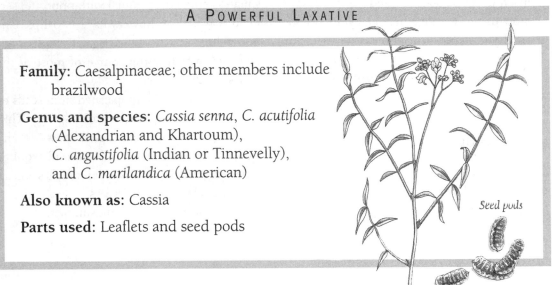

Family: Caesalpinaceae; other members include brazilwood

Genus and species: *Cassia senna, C. acutifolia* (Alexandrian and Khartoum), *C. angustifolia* (Indian or Tinnevelly), and *C. marilandica* (American)

Also known as: Cassia

Parts used: Leaflets and seed pods

Seed pods

Senna is a powerful laxative—so powerful, in fact, that many authorities call it a cathartic. Arab physicians first wrote of its bowel-stimulating action in the 9th century, but their descriptions suggest that it had been widely used for centuries from the Middle East to India. Senna was introduced into European herbal healing before the Crusades and has played a prominent role ever since.

Both senna and cinnamon come from trees with peelable bark—in Arabic, *quetsiah*, meaning "to cut." *Quetsiah* evolved into senna's genus name, *Cassia*. Although both senna and cinnamon are sometimes called cassia today, these two herbs have very different actions and should not be confused.

Healing History

Seventeenth-century English herbalist Nicholas Culpeper, who came close to prescribing every herb for every ill, could not resist claiming that senna "cleanses the stomach, purges melancholy and phlegm from the head, brain, lungs, heart, liver, and spleen, cleansing those parts of evil humour; strengthens the senses, procures mirth, purifies the blood [treats venereal disease], and is also good in chronic agues [fevers]." Other herbalists generally recommended senna only as a laxative.

Native Americans recognized the laxative action of the American form of senna but used the herb primarily to treat fever. The 19th-century Eclectics, forerunners of today's naturopaths, were influenced by Native American medicine and called senna "very useful in all forms of febrile [fever-producing] diseases in which laxative action is desired."

Contemporary herbalists tout senna's laxative action but warn of its terrible taste and side effects, primarily intestinal cramps.

Therapeutic Uses

Senna does not treat fever, nor does it "purge melancholy and procure mirth." Quite the contrary. If you're not careful with this herb, you'll live to regret using it.

Constipation. Like aloe, buckthorn, and cascara sagrada, senna contains anthraquinones, chemicals that stimulate the colon. The herb is an ingredient in many over-the-counter laxatives, including Correctol, Ex-Lax, Fletcher's Castoria, and Perdiem.

Senna and the other anthraquinone laxatives should be considered last resorts for constipation. First, increase your fiber intake, drink more fluids, and exercise more often. If that doesn't work, try the bulk forming laxative psyllium (see page 325). If that's not successful, try a gentler anthraquinone, cascara sagrada (see page 110). Finally, if you still need relief, try senna in consultation with your physician.

Commission E, the expert panel that evaluates herbal medicines for the German counterpart of the FDA, approves senna as a laxative.

Rx Recommendations

Because of senna's disgusting taste, herbalists generally discourage using the plant material. Instead, they recommend over-the-counter products containing it. Follow the package directions.

Those game enough to try the unprocessed herb can brew an infusion from 1 to 2 teaspoons of dried leaves per cup of boiling water. Steep for 10 minutes, then strain. Drink up to 1 cup a day in the morning or before bed for no more than a few days.

The taste of senna is nauseating. To make it more palatable, add sugar, honey, and lemon and mix senna with taste-masking herbs such as anise, fennel, peppermint, chamomile, ginger, coriander, cardamom, and licorice.

Some sources say the pods have milder action. Steep four pods in a cup of warm water for 6 to 12 hours. Drink up to 1 cup a day in the morning or before bed for no more than a few days.

As a tincture, use ½ to 1 teaspoon in the morning or before bed for no more than a few days.

Do not give senna to children under age 2. For older children and adults over age 65, start with low-strength preparations and increase the strength if necessary.

The Safety Factor

Senna's powerful action means that it should not be used by those with chronic gastrointestinal conditions such as ulcers, colitis, or hemorrhoids. Women who are pregnant or nursing should also avoid the herb.

You should never take senna for more than 2 weeks. Over time, it causes lazy bowel syndrome, an inability to have bowel movements without chemical stimulation.

Large amounts of senna cause diarrhea, nausea, and severe cramps with possible dehydration. Long-term use may cause enlargement of the fingertips (clubbing). An article in *Lancet* described this effect in a woman who had taken up to 40 senna laxative tablets a day for 15 years. Her fingers returned to normal when she stopped using the herb.

Senna leaves may cause a skin rash in people who are sensitive to the plant.

Wise-Use Guidelines

The FDA considers senna an herb of undefined safety. For adults who are not pregnant or nursing, are not taking other laxatives, and do not have chronic gastrointestinal conditions, senna is considered relatively safe when used only occasionally in the amounts typically recommended.

You should take medicinal amounts of senna only in consultation with your doctor. If it causes cramping, reduce the dosage or stop using it altogether. Let your doctor know if you experience unpleasant effects or if constipation does not improve significantly within 2 weeks.

Growing Information

Senna is not a garden herb in the United States. Native to Egypt and Sudan, it's a small, woody shrub that reaches 3 feet and has branching stems, pointed leaves, and seeds encased in a leathery pod. The species generally used in herbal medicine is grown in the Tennevelly region of India, near the subcontinent's southern tip. One species grows in the eastern United States.

Shepherd's Purse

Family: Cruciferae; other members include cabbage, broccoli, and cauliflower

Genus and species: *Capsella bursa-pastoris*

Also known as: Lady's purse, rattle pouches, and rattle weed

Parts used: Leaves and flowers

Shepherds never get much respect. In the ancient world, theirs was a humble calling. And in the Old West, cattle ranchers looked down on "sheep herders." So perhaps we should not be surprised that the herb named for shepherds has shared a similar fate.

More than 300 years ago, Nicholas Culpeper wrote, "Few plants possess greater virtues than this, and yet it is utterly disregarded." No one is interested, some authorities say, because shepherd's purse is a common weed that's medicinally worthless. But the few scientific studies done to date have revealed some intriguing possibilities for treating bleeding and inducing labor.

Healing History

Ancient Greek and Roman physicians recommended shepherd's purse seeds as a laxative. It was not widely used until the 16th century, however, when an Italian physician promoted it to stop bleeding, particularly to eliminate blood in the urine. Some physicians adopted the plant, but most dismissed it as worthless.

The Pilgrims introduced shepherd's purse into North America, where it quickly became a weed. Folk herbalists used it to stop bleeding, while physicians generally regarded it as useless.

America's 19th-century Eclectic physicians, forerunners of today's naturopaths, prescribed shepherd's purse to stop bleeding. Their text *King's American Dispensatory* (1898) attempted to explain the controversy over the herb's effectiveness by observing that "the fresh herb is decidedly more active than the dried." *King's* called shepherd's purse very efficient for treating bloody urine and recommended it to stop excessive menstrual flow and to relieve diarrhea, dysentery, and bleeding hemorrhoids.

During World War I, when other coagulants were in short supply, wounded soldiers were given shepherd's purse tea.

Contemporary herbalists recommend the internal use of dried shepherd's purse, not the fresh herb, for bloody urine, nosebleeds, heavy menstrual flow, and bleeding after childbirth. They also support the herb's external use as an astringent to treat wounds and hemorrhoids.

Therapeutic Uses

Shepherd's purse won't set the world of herbal medicine on fire, but it may help some women with heavy menstrual flow or pregnant women waiting to go into labor—if they can stomach its taste.

Bleeding. Shepherd's purse contains substances that hasten the coagulation (clotting) of blood, according to an article in the British scientific journal *Nature*. German medical herbalist Rudolph Fritz Weiss, M.D., writes that the herb "definitely has haemostatic [blood-stopping] properties . . . [but they are] not very great."

First-aid experts recommend treating bleeding with sustained pressure on the wound. Blood in phlegm, urine, or stool requires prompt professional treatment.

Although shepherd's purse is no substitute for standard medical care, people with ulcers, colitis, Crohn's disease, or bleeding disorders or women with heavy menstrual flow might try it in consultation with their physicians.

Commission E, the expert panel that evaluates herbal medicines for the German counterpart of the FDA, approves shepherd's purse as a treatment for persistent nosebleeds and menorrhagia (heavy menstrual flow).

Labor inducement. Shepherd's purse contains some substances that may help stimulate uterine contractions as effectively as the drug oxytocin (Pitocin), which is often given to trigger labor. Women who are trying to conceive or are pregnant should not use shepherd's purse, except at term and in consultation with their physicians.

Wounds. Shepherd's purse has some mild anti-inflammatory astringent action, lending some support to its traditional role as a treatment for wounds and hemorrhoids.

Rx Recommendations

To help stop bleeding or to hasten labor, use 1 teaspoon of dried herb per cup of boiling water. Steep for 10 minutes, then strain. Drink up to 2 cups a day. Shepherd's purse has a biting, unpleasant taste. To make it more palatable, add sugar, honey, and lemon or mix it with an herbal beverage blend.

As a homemade tincture, use ¼ to ½ teaspoon up to twice a day.

When using commercial preparations, follow the package directions.

Do not give shepherd's purse to children under age 2. For older children and adults over age 65, start with low-strength preparations and increase the strength if necessary.

To use shepherd's purse externally on wounds or hemorrhoids, soak a clean cloth in either an infusion or a tincture.

The Safety Factor

If shepherd's purse does in fact stop bleeding, no one is sure exactly how. It may strengthen blood vessel walls, or it may stimulate clotting. Blood clots may trigger heart attack or stroke. Anyone with a history of any of these conditions, and anyone taking anticoagulant (blood-thinning) medication, including low-dose aspirin, should not use shepherd's purse.

The medical literature contains no reports of harm from this herb.

Wise-Use Guidelines

For adults who are not pregnant or nursing, are not taking anticoagulant medication or supplements (vitamin E, for example), and have no history of heart attack, stroke, or thromboembolism, shepherd's purse is considered safe in the amounts typically recommended.

You should take medicinal amounts of shepherd's purse only in consultation with your doctor. If it causes minor discomfort, such as stomach upset or diarrhea, reduce the dosage or stop using it altogether. Let your doctor know if you experience any unpleasant effects or if the symptoms for which you're using the herb do not improve significantly within 2 weeks.

Growing Information

Shepherd's purse is a foul-smelling annual that reaches 18 inches. Its slender stem rises from a rosette of deeply toothed leaves similar to dandelion. The stem bears a few small leaves and terminates in small white flowers. The fruits are wedge-shaped seed pods containing literally thousands of yellow seeds, hence the herb's common names.

Shepherd's purse grows easily from seeds planted in spring under full sun. It prefers well-drained sandy loam but tolerates most North American soils.

If unchecked, shepherd's purse can become a garden and lawn pest. To avoid this, clip the seed pods before they open. The young leaves have a peppery taste and may be added to soups and stews or eaten like spinach. Harvest the leaves and flowers as the flowers open.

Slippery Elm

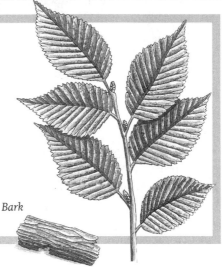

Family: Ulmaceae; other members include the elms

Genus and species: *Ulmus rubra* and *U. fulva*

Also known as: Red elm and Indian elm

Part used: Inner bark

Bark

No food or drug of today comes close to matching the place of honor that slippery elm held in 18th- and 19th-century America. Great elm forests covered the East, and even in cities, the versatile bark was always close at hand.

Soaked in water and wrapped around meats, slippery elm bark retarded spoilage in the days before refrigeration. Coarsely ground and mixed with water, it turned into a spongy mass and was molded into bandages to cover wounds and made into pill-like coverings for unpleasant-tasting medicines. Ground and mixed with water or milk, slippery elm bark turned into a soothing, nutritious gruel similar to oatmeal that was used to treat sore throats, coughs, colds, and gastrointestinal ailments and to feed infants and hospital patients. Slippery elm sore throat lozenges were a fixture in home medicine cabinets. The herb was the nation's leading home remedy for anything in need of soothing.

Slippery elm is still listed in the *National Formulary*, the pharmacists' reference, and health food stores still sell lozenges containing the herb. But our once-great elm forests have been decimated by Dutch elm disease, and both our landscapes and our herbal healing heritage are poorer as a result.

Healing History

The 1st-century Greek physician Dioscorides prescribed soaking in a European elm bath to speed the healing of broken bones. His prescription survived for more than 1,500 years.

In the 17th century, English herbalist Nicholas Culpeper wrote, "The decoction being bathed in, heals broken bones . . . [and] is excellent [for] places . . . burnt with fire. The leaves bruised, applied, and being bound thereon with its own bark heal wounds." Culpeper also claimed that elm root decoction restored hair on bald scalps.

Colonists found the Native Americans using American slippery elm bark as a food and treatment for wounds, sore throats, coughs, inflamed nipples (mastitis), and many other ailments. The colonists adopted these uses and developed many more, including applying slippery elm poultices to bring boils to a head.

Native American women inserted slippery elm sticks to induce abortion, and white women adopted the practice, which caused many deaths from uterine infection and hemorrhage. As a result, several state legislatures passed laws forbidding the sale of slippery elm bark in pieces longer than 1½ inches.

America's early 19th-century Thomsonian herbalists recommended slippery elm tea as a laxative gentle enough for children. Thomsonian midwives lubricated their hands with the slippery bark before performing internal examinations.

By the time of the Civil War, slippery elm was being used to treat syphilis, gonorrhea, and hemorrhoids. America's 19th-century Eclectic physicians, forerunners of today's naturopaths, deemed the herb very valuable and suggested that "a tablespoon of the powder boiled in milk affords a nourishing diet for infants newly weaned, preventing the bowel complaints to which they are subject. Some physicians consider the constant use of it, during and after the seventh month of gestation, as advantageous in facilitating an easy delivery."

Contemporary herbalists recommend slippery elm bark externally to cover wounds and soothe skin problems and internally as a tea to treat sore throats and coughs as well as diarrhea, ulcers, colitis, and other gastrointestinal complaints.

Therapeutic Uses

Even the FDA, which is usually critical of herbal medicines, calls slippery elm "an excellent demulcent" (soothing agent). The herb's bark is rich in a soluble fiber called mucilage that swells and becomes spongy and gelatinous when mixed with water.

Wounds. When applied to thoroughly washed wounds, slippery elm bark mucilage dries to form an herbal bandage.

Coughs, sore throats, and digestive problems. Slippery elm decoction helps soothe the throat and digestive tract. Besides providing mucilage, the herb stimulates production of digestive tract mucus, which also acts as a soother.

Women's health concerns. Slippery elm decoction has a long history of use by pregnant women, and the medical literature contains no reports of problems. The active constituent, mucilage, should not harm the fetus. If you have a history of problematic pregnancy, however, consult your physician before trying a slippery elm preparation.

Medicinal Myth

Slippery elm has never been shown to speed the healing of broken bones.

Rx Recommendations

For a poultice to bandage wounds, stir enough water into powdered bark to make a paste and apply to the affected area.

For a soothing decoction, use 1 to 3 teaspoons of powdered herb per cup of water. Blend a little water in with the powder first to prevent lumpiness. Bring to a boil and simmer for 15 minutes, then strain if you wish. Drink up to 3 cups a day. Slippery elm has only a slight taste and a mild aroma reminiscent of maple.

When using commercial preparations, follow the package directions.

You may give slippery elm cautiously to children under age 2.

The Safety Factor

Allergic reactions are possible. Otherwise, the medical literature contains no reports of slippery elm causing harm.

Wise-Use Guidelines

For adults, slippery elm is safe in the amounts typically recommended.

You should use medicinal amounts of slippery elm only in consultation with your doctor. Let your doctor know if you experience unpleasant effects or if the symptoms for which you're using the herb do not improve significantly within 2 weeks. If a wound becomes increasingly warm, red, painful, or inflamed, seek prompt medical care.

Growing Information

Slippery elm is a stately tree that reaches 60 feet. Its trunk bark is brown, but its branch bark is whitish. Its leaves are broad, rough, hairy, and toothed. Check local nurseries to see if this tree can be grown in your area.

Soybean

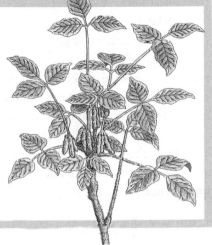

Family: Leguminosae; other members include beans and peas

Genus and species: *Glycine max*

Also known as: Soya

Parts used: Beans

Soybeans are the United States' fourth leading agricultural product, surpassed only by cattle, dairy products, and corn. An astonishing 70 million acres of American farmland are planted with soybeans, largely for cattle feed and export to Asia. The U.S soybean crop accounts for almost half of the world production and generates $14.6 billion a year in revenues.

Incredibly, soybeans never caught on in the American diet. That's slowly changing, however, as research continues to reveal more about soy's amazing health benefits.

Healing History

Soybeans were cultivated in China as early as 1200 B.C. They were that country's second most important crop, after rice. Soybeans served as a key source of protein for a culture that was largely vegetarian. The Chinese developed tofu around 200 B.C.

The ancient Japanese adopted soybeans and tofu. During the 18th century, soybeans were introduced into Europe, but they didn't arrive in the United States until Chinese immigrants brought them in the 1880s. Soybeans quickly became a major U.S. crop, raised almost entirely as cattle feed and for export to Asia. Tofu did not become widely used in this country until health foods became popular in the late 1960s.

From the 1970s through the 1980s, tofu was the food Americans loved to hate. The water-packed, spongy white blocks, resembling pressed cottage cheese, were the butt of countless put-downs by the hosts of late-night TV shows and others who considered health foods as bland and tasteless as, well, plain tofu.

During the 1990s, public opinion began to shift. Tofu and other soy foods have still not become national favorites, but the jokes have largely ceased, for two reasons. First, soy foods—in particular, soy-based textured vegetable protein—have become more familiar. Soy protein is now added to a large number of supermarket items, including soy dogs (a substitute for beef and pork franks) and soy burgers (a substitute for hamburgers).

Second, studies have now shown that tofu and other soy foods offer a remarkable number of health benefits—so many that the FDA now allows soy products to carry a health claim on their labels. Supplement companies have even packaged the bean's health-promoting compounds, isoflavones, into pills and capsules that are becoming quite popular.

Therapeutic Uses

The key isoflavones in soybeans are genistein and daidzein. The following chart shows how the various types of soy foods stack up in terms of their isoflavone content. (Incidentally, soy sauce is not a source of isoflavones.)

Soy Product	Portion	Isoflavones (mg)
Raw soybeans	½ cup (34 g)	176
Roasted soybeans (soy nuts)	½ cup (30 g)	167
Tempeh	4 oz. (19 g)	61
Soy protein	1 oz. (26 g)	57
Soy flour	¼ cup (8 g)	44
Tofu	4 oz. (18 g)	38
Textured soy protein	¼ cup (18 g)	28
Soy milk	8 oz. (10 g)	20

Soy and soy products have a remarkable number of health benefits. Here's what research has turned up so far.

High cholesterol. Many studies have shown that soy helps lower cholesterol. At Wake Forest University, researchers placed 156 men and women with high cholesterol on the low-fat diet recommended by the American Heart Association. In addition, the study participants were given one of five supplement drinks: a medically inactive placebo or four beverages containing varying amounts of soy isoflavones. After 9 weeks, those who received the placebo drinks showed no improvement in their cholesterol levels, but all of those who received the soy drinks showed reductions in cholesterol, with the greatest decrease occurring in the group whose beverage contained the most isoflavones.

Researchers at the Veterans Affairs Medical Center in Lexington, Kentucky, analyzed 38 other studies of soy protein's effect on cholesterol. They found that soy lowered cholesterol significantly. Study participants who consumed 47 grams (1.7 ounces) of soy protein a day saw their total cholesterol decline by 23 milligrams per deciliter of blood (mg/dl). The researchers concluded that substituting soy protein for animal protein significantly decreases cholesterol.

Because of all the research showing that soy protein helps cut cholesterol, in 1999, the FDA ruled that foods containing at least 6.25 grams of soy protein per serving may state on their labels that they reduce cholesterol and the risk of heart disease.

Commission E, the expert panel that evaluates herbal medicines for the German counterpart of the FDA, approves soy foods as a treatment for elevated cholesterol.

Hot flashes. Doctors prescribe estrogen-rich hormone replacement therapy (HRT) to relieve hot flashes. But HRT also increases the risk of breast cancer, which is one of the most common reasons why only a minority of women use it.

Soy isoflavones are plant estrogens (phytoestrogens). They're similar to human estrogen, but chemically weaker. Soy phytoestrogens are strong enough to prevent and relieve hot flashes but not so strong that they stimulate the growth of breast tumors. In fact, mounting evidence suggests that soy foods help prevent breast cancer (see below).

Italian researchers gave 104 postmenopausal women who had hot flashes either placebos or 76 milligrams of soy isoflavones a day. After 1 month, the women taking the soy reported significantly fewer hot flashes.

Breast cancer. Many studies have shown that compared with Americans, Asian women are substantially less likely to develop breast cancer. Epidemiologists used to believe that Asian women have a reduced risk because they eat a lower-fat diet than American women. Now, many scientists attribute the lower rate of breast cancer to the combination of less fat and more soy.

Human estrogen stimulates the growth of breast tumors. Weaker soy phytoestrogens attach to estrogen receptors on breast cells, effectively locking out the body's own estrogen and reducing its stimulating effect. In laboratory studies, breast cancer cells exposed to soy isoflavones had their growth reduced by 30 percent.

Australian researchers conducted diet surveys of 144 women newly diagnosed with breast cancer and 144 demographically similar women who were cancer-free. After accounting for other known risk factors (such as family history), the researchers determined that the women who were cancer-free consumed significantly more soy isoflavones than those with breast cancer.

Osteoporosis. Estrogen replacement is used to prevent osteoporosis in postmenopausal women. Animal studies have found that soy protein increases bone density, and recently, a human study produced the same results.

Researchers at the University of Illinois gave groups of postmenopausal women 40 grams of protein a day. In one group, the protein came from non-soy sources (meat and dairy products). In another group, the protein included moderate levels of soy isoflavones, and in a 3rd group, the protein included high levels of soy isoflavones. After 6 months, the women consuming the non-soy protein showed bone loss, while those eating the most soy isoflavones showed significantly increased bone mineral density.

Intriguing Possibility

There is some preliminary evidence that soy foods help prevent cancers of the colon and prostate.

Rx Recommendations

If you get your soy from foods, most experts recommend consuming about 5 ounces of tofu (about 1.5 servings) containing approximately 50 to 70 grams of soy protein weekly. If you have any of the conditions that may be prevented by soy, feel free to eat more.

Soy isoflavones are also available as supplements. Follow the label directions.

Because soybeans are such a major crop in

the United States, the soy trade organizations have had the financial resources to fund the studies showing soy's benefits. These results have not been duplicated for other beans, but according to research at the USDA, all edible beans contain isoflavones.

Soy contains the most isoflavones per serving, but it wouldn't take too many dishes made with other beans (burritos, baked beans, bean soups, or salads) to consume significant amounts of isoflavones. The chart below shows how various legumes compare in terms of isoflavone content (the figures are in parts per million).

The Safety Factor

Soy is safe for the vast majority of people, but allergies and other sensitivities are possible. If you develop any unusual symptoms after incorporating soy foods into your diet, eliminate those foods and see what happens. If your symptoms improve, that's a good indication of sensitivity. In that case, talk to your doctor about how to get soy's benefits without eating soy foods or taking soy supplements.

Growing Information

The soybean plant is an annual that grows from 1 to 5 feet tall. Its stems, leaves, and bean pods are covered with fine hairs that give the plant a fuzzy appearance and feel. The pods contain up to four seeds (beans).

Soybean is not a garden herb, but if you grow peas, you might grow soybeans. The beans can be roasted and eaten.

Legume	Genistein (ppm)	Daidzein (ppm)	Total (ppm)
Soybeans	24	38	62
Black beans	45	0	45
Pinto beans	22	23	45
Lima beans	40	0	40
Kidney beans	29	3	31
Red lentils	25	5	30
Fava beans	20	5	25
Great Northern beans	17	7	24
Black-eyed peas	23	0	23
Mung beans	22	0	22

Tarragon

Family: Compositae; other members include daisy, dandelion, and marigold

Genus and species: *Artemisia dracunculus*

Also known as: French or Russian tarragon, estragon, and dragon herb

Parts used: Leaves

Tarragon is best known as the main seasoning in bearnaise sauce. Like all aromatic herbs, it also has a long history in herbal healing.

Unlike most other aromatics, though, tarragon fell from healing fashion in the 17th century. Only recently has the herb been rediscovered as an oral anesthetic with some potential for preventing varicose veins.

Healing History

After discovering that chewing tarragon numbs the mouth, the ancient Greeks used the herb to treat toothache. They also decided that its anesthetic power and its wide-ranging root runners meant that it could help relieve the discomforts of traveling. The 1st-century Roman naturalist Pliny wrote that tarragon prevented fatigue on long journeys. During the Middle Ages, pilgrims placed tarragon sprigs in their shoes.

Oddly enough for an herb that numbs the mouth, around the 10th century, Arab physicians recommended tarragon as an appetite stimulant.

Under the Doctrine of Signatures, the medieval belief that an herb's appearance revealed its medicinal value, tarragon's serpentine roots were considered a sign that it could cure snakebite. Over the centuries, the belief expanded to include the bites of rabid dogs. But by the 17th century, this belief had faded. Nicholas Culpeper, who recommended dozens of herbs for the bites of "venomous creatures," did not mention tarragon in this regard. In fact, he hardly mentioned it at all.

After Culpeper, herbalists virtually abandoned tarragon because it loses most of its aromatic healing oil as it dries. Even America's 19th-century Eclectic physicians, forerunners of today's naturopaths, who prized botanical drugs, had no use for it.

Few contemporary herbalists value tarragon except in French cooking. Those who do recognize it reiterate its traditional uses as a diuretic, appetite stimulant, digestive aid, and toothache treatment.

Therapeutic Uses

While tarragon is no wonder herb, it deserves a place in herbal healing. Its active component is its oil, but drying largely destroys it. Either fresh or frozen leaves or comparatively large amounts of dried leaves must be used.

Toothache. Tarragon oil contains the same anesthetic compound, eugenol, as clove oil. This supports its age-old use for toothache. Tarragon provides only temporary relief of oral pain, however. If toothache persists, consult a dentist.

Infections. Like many culinary herbs, tarragon oil fights disease-causing bacteria in laboratory studies. You can use fresh leaves as garden first-aid for minor wounds.

Intriguing Possibilities

Tarragon oil contains rutin, a compound that strengthens blood vessel walls. Herbalists often recommend other herbs rich in rutin, notably violet and onion, for the treatment of varicose veins in the legs. These herbs may also help hemorrhoids, which are varicose veins in the anal area.

An animal study published in the *Journal of the National Cancer Institute* suggests that rutin has some anti-tumor activity.

Rx Recommendations

For temporary relief of oral pain, chew fresh leaves as needed.

For garden first-aid, apply fresh, crushed leaves to a cut or scrape until you can wash and bandage it.

For a pleasant, licorice-flavored infusion that may help prevent varicose veins and hemorrhoids, use 1 to 2 teaspoons of fresh or frozen herb per cup of boiling water. Steep for 10 to 15 minutes, then strain. Drink up to 3 cups a day.

As a homemade tincture, use $\frac{1}{2}$ to 1 teaspoon up to three times a day.

When using commercial preparations, follow the package directions.

Do not give medicinal amounts of tarragon to children under age 2. For older children and adults over age 65, start with low-strength preparations and increase the strength if necessary.

The Safety Factor

Large amounts of estragole, a compound in tarragon, produce tumors in mice. Tarragon has never been associated with human cancer, but until its effects are clarified, people with a history of cancer should probably not use the herb in medicinal amounts.

Otherwise, the medical literature contains no reports of tarragon causing harm.

Wise-Use Guidelines

Tarragon is included in the FDA list of herbs generally regarded as safe. For adults who are not pregnant or nursing, tarragon is considered safe when used in the amounts typically recommended.

You should take medicinal amounts of tarragon only in consultation with your doctor. If it causes minor discomfort, such as stomach upset or diarrhea, reduce the dosage or stop using it altogether. Let your doctor know if you experience unpleasant effects or if the symptoms for which you're taking the herb do not improve significantly within 2 weeks.

Growing Information

Tarragon comes in two varieties, Russian and French. The former has less oil—and therefore, less flavor and medicinal value—so a mention of tarragon almost always refers to the French plant.

Russian tarragon may be grown from seeds, but the more desirable French variety must be propagated from cuttings or root divisions. Divide the roots in spring and plant 1-inch pieces of their tips, or take cuttings in summer. Thin plants to 2-foot spacing.

French tarragon is a perennial with a creeping, serpentine root and stems that reach 2 feet. Its leaves look like a larger version of rosemary. This herb rarely flowers, and if it does, the fruits are sterile.

Tarragon grows best in rich, well-drained soil under full sun. Make sure the roots do not become waterlogged. If your winter temperatures drop below the teens, mulch well each fall. Divide tarragon roots every few years to retain the plants' vigor.

Tarragon leaves bruise easily. Harvest them carefully in early summer. Because it loses medicinal value when dried, freeze the fresh herb or preserve it in vinegar

Tea

Family: Theaceae; other members include camellia

Genus and species: *Camellia sinensis*

Also known as: Green tea and black tea

Parts used: Leaves

Tea is the world's second most popular beverage (water ranks as number one). Most Americans and Europeans drink it only as a mild stimulant, but this is changing as people learn more about tea's many antioxidant benefits. The fact is, a few cups of tea—specifically, green tea—a day can help prevent many serious conditions associated with aging, notably cancer and heart disease.

Many people, including some herbalists, use the term *tea* to describe any herbal beverage made by steeping plant material in hot water. This works colloquially, but in herbal medicine, it becomes confusing. For example, using the colloquial definition, coffee is a tea because it's a hot-water extract of plant material.

Technically, herbal hot-water extracts are not teas but infusions. In herbal medicine, *tea* refers to an infusion made with the leaves of the tea bush (*Camellia sinensis*).

Few herbals mention tea. In fact, most people don't even consider tea an herb. They typically ask, "Would you like coffee, tea, or herb tea?" Of course, coffee and tea are both herbs, so all of these beverages are herbal teas. In the context of the previous question, "herb tea" typically means a noncaffeinated herbal beverage.

There are three types of tea: green, black, and oolong. All begin as leaves of *Camellia sinensis*. Green tea, the type preferred in Japan and China, is simply tea leaves that are dried and crumbled. Green tea is the most medicinally beneficial variety. For black tea, preferred in Great Britain, Europe, and the United States, tea leaves are dried and then fermented, a process that gives it a darker color and richer, fuller-bodied flavor. Oolong tea is semi-fermented. Tea may also be named for the place it was grown (for example, Ceylon and Darjeeling).

Tea is different from tea tree (*Melaleuca alterniflora*), an Australian herb whose oil is a powerful topical antiseptic (see page 388).

Healing History

Tea has been used in Chinese medicine for at least 3,000 years to treat headache, diarrhea, dysentery, colds, coughs, asthma, and other respiratory problems. The Chinese also view tea as a grease cutter and recommend drinking it with fatty meals.

By the 8th century, tea was a favorite in India and Indonesia. The Dutch East India Company introduced tea into Holland in 1610, and by 1640, black tea had become popular with the English upper class. They drank it as an afternoon stimulant around 4 o'clock, which is still known as tea time.

The Chinese called black tea *pek-ho*, and the British adopted the term as *pekoe*. They considered the beverage so divine that they took the name tea from the Greek *thea*, meaning "goddess."

Demand for tea spurred England's colonization of India, Sri Lanka (formerly Ceylon), and Hong Kong. By the late 18th century, tea was an integral part of British culture and around the world, the English simply would not tolerate any threat to their tea supply. So in 1773, when the British Parliament levied a tax on tea imported into the North American colonies, outraged tea-loving colonists rioted in Massachusetts. They stormed the tea ships in Boston Harbor and dumped enormous quantities of the herb overboard. The Boston Tea Party helped trigger the American Revolution.

In Europe and North America, tea has always been used primarily as a stimulant beverage. Traditional herbalists and folk healers have also recommended it for diarrhea, colds, coughs, and other respiratory problems.

Therapeutic Uses

Tea contains three stimulant compounds: caffeine, theobromine, and theophylline. These account for the herb's effectiveness in treating respiratory problems. It also contains astringent tannins.

It's green tea's powerfully antioxidant polyphenols, however, that have rocketed the herb into medicinal prominence in recent years. Japanese scientists discovered that tea has polyphenols in the early 1980s. Like all antioxidants, these compounds help prevent and repair the cell damage that sets the stage for heart disease, most cancers, and many other degenerative conditions associated with aging, including cataracts and macular degeneration.

Cancer. Green tea was shown to have cancer-preventive value in laboratory animals in the early 1980s. The first study to find the same benefit in humans was published in 1988.

For the study, researchers in Kyushu, Japan, compared the diets and lifestyles of 139 people with stomach cancer and 2,852 people who were cancer-free. After accounting for other variables, the researchers determined that as green tea consumption increased, stomach cancer risk decreased. The greatest protective benefit was conferred on those who drank at least 10 cups a day.

Since then, green tea has been shown to reduce the risk of several other cancers, including esophageal, colorectal, pancreatic, lung, and breast cancers. The breast cancer study, from

Japan, is particularly intriguing. Compared with women with breast cancer who drank little or no green tea, women who regularly drank a lot (8 to 10 cups a day) had milder cases of breast cancer at diagnosis (fewer positive lymph nodes), a greater likelihood of estrogen-positive disease (which correlates with improved prognosis), less risk of metastasis (spread to other areas of the body), less risk of recurrence, and a better rate of survival.

Heart disease. The antioxidants in green tea help prevent heart disease. University of Kansas researchers have found that some of the antioxidants in green tea are 25 times as powerful as vitamin E, an antioxidant nutrient that's been shown in many studies to reduce heart attack risk. A Dutch study concluded that compared with people who drink no tea, those who drink 1 to 2 cups a day have significantly less atherosclerotic narrowing of their arteries, the underlying cause of heart disease and most strokes.

Respiratory problems. All of the stimulants in tea are bronchodilators that ease breathing by opening the bronchial passages, thus supporting the herb's traditional use as a remedy for respiratory problems. Until recently, physicians often prescribed pharmaceutical preparations of theophylline, one of the stimulant compounds in tea, to treat asthma.

Diarrhea. The astringent tannins in tea help account for the herb's binding action in diarrhea. Tea is one component of the BRATT diet, a popular home remedy for diarrhea that consists of bananas, rice, applesauce, tea, and toast.

Tooth decay. Tea is a good source of fluoride, which helps prevent tooth decay. Both green and black teas contain more fluoride than fluoridated water. The tannins in tea may also help fight the bacteria that cause tooth decay.

Intriguing Possibility

An animal study published in the *Journal of Nutrition Science* shows that tea lowers cholesterol. The herb may have a similar effect in people.

Tannins have some antiviral action, and Chinese reports claim that tea helps treat hepatitis. Hepatitis is a serious disease that requires professional care, but during convalescence, tea does no harm, and it may do some good.

Rx Recommendations

The specific antioxidant that's believed to account for tea's value in preventing cancer and heart disease is epigallocatechin gallate (EGCG). It is present in all forms of tea, but unfermented green tea has much higher concentrations. In laboratory studies, black tea has been shown to have only $\frac{1}{10}$ to $\frac{1}{100}$ of green tea's antioxidant punch.

Some studies, including the Dutch trial mentioned earlier, have found that black tea confers health benefits. A different Dutch study, however, involving 58,279 men and 62,573 women who were tracked for more than 4 years, showed that black tea had no value in protecting against lung, breast, or colorectal cancers, three diseases that green tea has been shown to help prevent.

The bottom line: Green tea is best for the prevention of cancer and cardiovascular disease. Black and oolong teas contain significantly less of the antioxidants found in green tea but are not entirely devoid of them.

If you're used to the rich, full-bodied flavor of black tea, green tea may taste thin and watery at first. But over time, you may come to appreciate its delicate flavor.

How strong a brew is necessary to maximize green tea's antioxidant benefits? University of Hawaii researchers steeped green tea for 2, 5, and 10 minutes, then ran laboratory tests to determine each brew's antioxidant activity. They all packed about the same antioxidant punch. Apparently, the antioxidant compounds in green tea are released quickly, and steeping longer than about 3 minutes does not appreciably increase their concentration.

For a pleasantly bitter infusion, use 1 tea bag or 1 to 2 teaspoons of dried herb per cup of boiling water. Steep for 10 to 15 minutes and strain (if you use loose tea).

In the studies showing tea's cancer-preventive benefit, participants drank more than 5 cups a day, and sometimes more than 10. That might expose you to more caffeine than you can comfortably tolerate. When steeped for around 3 minutes, a typical cup of tea contains about 40 milligrams of caffeine, compared with 100 milligrams in a cup of brewed coffee. Ten cups of tea would contain approximately as much caffeine as 4 cups of brewed coffee.

You may give weak tea preparations cautiously to children under age 2. For older children and adults over age 65, start with low-strength preparations and increase the strength if necessary.

The Safety Factor

Caffeine is a classically addictive drug that causes nervousness, restlessness, insomnia, and many other potentially problematic effects. (For more information, see Coffee on page 144.)

Caffeine has been linked to an increased risk of birth defects, so pregnant women should not consume it.

Large amounts of tea may cause gastrointestinal upset.

Wise-Use Guidelines

For adults who are not pregnant or nursing, tea is safe in the amounts typically recommended.

You should use medicinal amounts of tea only in consultation with your doctor. If it causes minor discomfort, such as stomach upset, reduce or eliminate it. Let your doctor know if you experience unpleasant effects or if the symptoms for which you're drinking tea do not improve significantly within 2 weeks.

Growing Information

Tea is not a garden herb in North America. It is cultivated primarily in India, Sri Lanka, and Indonesia.

The tea tree is a small evergreen that grows to 30 feet in the wild. In cultivation, however, it is pruned into a bushy shrub to allow easier harvesting of the leaves.

Tea Tree

Family: Myrtaceae; other members include eucalyptus, myrtle, and clove

Genus and species: *Melaleuca alternifolia*

Also known as: Teatree oil and Australian teatree

Parts used: Leaf oil

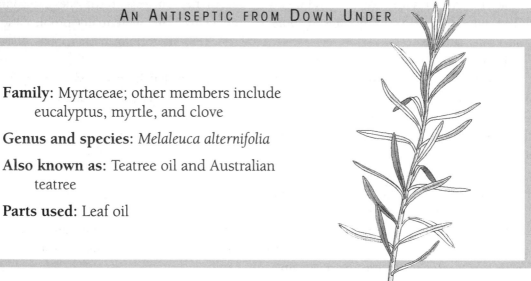

Don't confuse tea tree with *Camellia sinensis*, the plant whose leaves give us the tasty, mildly stimulating beverage known as tea (see page 384). Tea tree, *Melaleuca alternifolia*, has some impressive therapeutic powers of its own.

Healing History

When the British explorer Captain James Cook first arrived in Australia in 1777, he found the aborigines treating skin infections with crushed tea tree leaves. White settlers adopted the plant and used its leaves to make a beverage tea, hence the name tea tree. They also used the leaves to flavor beer. Australian physicians introduced tea tree's medicinal benefits to Europe and the United States.

During the 1920s, tea tree oil was used as an antiseptic in surgery and dentistry. During World War II, it was used to disinfect wounds.

Today, tea tree oil is an ingredient in some antiseptic soaps, creams, acne products, deodorants, toothpastes, mouthwashes, and antifungal creams and vaginal suppositories.

Therapeutic Uses

Modern science has discovered that the essential oil liberated by crushing tea tree leaves is a powerful antiseptic.

Wounds. A study at the University of Western Australia found that tea tree oil kills many microorganisms that can cause infection, including the yeast fungus *Candida albicans* and several bacteria—*Escherichia coli*, *Staphylococcus aureus*, and *Pseudomonas aeruginosa*. Another study at the same university showed that even when staphylococcus bacteria are resistant to pharmaceutical antibiotics, tea tree oil kills them.

Tea tree oil can also be used to treat insect bites and stings. It even has a reputation for relieving the pain of fire ant bites.

Athlete's foot. Australian researchers gave people with athlete's foot one of the following treatments: a medically inactive placebo cream; a cream containing 1 percent tolnaftate, a standard pharmaceutical (used in Aftate, Desenex, and Tinactin); or a cream containing 10 percent tea tree oil. The herb was as effective as the tolnaftate.

Acne. At Royal Prince Alfred Hospital in Australia, researchers gave 124 people with mild to moderate acne either an over-the-counter 5 percent benzoyl peroxide lotion or a lotion containing tea tree oil. The benzoyl peroxide lotion worked faster, but by the end of the study, both treatments were equally effective. The tea tree oil caused fewer side effects such as skin irritation.

Fungal toenail infections. Stubborn, hard-to-treat fungal toenail infections discolor and thicken toenails. At the University of Rochester School of Medicine, researchers had 117 people with fungal toenail infections apply either a standard pharmaceutical (1 percent clotrimazole) or tea tree oil (100 percent) twice a day for 6 months. Both treatments produced the same results—60 percent of the people in each group experienced improvements in their symptoms, if not complete cure.

Yeast infections. Tea tree oil's activity against the yeast fungus has led to its use in treating vaginal yeast infections.

Intriguing Possibility

Added to baths or vaporizers, tea tree oil may help treat respiratory infections. Australians also use tea tree oil to treat scabies and head lice.

Rx Recommendations

Use a cotton ball or cotton swab to apply 100 percent tea tree oil to affected skin or toenails twice a day.

If you've been diagnosed with a vaginal yeast infection, try placing a few drops of tea tree oil on a tampon and inserting it. Leave it in place for 24 hours, then remove it. If continued treatment is necessary, use a new tampon.

The Safety Factor

Do not ingest tea tree oil. Swallowing as little as a few teaspoons can be fatal.

Anyone may use tea tree oil topically, including pregnant or nursing women, children, and the elderly. For those with sensitive skin (children and people with fair complexions), the oil should be diluted in vegetable oil before it's applied.

Wise-Use Guidelines

You should use medicinal amounts of tea tree oil only in consultation with your doctor. If the oil causes a rash, itching, or skin irritation, use less or stop using it completely. Let your doctor know if you experience any unpleasant effects or if the symptoms for which you're using the herb do not improve significantly within 2 weeks.

Growing Information

Native to the swampy lowlands of New South Wales, Australia, tea tree is an evergreen that can reach 40 feet. It has narrow, needlelike leaves that release the plant's antiseptic, aromatic oil when crushed. Its white flowers bloom in summer.

Thyme

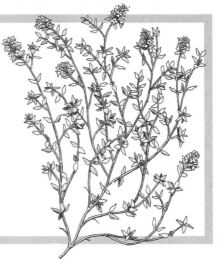

Family: Labiatae; other members include mints

Genus and species: *Thymus vulgaris* and *T. serpyllum*

Also known as: Common or garden thyme (*T. vulgaris*); wild thyme, creeping thyme, mother thyme, and mother of thyme (*T. serpyllum*)

Parts used: Leaves and flowers

Parsley, sage, rosemary, and . . . Listerine? Or perhaps Vicks VapoRub?

Thyme is commonly found in kitchen spice racks, but without realizing it, millions of Americans stock the herb's oil in their medicine chests as well. Its inclusion in mouthwashes and decongestants is no coincidence. Thyme has a long history of use as an antiseptic, cough remedy, and digestive aid.

Healing History

Both the Roman poet Virgil and his naturalist countryman Pliny mention thyme as a meat preservative. The herb was sprinkled on sacrificial animals to make them more acceptable to the gods.

Like so many other aromatic herbs, thyme was introduced into cooking as an offshoot of its meat-preserving action. The Romans also used it medicinally as a cough remedy, digestive aid, and treatment for intestinal worms.

The emperor Charlemagne ordered thyme grown in all of his imperial gardens for both its culinary and medicinal value. The 12th-century German abbess/herbalist Hildegard of Bingen considered it the herb of choice for skin problems, anticipating its later use as an antiseptic.

During the Middle Ages, thyme became linked to courage. It was fashionable for noblewomen to embroider sprigs of thyme on scarves and give them to favorite knights departing for the Crusades.

As the centuries passed, thyme was used as an antiseptic during plagues. Those troubled by "melancholia" (depression) were advised to sleep on thyme-stuffed pillows.

Medieval anatomists named the lymph gland in the chest the thymus because it reminded them of a thyme flower.

Sixteenth-century British herbalist John Gerard recommended thyme for leprosy and to "cure sciatica . . . pains in the head . . . [and] falling sickness [epilepsy]."

In the 17th century, Nicholas Culpeper called thyme "excellent for nervous disorders . . . headaches . . . and a certain remedy for that troublesome complaint, the nightmare." He claimed that the herb "provokes the terms [menstruation], gives safe and speedy delivery to women in travail [labor], and brings away the after-birth." Culpepper also recommended thyme as "a noble strengthener of the lungs . . . an excellent remedy for shortness of breath. . . . It purges the body of phlegm . . . comforts the stomach much and expels wind."

By the late 17th century, apothecary shops were selling thyme oil as a topical antiseptic under the name "oil of origanum." In 1719, German chemist Caspar Neumann extracted thyme oil's active constituent, which he called "camphor of thyme." In 1853, French chemist M. Lallemand named it thymol, as it is called today.

From the mid-19th century through World War I, thymol enjoyed great popularity as an antiseptic. America's Eclectic physicians, forerunners of today's naturopaths, extolled it in their textbook *King's American Dispensatory* (1898): "Thymol is considered by many to be superior to carbolic acid [the antiseptic made famous in 1867 by the father of antiseptic surgery, Joseph Lister]. It prevents putrefaction and arrests it when it has commenced. . . . Dissolved in water, it forms an invaluable disinfectant [for] sick rooms." The Eclectics also prescribed thyme infusion for headache, gastrointestinal upsets, "hysteria" (menstrual cramps), and as a menstruation promoter.

World War I caused a major thymol crisis. Most of the world's supply was distilled in Germany. When the British and French declared war on Germany, they had to scramble to overcome a terrible shortage of the suddenly vital battlefield antiseptic.

Although thymol has since been replaced by more potent germ fighters, it remains an ingredient in several antiseptic mouthwashes, including Listerine.

Contemporary herbalists recommend thyme externally for disinfecting wounds and internally for indigestion, sore throats, laryngitis, coughs, whooping cough, and nervousness.

Therapeutic Uses

Thyme's aromatic oil contains two compounds, thymol and carvacol, that account for its medicinal value. Both chemicals have preservative, antibacterial, and antifungal properties. They also have expectorant properties and may be useful as digestive aids.

Infections. In laboratory studies, thyme fights several disease-causing bacteria and fungi, supporting the herb's traditional role as an antiseptic. Infusions of the dried herb are nowhere near as powerful as the oil or distilled thymol, but you can use fresh leaves as garden first-aid for minor wounds.

Coughs. German researchers have lent support to thyme's traditional role as a phlegm loosener (expectorant). In Germany, where herbal medicine is considerably more mainstream than in the United States, thyme preparations are frequently prescribed to relax the respiratory tract and treat coughs, whooping cough, and emphysema.

German medical herbalist Rudolph Fritz

Weiss, M.D., writes, "Thyme is to the trachea [windpipe] and the bronchi what peppermint is to the stomach and intestines." Commission E, the expert panel that evaluates herbal medicines for the German counterpart of the FDA, approves thyme as a treatment for cold-related coughs, bronchitis, and whooping cough.

Digestive problems. Thymol and carvacol relax the smooth muscle tissue of the gastrointestinal tract, making thyme an antispasmodic. The action of these chemical constituents lends support to its traditional role as a digestive aid.

Women's health concerns. Antispasmodics relax not only the digestive tract but also other smooth muscles, such as the uterus. Small amounts may help relieve menstrual cramps, lending credence to the Eclectic physicians' use of thyme.

In large amounts, thyme oil and thymol are considered uterine stimulants. Pregnant women may use thyme as a culinary spice, but they should avoid large amounts and not ingest the oil.

Intriguing Possibility

In a laboratory study, Israeli scientists have found that thyme infusion inhibits the growth of *Helicobacter pylori*, the bacteria that cause most gastrointestinal ulcers. It's too early to call thyme an ulcer treatment, but if you have ulcers, you may want to try drinking thyme tea.

Rx Recommendations

For garden accidents, crush fresh leaves into minor wounds until you can wash and bandage them. After you have thoroughly washed them, apply a few drops of thyme tincture as an antiseptic.

For an infusion to help settle the stomach, soothe a cough, or possibly help relieve menstrual symptoms, use 2 teaspoons of dried herb per cup of boiling water. Steep for 10 minutes, then strain. Drink up to 3 cups a day. Thyme tastes pleasantly aromatic, with a faint clovelike aftertaste.

As a homemade tincture, take ½ to 1 teaspoon up to three times a day.

When using commercial preparations, follow the package directions.

Do not give medicinal preparations of thyme to children under age 2. For older children and adults over age 65, start with low-strength preparations and increase the strength if necessary.

The Safety Factor

Use the herb, not its oil. Even a few teaspoons of thyme oil can be toxic, causing headache, nausea, vomiting, weakness, thyroid impairment, and heart and respiratory depression.

One animal study showed that thyme suppresses thyroid activity in rats. People with thyroid conditions should consult their physicians before taking medicinal doses.

Thyme and thyme oil may cause a rash in people who are sensitive to them.

Wise-Use Guidelines

The FDA includes thyme in its list of herbs generally regarded as safe. For adults who are not pregnant or nursing and do not have thyroid problems, thyme is considered safe when used in the amounts typically recommended.

You should take medicinal amounts of thyme only in consultation with your doctor. If it causes minor discomfort, such as headache or nausea, reduce the dosage or stop using it altogether. Let your doctor know if you experience unpleasant effects or if the symptoms for which you're using the herb do not improve significantly within 2 weeks.

Growing Information

Thyme is an aromatic, perennial, many-branched, groundcover shrub that reaches about 12 inches. It has small, opposite, virtually stalkless leaves and lilac or pink flowers that bloom in midsummer.

This hardy herb can be propagated from seeds, cuttings, and root divisions. Seeds require a temperature around 70°F to germinate and often do best when started indoors. For cuttings, snip 3-inch pieces from stems with new growth and place them in wet sand. Roots should appear in about 2 weeks.

The best time for root division is in spring. Uproot a plant carefully, preserving as much of its root soil as possible. Divide it in half or thirds and replant the divisions 12 inches apart in moist soil.

Once established, thyme requires little care. It prefers well-drained, slightly dry soil. Wetting thyme leaves during watering reduces their fragrance.

Clumps tend to become woody after a few years. To prevent this, roots should be divided periodically.

Thyme survives frost, but in areas with cold winters, use mulch. Thyme may be killed if winter temperatures drop below 10°F.

Harvest the leaves and flowers just before the flowers bloom. Dry and store them in airtight containers to preserve the herb's oil.

Turmeric

Family: Zingiberaceae; other members include ginger

Genus and species: *Curcuma longa*

Also known as: Curcuma

Parts used: Rhizomes and roots

Turmeric is a fairly recent addition to most American spice racks, but it's been a mainstay in Indian curries for thousands of years. Its arrival here is good news for our palates and our health.

Turmeric has not been well-researched in humans. Studies with animals show that the herb has an impressive array of medical uses—as an immune stimulant, as a treatment for arthritis, digestive problems, and scabies, and as a preventive for cataracts, cancer, heart disease, and liver problems.

Healing History

Turmeric gives curry blends their yellow color. In addition to its role in cooking, the herb held a place of honor in India's traditional Ayurvedic medicine. A symbol of prosperity, it was considered a cleanser for the whole body. Medically,

it was used as a digestive aid and as a treatment for fever, infections, dysentery, arthritis, and jaundice and other liver problems.

Traditional Chinese physicians prescribed turmeric to treat liver and gallbladder problems, stop bleeding, and relieve chest congestion and menstrual discomforts.

The ancient Greeks were well-aware of turmeric, but unlike its close botanical relative, ginger, it never caught on in the West as either a culinary or a medicinal herb. It was, however, used to make orange-yellow dyes.

In the 1870s, chemists noticed that turmeric's orange-yellow root powder turned reddish brown when exposed to alkaline chemicals. This discovery led to the development of "turmeric paper," thin strips of tissue brushed with a decoction of turmeric, then dried. During the late 19th century, turmeric paper was used in laboratories around the world to test for alkalinity. Eventually, it was replaced by litmus paper, which is still used today.

American chemists used turmeric paper, but not even the botanically oriented 19th-century Eclectic physicians, forerunners of today's naturopaths, had much use for turmeric itself, except to add color to medicinal ointments.

In the 1930s, Maude Grieve's influential *Modern Herbal* said that turmeric was "once a cure for jaundice," then dismissed it as "seldom used in medicine except as a coloring."

Today's naturopaths may be the intellectual heirs of Eclectic medicine, but they've parted company with their predecessors when it comes to turmeric. They extol the herb as an anti-inflammatory. "Turmeric is one of nature's most potent anti-inflammatory agents," says Joseph Pizzorno, N.D., coauthor of *The Textbook of Natural Medicine* and former president of Bastyr University, the naturopathic medical school near Seattle.

Naturopaths also recommend turmeric for the prevention and treatment of degenerative conditions that respond to antioxidants, including cancer and heart disease.

Therapeutic Uses

Because Western scientists and herbalists didn't show much interest in turmeric until recently, the vast majority of research involving the herb has been done in India. The yellow pigment in turmeric, curcumin, is its most medicinally active compound. Curcumin is an immune stimulant with antimicrobial, stomach-soothing, anti-inflammatory, antioxidant, and liver- and heart-protecting action.

Enhanced immunity. Indian researchers tested the immune function of laboratory animals, then fed them a curcumin-enriched diet for 5 weeks. Subsequent retesting showed significant improvement in some measures of immune function.

Wounds. Like many culinary herbs, turmeric helps retard food spoilage because it has antibacterial action. It may also help prevent bacterial wound infections.

Food poisoning. Turmeric is notably effective against salmonella bacteria, a frequent cause of food poisoning (also called gastroenteritis and stomach flu). The herb also fights protozoa in laboratory tests, lending some credence to its traditional use in treating amoebic dysentery.

Digestive problems. Turmeric stimulates the flow of bile, which helps digest fats. This validates the herb's traditional role as a digestive aid. Commission E, the expert panel that evaluates herbal medicines for the German counterpart of the FDA, approves turmeric for indigestion.

Scabies. In an Indian study, 814 people infested with tiny, itchy scabies mites were treated with a combination of turmeric and another Indian herb, neem. Almost all of the study participants (97 percent) reported that the infestation disappeared in 3 to 15 days. The treatment was cheaper than standard medical scabicides and caused no adverse reactions.

Arthritis. Many animal studies show that turmeric and curcumin exhibit anti-inflammatory action with no significant gastrointestinal side effects. In some studies, curcumin has been found to be as effective an anti-inflammatory as ibuprofen or cortisone.

Several Indian studies have tested turmeric and curcumin as treatments for osteoarthritis and rheumatoid arthritis, with positive results. In one study, the herb relieved the morning stiffness and joint swelling of rheumatoid arthritis as well as a prescription nonsteroidal anti-inflammatory drug (NSAID). But unlike NSAIDs, turmeric caused no significant abdominal distress.

Pharmaceutical manufacturers have now introduced a new class of anti-inflammatory drugs, the COX-2 inhibitors. They deliver the same benefits as NSAIDs but with fewer side effects. It turns out that curcumin is a natural COX-2 inhibitor.

Cataracts. Cataracts are caused by oxidative damage to the lens of the eye, the type of damage that antioxidants help prevent. In one study, animals were fed a diet enriched with either corn oil or turmeric for 14 days, then exposed to conditions that produce cataracts. The animals that were fed turmeric developed significantly fewer cataracts.

Cancer. Antioxidants help prevent the cell damage that sets the stage for cancer. Many laboratory studies have shown that curcumin has anti-cancer activity. Reports published in journals such as *Cancer Letters*, *Cancer Research*, and *Carcinogenesis* say that the compound inhibits the growth of several cancers, among them colon cancer and lymphoma.

So far, very few human trials have examined the effects of curcumin on cancer. In one of them, an Indian study published in the journal *Mutagenesis*, smokers had their urine tested for compounds that cause genetic mutations (mutagens), a marker for cancer-causing biochemical activity. Then they were given 1.5 grams of turmeric (about a teaspoon) for 30 days. Even though they didn't change their smoking habits, the number of mutagens in their urine decreased significantly.

Heart disease. Turmeric's close botanical relative, ginger, reduces cholesterol, lowers blood pressure, and helps prevent the blood clots that trigger heart attacks and most strokes. Animal studies show similar benefits from turmeric.

Few human trials have explored turmeric's effects on the heart and cardiovascular system. In one pilot study, Indian researchers measured the cholesterol levels of 10 adults, then asked them to take 500 milligrams of curcumin every day for 10 days. Their cholesterol levels fell significantly.

Liver damage. Several animal studies suggest that turmeric protects the liver from the damaging effects of many toxic compounds, including alcohol, aflatoxin, and carbon tetrachloride. These findings lend credence to the herb's traditional use in liver ailments.

If you regularly drink alcohol and/or regularly take certain pharmaceuticals, including large doses of the common pain reliever acetaminophen, you may be at risk for liver damage. Ask your physician about taking turmeric to help protect your liver.

Intriguing Possibilities

Animal studies suggest that turmeric helps prevent and heal ulcers and helps prevent gallstones. The herb also lowers blood sugar (glucose) levels, suggesting that it may help control diabetes.

Medicinal Myth

The Chinese used turmeric to stimulate menstruation. To date, no research has confirmed that the herb has any effect on the uterus.

Rx Recommendations

To treat minor wounds, wash them with soap and water, then sprinkle on some powdered turmeric before applying a bandage.

For an infusion to help aid digestion, use 1 teaspoon of turmeric powder per cup of warm milk. Drink up to 3 cups a day. Turmeric tastes pleasantly aromatic, but in large amounts, it becomes somewhat bitter.

To treat arthritis, it's best to buy curcumin supplements. Dr. Pizzorno recommends 400 milligrams of curcumin three times a day, or you can follow the package directions on the product you choose.

Do not give medicinal turmeric preparations to children under age 2. For older children and adults over age 65, start with low-strength preparations and increase the strength if necessary.

The Safety Factor

One animal study has shown that turmeric reduces fertility. This experiment has not been replicated, and its implications for human fertility, if any, remain unclear. Nevertheless, people who are trying to conceive and those with fertility problems should probably not use medicinal amounts.

Turmeric's potential anti-clotting effect may cause problems for those with clotting disorders. If you have a blood-clotting problem, discuss the herb with your physician before using medicinal preparations.

Unusually large amounts of turmeric may cause stomach upset.

Wise-Use Guidelines

Turmeric is on the FDA list of herbs generally regarded as safe. For adults who are not pregnant or nursing, do not have clotting disorders, and are not taking anticoagulant (blood-thinning) medications or supplements (vitamin E, for example), turmeric is considered safe when used in the amounts typically recommended.

You should take medicinal amounts of turmeric only in consultation with your doctor. If it causes minor discomfort, such as heartburn or stomach upset, reduce the dosage or stop using it altogether. Let your doctor know if you experience unpleasant effects or if the symptoms for which you're using the herb do not improve significantly within 2 weeks.

Growing Information

Turmeric is not a garden herb in North America. Grown from India to Indonesia, it's a perennial with a pulpy, orange, tuberous rhizome (underground stem) that grows to about 2 feet in length. The aerial parts, which reach 3 feet, include large, lily-like leaves; a thick, squat, central flower spike; and funnel-shaped yellow flowers.

Uva-Ursi

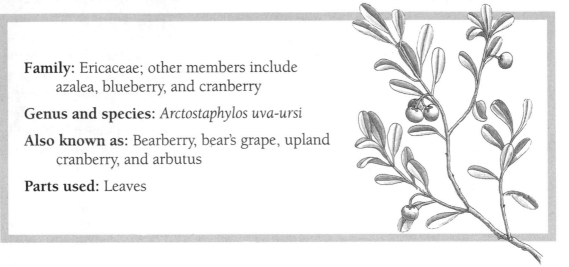

Family: Ericaceae; other members include azalea, blueberry, and cranberry

Genus and species: *Arctostaphylos uva-ursi*

Also known as: Bearberry, bear's grape, upland cranberry, and arbutus

Parts used: Leaves

Uva-ursi has been used as a diuretic and urinary antiseptic for more than 1,000 years by cultures as widely separated as the Chinese and Native Americans. Today, it is an ingredient in most herbal diuretics and urinary remedies and in many weight-loss formulas. Even herbal conservative Varro E. Tyler, Ph.D., describes uva-ursi as "a modestly effective urinary antiseptic and diuretic."

Uva-ursi may not be effective if it's taken in combination with certain foods, however. This is crucial information that some herbals fail to mention.

Healing History

The Roman physician Galen used uva-ursi's astringent leaves to treat wounds and stop bleeding, but the herb was largely ignored by Western herbalists until the 13th century. Then,

Marco Polo reported that Chinese physicians prescribed it as a diuretic to treat kidney and urinary problems. Polo's famous travelogue made uva-ursi popular in Europe as a urinary and kidney remedy.

Uva-ursi's association with the kidney was strengthened by the medieval Doctrine of Signatures, the belief, once widely held, that a plant's physical appearance revealed its healing virtues. The herb grew in rocky, gravelly places, and at the time, kidney stones were called "gravel."

North American colonists found that Native Americans had independently discovered uva-ursi's benefit as a urinary remedy. They also mixed its leathery leaves with tobacco and created the smoking mixture kinnikinnik.

Uva-ursi was incorporated into the *U.S. Pharmacopoeia*, a standard drug reference, as a urinary antiseptic in 1820 and remained there until 1936. Chemists isolated the herb's major active compound, arbutin, in 1852.

The 19th-century Eclectics, forerunners of today's naturopaths, recommended uva-ursi for diarrhea, dysentery, gonorrhea, bed-wetting, and "chronic affections of the kidneys and urinary passages."

Today, homeopaths recommend a microdose of uva-ursi for incontinence, blood in the urine, and kidney and urinary tract infections.

Contemporary herbalists continue to recommend uva-ursi for kidney and urinary problems.

Therapeutic Uses

According to several studies, the arbutin in uva-ursi is chemically transformed into an antimicrobial antiseptic, hydroquinone, in the urinary tract. In addition, the herb contains several diuretic chemicals (including ursolic acid), powerful astringents (tannins), and allantoin, a chemical that helps promote the growth of healthy new cells.

Urinary problems. The actions of uva-ursi's active compounds support its age-old use in urinary tract infections (UTIs) and other urinary ailments. The herb is notably effective against *Escherichia coli*, the most frequent cause of UTIs. Some herbalists report that uva-ursi has cured UTIs that were unresponsive to pharmaceutical antibiotics. This is certainly possible, but scientific sources say that pharmaceutical antibiotics are generally more effective.

For mild urinary symptoms, try uva-ursi as herbal first-aid. For urinary problems that require professional care, use the herb in addition to standard therapies. Commission E, the expert panel that evaluates herbal medicines for the German counterpart of the FDA, approves uva-ursi for urinary tract ailments.

There's an important catch to using uva-ursi. To receive the greatest antiseptic benefit, the urine must be alkaline. This means that you must avoid acidic foods and supplements, such as sauerkraut, citrus fruits and their juices, and vitamin C, while taking the herb.

Women's health concerns. Diuretics may provide relief from the premenstrual bloating that bothers many women. Pregnant and nursing women should not take diuretics, however. Uva-ursi also stimulates uterine contractions in animal studies, making it even more off-limits to women who are pregnant or trying to conceive.

High blood pressure. Physicians often prescribe diuretics to treat high blood pressure. High blood pressure is a serious condition that requires professional care, so if you have it and would like to include uva-ursi in your overall treatment plan, discuss it with your physician.

Diuretics deplete the body of potassium, an essential nutrient. If you use uva-ursi regularly, be sure to eat more potassium-rich foods such as bananas and fresh vegetables.

Congestive heart failure. Physicians often prescribe diuretics to treat congestive heart failure, which involves serious fatigue of the heart. This condition requires professional care. If you would like to include uva-ursi in your overall treatment plan, discuss using it with your physician.

Wounds. When applied topically, uva-ursi's allantoin may help spur wound healing. Allantoin is the active ingredient in Derma-Heal, an over-the-counter skin cream.

Diarrhea. The astringent tannins in uva-ursi are binding and help relieve diarrhea.

Intriguing Possibility

Uva-ursi appears to have some anti-inflammatory action and may help heal dermatitis. In animal studies, the herb has helped treat hepatitis.

Rx Recommendations

To treat wounds, apply fresh, crushed leaves to minor cuts and scrapes after thoroughly washing them with soap and water. You can also dip a clean cloth in a decoction and apply the compress to the affected area.

To minimize the unpleasantly astringent taste of this high-tannin herb, soak the leaves in cold water overnight. Then, to prepare a decoction for relief from urinary symptoms or diarrhea, simmer 1 teaspoon per cup of boiling water for 10 minutes, then strain. Drink up to 3 cups a day.

As a homemade tincture, use ¼ to 1 teaspoon up to three times a day.

When using commercial preparations, follow the package directions.

Do not give uva-ursi to children under age 2. For older children and adults over age 65, start with low-strength preparations and increase the strength if necessary.

The Safety Factor

Uva-ursi often turns urine a dark green. This is harmless and should be no cause for alarm.

Herbal weight-loss formulas typically contain diuretics, with uva-ursi being among the common ingredients. Because diuretics boost urine production, they temporarily eliminate some water weight. Any pounds lost with help from diuretics almost invariably return, and weight-loss experts advise against using diuretics. The keys to permanent weight control include a low-fat, high-fiber diet and regular aerobic exercise.

Some herb conservatives warn against using uva-ursi because they say it causes vomiting, ringing in the ears, and convulsions. The source of this warning is one study reported in 1949, which did not use bulk uva-ursi but rather very large amounts of its isolated antiseptic chemical, hydroquinone. Recommended doses of the whole herb are considered safe, but if you experience nausea or ringing in the ears, reduce the dosage or stop using the herb.

Because uva-ursi is astringent, it can help treat diarrhea. The main medical hazard of diarrhea is dehydration, and because uva-ursi is a diuretic, it may contribute to dehydration. If you use uva-ursi to treat diarrhea, be sure to drink plenty of water and other nonalcoholic fluids.

Uva-ursi has such high levels of tannins that it has been used to tan leather. Large doses of tannins may cause stomach upset.

Tannins also have both pro- and anticancer action. Some authorities warn against their use, but tannins' role in human cancers, if any, remains unclear. That said, people who have a history of cancer should either add milk, which appears to neutralize tannins, or not use uva-ursi in large amounts.

Wise-Use Guidelines

The FDA lists uva-ursi as an herb of undefined safety. For adults who are not pregnant or nursing, uva-ursi is considered relatively safe in the amounts typically recommended.

You should use medicinal amounts of uva-ursi only in consultation with your doctor. If it causes minor discomfort, such as nausea, reduce the dosage or stop using it altogether. Let your doctor know if you experience unpleasant effects or if the symptoms for which you're using the herb do not improve significantly within 2 weeks.

Growing Information

Ancient Mediterranean bears must have loved the bright red, mealy, currant-size berries of this delicate, branching, perennial groundcover. Both its Greek genus name, *Arctostaphylos*, and its Latin-rooted species name, *uva-ursi*, mean bear's berry. The plant is often called bearberry in English. It's the leaves, however, not the berries, that are used in herbal healing.

Uva-ursi grows throughout the temperate world. It has a long, fibrous root; woody stems and branches; inch-long, leathery, evergreen, paddle-shaped leaves; and tiny white flowers tinged with red. The plant rarely grows taller than a few inches and prefers a dry, rocky, or sandy habitat.

Uva-ursi is typically propagated from cuttings. Be patient. This plant takes an unusually long time to root. It's more convenient simply to buy small plants from a specialty herb nursery.

Uva-ursi does poorly in rich soil. It prefers poor, gravelly, acidic soil, under full sun or partial shade. Keep your uva-ursi patch well-weeded until the plants have become established. It does not transplant well. Once established, uva-ursi spreads to become a hearty, attractive groundcover that can survive temperatures of $-50°F$.

Harvest leaves in autumn before the first frost. Because of their leathery texture, they are difficult to air-dry. Spread them in a single layer and dry them in the oven.

Valerian

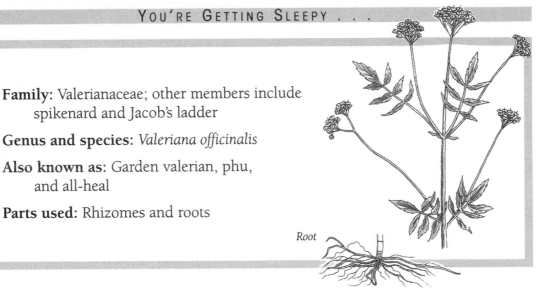

Family: Valerianaceae; other members include spikenard and Jacob's ladder

Genus and species: *Valeriana officinalis*

Also known as: Garden valerian, phu, and all-heal

Parts used: Rhizomes and roots

Root

Back in the 13th century, the elders of Hamelin, Germany, decided to rid their town of rats. They contracted with an itinerant flute player, one Pied Piper, whose music attracted the rodents, allowing him to lead them out of town. But when the Pied Piper returned for his fee, the elders of Hamelin refused to pay him. In revenge, he used his flute to charm Hamelin's children away forever.

In modern versions of this story, the Pied Piper's powers are entirely musical, but early German folklore credits him with being an accomplished herbalist as well. In addition to his hypnotic flute playing, the Pied Piper charmed both the rats and the children with hypnotic valerian root.

Valerian can, indeed, charm rats—and cats. The herb contains chemicals similar to those in catnip.

Healing History

Valerian has such a disagreeable odor that ancient Greek and Roman authorities, including Dioscorides, Pliny, and Galen all called it fu. The term *Valeriana* first appeared around the 10th century, derived from the Latin *valere*, to be strong.

Dioscorides recommended valerian as a diuretic and antidote to poisons. Pliny considered it a pain reliever. Galen prescribed it as a decongestant.

By the time the plant's name became valerian, early European herbalists considered it a panacea and also called it all-heal. The 12th-century German abbess/herbalist Hildegard of Bingen recommended the herb as a tranquilizer and sleep aid about 100 years before the Pied Piper used it as a hypnotic.

During the late 1500s, valerian's popularity grew after an Italian physician claimed that the herb cured him of epilepsy. In 1597, British herbalist John Gerard wrote that in Scotland "no broth or physic [medicine] . . . be worth anything" if it did not include valerian. Gerard recommended the herb enthusiastically for chest congestion, convulsions, bruises, and falls.

Seventeenth-century English herbalist Nicholas Culpeper added several of his own recommendations: "The decoction of the root . . . is of special virtue against the plague. . . . [It] provokes women's courses [menstruation] . . . is singularly good for those troubled with cough . . . is excellent [for] any sores, hurts, or wounds. . . ." Later, European herbalists considered the herb a digestive aid and treatment for "hysteria" (menstrual discomforts).

Early colonists discovered several Native American tribes using the pulverized roots of the American form of valerian to treat wounds. This use of the herb brought it to the attention of Samuel Thomson, the founder of Thomsonian medicine, which was popular before the Civil War. Thomson called valerian "the best nervine [tranquilizer] known."

Valerian entered the *U.S. Pharmacopoeia*, a standard drug reference, as a tranquilizer in 1820 and remained there until 1942. It was listed in the *National Formulary*, the pharmacists' guide, until 1950.

America's 19th-century Eclectic physicians, forerunners of today's naturopaths, prescribed valerian as a "calmative . . . for epilepsy . . . mild spasmodic affections . . . [and] hypochondria." But the Eclectic text *King's American Dispensatory* (1898) warned against using large doses because they caused "restlessness, agitation, giddiness, nausea, and visual illusions."

During World War I, Europeans afflicted with "overwrought nerves" from artillery bombardment frequently took valerian.

Contemporary herbalists generally agree with David Hoffmann's *Holistic Herbal*, which deems valerian "one of the most useful relaxing herbs." Today's herbalists recommend it for nervousness, anxiety, insomnia, headache, and intestinal cramps.

In Germany, where herbal medicine is considerably more mainstream than in the United States, valerian is the active ingredient in more than 100 over-the-counter tranquilizers and sleep aids. Some are specially formulated for children, a use the Pied Piper would probably endorse.

Therapeutic Uses

All parts of valerian contain valepotriates, compounds with sedative properties. They occur in highest concentration in the roots.

Insomnia. Many studies have found valerian to be an effective sedative.

In one study, German researchers gave 128 people with insomnia either medically inactive placebos or 400 milligrams of valerian root extract. Those who took the herb showed significant improvement in sleep quality without morning grogginess or other significant side effects.

In another German study, 68 adults with chronic insomnia were given either twice-daily placebos or sleep aids containing 320 milligrams of valerian root extract and 160 milligrams of an extract of lemon balm leaf, also an herbal tranquilizer (see page 266). Those taking the herbal medicine fell asleep significantly faster, enjoyed significantly longer periods of sleep, and reported significantly greater overall feelings of well-being. The herbal preparation caused no morning hangover.

Swiss researchers repeated this study using a slightly different formula: 360 milligrams of valerian and 240 milligrams of lemon balm once a day, 30 minutes before bedtime. Once again, those who took the herbal combination reported significantly better sleep quality with no side effects.

A third German study used standard physiological tests to measure the depth of sleep in 14 elderly people with insomnia. Compared with those who took placebos, the study participants who took valerian passed more quickly from light stage 1 sleep into deeper sleep. Other studies have reported similar results.

Some researchers have compared valerian with benzodiazepines such as diazepam (Valium) and triazolam (Halcion). Valerian is a much milder and safer sedative, for the following xreasons.

• The benzodiazepines can cause dependence and addiction. Regular users may develop a tolerance and require increasing amounts to obtain the desired effect. When the drug is stopped, they may develop withdrawal symptoms, including restlessness, insomnia, headache, nausea, and vomiting. Although a psychological dependence may develop, valerian is not addictive and discontinuation produces no withdrawal symptoms.
• The benzodiazepines' sedative effects increase substantially with simultaneous use of alcohol or barbiturates. The combination is often used in suicide attempts. Valerian's sedative effect increases less with alcohol or barbiturates.
• The benzodiazepines often cause morning grogginess. Unusually large amounts of valerian may cause morning grogginess, but recommended amounts do not.
• Children born to women who used Valium while pregnant are at increased risk for cleft palate. Valerian has not been linked to birth defects.

Commission E, the expert panel that evaluates herbal medications for the German counterpart of the FDA, endorses valerian for sleep problems.

High blood pressure. Animal studies have found that valerian reduces blood pressure. Of course, what occurs in animals does not necessarily apply to people, but if you have high blood pressure and want to incorporate valerian into your overall treatment plan, discuss it with your physician.

Intriguing Possibilities

Animal studies suggest that valerian has anticonvulsant effects, lending some credence to its traditional use in treating epilepsy.

Several reports show that the herb has some anti-tumor effects similar to those of nitrogen mustard. One day, valerian may play some role in cancer treatment.

Rx Recommendations

As a sleep aid, buy a commercial valerian root extract or tincture and follow the label directions. Herbalists discourage using valerian infusions because they taste foul.

Do not give valerian to children under age 2. For older children and adults over age 65, start with low-strength preparations and increase the strength if necessary.

The Safety Factor

Unusually large amounts of valerian may cause headache, giddiness, blurred vision, restlessness, nausea, and morning grogginess.

In 1998, a case report in the *Journal of the American Medical Association* suggested that withdrawal from valerian might have contributed to serious complications in one man who was hospitalized for congestive heart failure. It's possible, but this man was taking almost a dozen pharmaceutical drugs, had undergone two invasive procedures (lung biopsy and cardiac catheterization) under anesthesia, and had taken up to 2 grams of valerian a day for several years—many times the recommended dose.

The Duke University physicians who reported the case concluded: "Valerian root may be associated with serious withdrawal symptoms following abrupt discontinuation." Given the man's situation, this seems extremely unlikely for healthy people who take valerian in the recommended amounts.

Harm from valerian overdose seems unlikely. The journal *Veterinary and Human Toxicology* reported the case of a woman who tried to commit suicide by taking 40 capsules of valerian root extract, each containing 470 milligrams of the herb. She experienced fatigue, abdominal cramps, tightness in her chest, lightheadedness, dilated pupils, and hand tremors, all of which cleared up without medical treatment in 24 hours. Medical tests, including liver function tests, were all normal.

Wise-Use Guidelines

Valerian appears in the FDA list of herbs generally regarded as safe. For adults who are not pregnant or nursing and are not taking other tranquilizers or sedatives, valerian is considered safe when used in the amounts typically recommended.

You should take medicinal amounts of valerian only in consultation with your doctor. If it causes minor discomfort, such as headache or stomach upset, reduce the dosage or stop using it altogether. Let your doctor know if you experience unpleasant effects or if the symptoms for which you're taking the herb do not improve significantly within 2 weeks.

Growing Information

Medicinal valerian is a hardy perennial that reaches about 5 feet. Its medicinal roots consist of long, cylindrical fibers issuing from its rhizome. Its stem is erect, grooved, and hollow. Valerian leaves are fernlike. Tiny white, pink, or lavender flowers develop in umbrella-like clusters and bloom from late spring through summer. When dried, valerian roots have an unpleasant odor, once described by American herbalist Michael Moore as the smell of dirty socks.

Valerian may be propagated from seeds or root divisions. Seeds have limited viability. When viable, they germinate in about 20 days. Roots may be divided in spring or fall. Thin plants to 12-inch spacing. Valerian grows in many soils but does best in rich, moist, well-drained loam under full sun or partial shade. Once established, the plants self-sow and spread by root runners. Older plants become weedy and overcrowded and lose vitality. Thin them when harvesting their roots.

Valerian has an effect on cats similar to that of catnip. Intoxicated felines have been known to destroy plants; use chicken-wire fencing if necessary. Harvest roots in the fall of their 2nd year, and split thick roots to speed drying.

Vervain

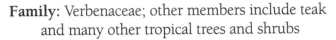

Family: Verbenaceae; other members include teak and many other tropical trees and shrubs

Genus and species: *Verbena officinalis* (European); *V. hastata* (American)

Also known as: Simpler's joy, blue vervain, verbena, herb-of-the-cross, enchanter's herb, and Indian hyssop

Parts used: Leaves, flowers, and roots

During the Middle Ages, healing herbs were often called simples, and herbalists were known as simplers. Vervain was prescribed so frequently for so many conditions that it became known as simpler's joy.

The name has some basis in fact. Vervain appears to act like mild aspirin, helping to relieve minor pain and inflammation.

Healing History

In Egyptian mythology, vervain grew from the tears of Isis, goddess of fertility, as she grieved for her murdered brother-husband, Osiris. A thousand years later, vervain entered Christian mythology as the herb pressed into Christ's wounds to stanch his bleeding, hence its name herb-of-the-cross.

Hippocrates recommended vervain for fever and plague. The court physician to Roman emperor Theodosius the Great prescribed it for tumors of the throat (probably goiters). His fanciful prescription advised cutting vervain root into two pieces, then tying one around the patient's throat and hanging the other over a fire. As the heat and smoke shriveled the hanging root, the tumor was supposed to shrink.

The Romans spread vervain throughout Europe, where it became especially popular among the Druids of pre-Christian England. They used the herb in magic spells, hence its name enchanter's herb.

The 12th-century German abbess/herbalist Hildegard of Bingen prescribed a decoction of vervain and vermouth for "toxic blood [infections], toothache, [and] discharges from the brain to the teeth."

Our word *vervain* comes from the Celtic *ferfaen*, from *fer*, to drive away, and *faen*, a stone. This is a reference to the herb's traditional role in treating kidney stones.

During the Middle Ages, vervain became a popular acne remedy. People who had pimples stood outside at night holding a handful of the herb wrapped in a cloth. When a shooting star passed, they rubbed the cloth over their pimples and the blemishes were supposed to disappear.

From a remedy for acne, vervain evolved into a treatment for other skin problems. Seventeenth-century herbalist Nicholas Culpeper wrote, "The leaves bruised, or the juice mixed with vinegar, does wonderfully cleanse the skin, and take away morphew [dandruff]." Culpeper recommended vervain to treat jaundice, gout, cough, wheezing, bleeding gums, shortness of breath, fever, plague, gravel (kidney stones), and dropsy (congestive heart failure). He also said that "used with hog grease, it helps with swellings and pains of the secret parts [genitals]."

Colonists introduced European vervain into North America, and it quickly went wild. They also found Native Americans using the American form of vervain, also known as Indian hyssop, to treat fever and gastrointestinal complaints and to clear cloudy urine.

During the Revolutionary War, military physicians relied on vervain to relieve pain, loosen bronchial mucus, and induce vomiting. More than a century later, the Eclectics, forerunners of today's naturopaths, recommended it as a treatment for fever, colds, coughs, intestinal worms, menstrual irregularity, and bruises, and as a tonic "during convalescence from acute diseases."

Contemporary herbalists recommend vervain as a tranquilizer, expectorant, menstruation promoter, and treatment for headache, fever, depression, seizures, wounds, dental cavities, and gum disease.

Therapeutic Uses

The standard prescription to "take two aspirin and call me in the morning" has long been attributed to physicians. But an herbalist might say the same thing, substituting vervain for aspirin. No wonder they called this herb simpler's joy.

Pain and inflammation. Chemically, vervain is quite different from aspirin, but German and Japanese studies suggest that it has similar effects, combining mild pain relief with some ability to reduce inflammation. These findings support vervain's traditional use in treating headache, toothache, wounds, and kidney stones.

Constipation. One study suggests that vervain has a mild laxative effect.

Medicinal Myth

Vervain has never been shown to treat dandruff, induce vomiting, promote menstruation, or remove kidney stones. Its primary benefit is its ability to provide mild pain relief.

Rx Recommendations

For a very bitter infusion to help treat headache, mild arthritis, and other minor pains, use 2 teaspoons of dried herb per cup of boiling water. Steep for 10 to 15 minutes, then strain. Drink up to 3 cups a day. Mask vervain's bitterness with sugar, honey, and lemon or mix the herb with an herbal beverage tea.

As a homemade tincture, use ½ to 1 teaspoon up to three times a day.

When using commercial preparations, follow the package directions.

Do not give medicinal doses of vervain to children under age 2. For older children and adults over age 65, start with low-strength preparations and increase the strength if necessary.

The Safety Factor

European animal studies have found that vervain depresses the heart rate, constricts the bronchial passages, and stimulates the intestines and uterus. Because it may slow heart rate, it should not be used by anyone with congestive heart failure or a history of heart disease. The possibility of bronchial constriction may cause problems for people with asthma and other respiratory conditions. Intestinal stimulation may aggravate chronic gastrointestinal conditions, such as colitis or Crohn's disease.

Because of vervain's potential stimulating effect on the uterus, pregnant women should steer clear of the herb, except possibly at term and under the supervision of a physician to help induce labor.

Wise-Use Guidelines

Although both vervain species have similar effects, the FDA includes *Verbena officinalis* among herbs generally regarded as safe but considers *V. hastata* an herb of undefined safety.

For adults who are not pregnant or nursing and do not have a history of the conditions mentioned above, both vervains are considered relatively safe in the amounts typically recommended.

You should use medicinal amounts of vervain only in consultation with your doctor. If it causes minor discomfort, such as stomach or intestinal distress, reduce the dosage or stop using it altogether. Let your doctor know if you experience unpleasant effects or if the symptoms for which you're using the herb do not improve significantly within 2 weeks.

Growing Information

Vervain is a 3-foot perennial with thin, erect, stiff stems. Its opposite leaves are oblong and toothed near the ground and lance-shaped and deeply lobed higher up. The plant develops slender flower spikes that bear small blue or lilac flowers from early summer through mid-fall. The herb's bluish flowers gave it the name blue vervain.

Vervain grows easily from seeds planted in spring after the danger of frost has passed. Although it's a perennial, the herb is rather short-lived, but it does self-sow. Vervain prefers rich, moist loam under full sun. Harvest the leaves and flowers as the plants flower.

White Willow

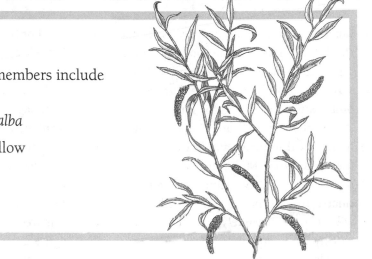

Family: Salicaceae; other members include poplar

Genus and species: *Salix alba*

Also known as: Salicin willow

Part used: Bark

Look at a white willow, and what do you see? Most people see only a stately shade tree—but herbalists also see the potent pain reliever, aspirin.

In fact, aspirin was originally created from a compound in white willow bark called salicin. It gets its name from the herb's genus, *Salix*.

White willow grew on the banks of the Nile, and the ancient Egyptians considered it a symbol of joy. The Hebrews adopted the beautiful tree. In Leviticus (23:40), God commanded them to celebrate the autumn harvest festival by setting up temporary shelters covered with willow boughs: "Ye shall take . . . boughs of willow . . . and rejoice seven days."

But the willow became a symbol of sorrow after the destruction of the first Temple in Jerusalem, which began the Jews' Babylonian exile. Consider the willow's transformation in Psalm 137: "By the rivers of Babylon, where we sat down, and there we wept, when we remembered Zion, upon the willows, we hanged up our harps, for they that led us there captive asked of us . . . song." Since that time, the graceful tree has been known as weeping willow.

Healing History

Chinese physicians have used white willow bark to relieve pain since 500 B.C. That application took 5 centuries to find its way to Europe. The 1st-century Greek physician Dioscorides was the first Westerner to recommend willow bark for pain and inflammation, but his prescription did not catch on. A century later, the Roman doctor Galen recommended the herb only for the vague purpose of "drying up humors."

As the centuries passed, herbalists prescribed white willow bark for many ailments, including suppressing sexual desire. Seventeenth-century English herbalist Nicholas Culpeper noted, "The leaves, bark, and seed are used to stanch bleeding . . . stay vomiting . . . provoke urine . . . take away warts . . . and clear the face and skin from spots and discolourings. . . . The leaves bruised and boiled in wine stays the heat of lust in man or woman, and quite extinguishes it if it be long used."

At the time, white willow was not commonly used to treat pain, but Culpeper touted the work of one Mr. Stone, who demonstrated its "great efficacy . . . in intermittent fever [malaria]." Culpeper concluded that white willow bark "is likely to become an object worthy of . . . attention."

He was referring to the research of Rev. Edmund Stone, a physician-minister in Chipping-Norton in Oxfordshire, England. Stone was looking for a substitute for cinchona, the bark of the South American cinchona tree, which had been brought to Europe from the New World a century earlier. Cinchona was the first effective treatment for malaria, a scourge throughout Europe since ancient times, but it was extremely expensive.

In 1757, Stone collected some white willow bark for the medicinal uses that Culpeper had described, and he happened to taste it. He was surprised at its bitterness, which reminded him of cinchona. Stone wondered if willow bark might be a poor person's cinchona for fever and chills.

From the perspective of the Doctrine of Signatures, the medieval belief that a plant's physical appearance pointed to its medicinal uses, the signs looked promising. Willows grew along cool, damp riverbanks and in swampy lowlands, exactly the environments that physicians of Stone's era (wrongly) believed produced malaria and other illnesses marked by fever, or "ague."

For 6 years, Stone pulverized white willow bark, brewed a bitter tea with the powder, and gave his experimental medicine to 50 people with fevers. According to Stone, most of his patients' agues and chills disappeared shortly after drinking his concoction.

Stone wrote a report, "An Account of the Success of the Bark of the Willow in the Cure of Agues," in which he touted white willow bark as a cheap substitute for cinchona: "As this tree delights in a moist or wet soil where agues chiefly abound, the general maxim that many natural maladies carry their cures along with them, or that their remedies lie not far from the cause was so very [appropriate] to this particular case that I could not help applying it."

On April 25, 1763, Stone sent his report to the Royal Society, England's most prestigious scientific organization. Its publication in the society's journal, *Philosophical Transactions*, later that year finally popularized white willow bark in the West as a treatment for fever—more than 2,000 years after the Chinese had first touted it for that purpose.

Alas, white willow was no cinchona. It contains no quinine, the drug that treats malaria. Nonetheless, it brought down other fevers and quickly became Europe's drug of choice for fever, pain, and inflammation.

Early colonists introduced the tree into North America and found many Native American tribes using the bark of native willows to treat pain, chills, and fever.

From Salicin to Aspirin

Around 1828, French and German chemists extracted white willow bark's active compound, salicin. Ten years later, an Italian chemist isolated salicin's aspirin precursor, salicylic acid. Although this potent pain reliever was first discovered in white willow, chemists made the first aspirin from another herb that contains the same chemical—meadowsweet. Salicin was discovered in meadowsweet in 1839.

During the mid-19th century, researchers that showed both salicin and salicylic acid reduce fever and relieve pain and inflammation. Unfortunately, they also have unpleasant—and potentially hazardous—side effects: nausea, diarrhea, bleeding, stomach ulceration, ringing in the ears (tinnitus), and at high doses, respiratory paralysis and death.

Chemists began tinkering with salicylic acid, hoping to preserve its benefits while minimizing its side effects. In 1853, German chemists added a molecular acetyl group to an extract of meadowsweet to create acetylsalicylic acid. The new compound still had some of salicylic acid's side effects, but it was able to cross the blood-brain barrier, which made it more potent.

"Acetylsalicylic acid" was quite a mouthful, so the scientists who synthesized it took the "a-" from *acetyl* and "-spirin" from meadowsweet's genus name, *Spirea*, to create the word *aspirin*.

News of aspirin's synthesis was published in an obscure German medical journal and forgotten for 50 years. Then in the late 1890s, a German chemist, Felix Hoffman, got upset that his father's rheumatoid arthritis medications brought him so little relief. Hoffman, an employee of Fredrich Bayer and Company, began looking for a better pain reliever. He delved into the journals and found the old reports of aspirin. Hoffman prepared the drug, and his father's condition improved significantly.

At first, Hoffman's superiors at Bayer were not interested in aspirin, but eventually, they got behind it. In 1899, they released it in Europe and North America under the brand name Aspirin.

Aspirin quickly became the household drug of choice for a broad range of everyday ailments. Then, in a landmark trademark-protection battle, Bayer lost its trademark on Aspirin. The court ruled that the term had already passed into general usage.

Contemporary herbalists recommend white willow bark for headache, fever, arthritis, and other pain and inflammation. Increasingly, the herb is used to prevent heart attack.

Therapeutic Uses

Contrary to Culpeper's opinion, white willow bark won't cure malaria. But it is indeed herbal "aspirin." It contains more salicylates than meadowsweet, making it a more potent natural healer.

Fever, pain, and inflammation. Try white willow any time that you think you need aspirin. Aspirin is a more concentrated source of salicylates, the active chemicals in white willow, so don't expect the herb to be as potent.

On the other hand, compared with the little white pills, white willow bark causes fewer side effects.

Commission E, the expert panel that evaluates herbal medicines for the German counterpart of the FDA, approves white willow bark for the treatment of fever, headaches, and muscle and joint pain.

Heart attack and stroke. Low-dose aspirin, one-half to one standard tablet a day, has become a standard preventive and first-aid for heart attack. Aspirin helps prevent and dissolve the blood clots that trigger heart attack and most strokes. A cup of willow bark tea contains a similar low dose of aspirin-like salicin.

There have been no studies on willow bark as an aspirin substitute for heart attack prevention, but biochemically, the herb should be expected to have similar value. If you've been advised to take low-dose aspirin regularly, ask your physician about including willow bark in your regimen.

Women's health concerns. Like aspirin, white willow contains enough salicylate to suppress the action of compounds called prostaglandins that are involved in menstrual cramps. If you have mild cramps, the herb may help.

Pregnant women should not use white willow. In animal studies, aspirin is associated with an increased risk of birth defects. The herb is not as powerful, but it's better to be safe than sorry.

Intriguing Possibilities

One laboratory study suggested that white willow may reduce blood sugar (glucose) levels. The herb's effect on diabetes in humans, if any, remains unclear.

Regular aspirin use has also been associated with reduced risk of digestive tract cancers, including colon cancer. White willow bark may provide similar preventive benefits.

Rx Recommendations

For a decoction to relieve pain, fever, and inflammation, use 1 teaspoon of powdered bark per cup of cold water and soak for 8 hours, then strain if you wish. Drink up to 3 cups a day. White willow tastes bitter and astringent. You can add honey and lemon or mix the herb with an herbal beverage tea.

To help prevent heart attack and stroke, drink 1 or 2 cups a day.

When using commercial preparations, follow the package directions.

Do not give white willow to children under age 2. For other children and adults over age 65, start with low-strength preparations and increase the strength if necessary.

In children under age 16 with fevers related to colds, flu, or chickenpox, aspirin may cause Reye's syndrome, a rare but potentially fatal condition. White willow has never been linked to Reye's syndrome, but because of its aspirin-like action, do not give it to children with those illnesses.

The Safety Factor

Aspirin upsets some people's stomachs. White willow bark is less potent and rarely causes this problem, but stomach upset is still possible in those who are sensitive to aspirin. If stomach upset, nausea, or tinnitus develops, reduce your dose or stop using the herb.

People with chronic gastrointestinal conditions, such as ulcers and gastritis, should not use the herb.

Aspirin also triggers asthma attacks in some people. If you are aspirin-sensitive, do not use white willow bark.

Wise-Use Guidelines

For adults who are not pregnant or nursing, are not taking aspirin or other salicylate medications, and do not have chronic gastrointestinal conditions or asthma, white willow bark is considered relatively safe in the amounts typically recommended.

You should use medicinal amounts of white willow only in consultation with your doctor. If it causes minor discomfort, such as stomach upset or ringing in the ears, reduce the dosage or stop using it altogether. Let your doctor know if you experience unpleasant effects or if the symptoms for which you're using the herb do not improve significantly within 2 weeks.

Growing Information

Throughout history, many of the 500 willow species have been used in herbal healing. For the last 200 years, however, only white willow has been commonly used. It reaches 75 feet and has rough, grayish brown bark and long, thin leaves on flexible branches, which give the tree a graceful beauty.

White willows grow in almost any moist garden soil under full sun. Buy saplings at nurseries or propagate them from first-year branches several feet in length rooted in water or from foot-long hardwood cuttings taken in spring or fall and rooted the same way. Do not transplant willows.

Willows grow quickly and must be pruned regularly. Harvest the bark from older branches during pruning and dry it.

Witch Hazel

A COOLING, SOOTHING ASTRINGENT

Family: Hamamelidaceae; no other members

Genus and species: *Hamamelis virginiana*

Also known as: Winterbloom, snapping hazelnut, and hamamelis

Parts used: Leaves and bark

The next time someone you know pooh-poohs herbal healing, ask what the person thinks of witch hazel. The clear, pungent liquid extract of this bushy herb is a standard home remedy for cuts, bruises, hemorrhoids, and other minor skin conditions. More than 1 million gallons of witch hazel are sold each year in the United States, making it one of the nation's most widely used healing herbs.

The "hazel" in the herb's name comes from its similarity to the common hazelnut. As for the "witch," some say that early colonists used the shrub to make brooms, witches' favorite form of transportation. Others trace it to witch hazel's winter flowering and the loud "pop" when it disperses its seeds, supposedly evidence of occult influence. Still others claim that the shrub's forked branches were used by dousers looking for water and that dousing was once associated with witchcraft.

For the record, the herb's name has nothing to do with witchcraft. In medieval Middle English, "witch" had another meaning. It was spelled *wych* or *wyche*, and it meant "pliant" or "flexible." Witch hazel's branches are, indeed, flexible—so springy, in fact, that Native Americans used them to make bows.

Healing History

Witch hazel was highly valued in Native American medicine. Many tribes rubbed a decoction of the herb on cuts, bruises, insect bites, aching joints, sore muscles, and sore backs. They also drank witch hazel tea to stop internal bleeding, prevent miscarriage, and treat colds, fevers, sore throats, and menstrual pain.

The colonists adopted witch hazel, but the herb was not very popular until the 1840s, when an Oneida medicine man reportedly introduced the plant to Theron T. Pond of Utica, New York. Pond was impressed with the plant's astringent properties and its ability to treat burns, boils, wounds, and hemorrhoids. In 1848, he began marketing witch hazel extract as Pond's Golden Treasure. Later, the name was changed to Pond's Extract, which became a big hit. Witch hazel water has been with us ever since.

Early witch hazel water was simply a strained decoction of the shrub's leaves and twigs that contained tannins, which made the extract highly astringent. By the late 19th century, manufacturers switched to steam distillation, a simpler process but one that left the resulting water with little if any of the plant's astringent tannins. That's when the controversy erupted.

King's American Dispensatory (1898), the text used by the Eclectics, forerunners of today's naturopaths, asserted: "The decoction is very useful in hemorrhage, diarrhea, dysentery, swellings, inflammations, tumors, hemorrhoids, epistaxis [nosebleed], and uterine hemorrhage following delivery. . . . [However] since the introduction of the distilled extract [witch hazel] has been largely abandoned. . . . The fluid extract has little to recommend it."

Nonetheless, witch hazel was listed as an astringent and anti-inflammatory in the *U.S. Pharmacopoeia*, a standard drug reference, from 1862 through 1916 and in the *National Formulary*, the pharmacists' reference, from 1916 to 1955. The *National Formulary* finally dropped it because in 1947, the 24th edition of *The Dispensatory of the United States* stated that witch hazel "is so nearly destitute of medicinal virtues, it scarcely deserves official recognition. . . . [Its continued use serves only to fill] the need in American families for an embrocation [liniment] which appeals to the psychic influence of faith."

Yet today, witch hazel can be found on the shelves of every pharmacy. Contemporary herbalists sidestep the controversy by recommending only the decoction of witch hazel bark, which contains astringent tannins. They are unanimous in their praise of the herb's cooling, astringent action when used externally for cuts, burns, scalds, bruises, inflammation, and hemorrhoids. They recommend it as a gargle for sore throat and sores in the mouth and internally to treat diarrhea.

Therapeutic Uses

Wouldn't it be ironic if this widely used herbal remedy turned out to be worthless? Fortunately, that does not appear to be the case. While it's true that witch hazel water contains no astringent tannins, several studies show that it still retains astringent action, presumably from other compounds in the plant.

Hemorrhoids and skin problems. Commercial witch hazel water may not have tannins, but it contains other compounds with reported antiseptic, anesthetic, astringent, and anti-inflammatory action. Witch hazel water is an ingredient in Fleet Medicated Wipes for hemorrhoids, Tucks pads, and several over-the-counter treatments for poison ivy, oak, and sumac.

Commission E, the expert panel that evaluates herbal medicines for the German counterpart of the FDA, approves witch hazel for hemorrhoids and skin inflammations.

Sunburn. German researchers gave 30 people with sunburn one of three treatments: a medically inactive placebo cream, a skin cream containing aloe gel and vitamin E (both recommended for skin problems), or a lotion containing 10 percent witch hazel distillate. Participants applied their treatments three times over a 48-hour period. Although differences in redness were not clearly visible to the naked eye, they were to an instrument called a chromameter—and the witch hazel lotion reduced redness best.

Another German study compared witch hazel with a chamomile preparation and hydrocortisone, an over-the-counter anti-inflammatory drug, in 24 people with sunburn. The hydrocortisone worked best, but witch hazel was almost as effective and "clearly superior" to the chamomile lotion.

Rx Recommendations

It's most convenient to use commercial witch hazel water, which is available in pharmacies.

If you'd like to make an astringent decoction, boil 1 teaspoon of powdered leaves or twigs per cup of water for 10 minutes. Strain and cool. Apply the liquid directly or mix it into a skin lotion.

For a bitter, astringent gargle, use 1 teaspoon of bark per cup of boiling water. Steep for 10 minutes, then strain.

You may use witch hazel externally on anyone, but dilute it for use on children under age 2.

The Safety Factor

The medical literature contains no reports of harm from using witch hazel externally or as a gargle, but most experts advise against ingesting preparations of this herb.

Wise-Use Guidelines

Witch hazel is considered safe in the amounts typically recommended.

If it causes minor discomforts, such as skin irritation, dilute it before using or stop using it altogether. Let your doctor know if you experience unpleasant effects or if the symptoms for which you're using the herb do not improve significantly within 2 weeks.

Growing Information

Witch hazel's Latin name refers to Virginia, but the shrub grows all over the eastern United States. Most commercial witch hazel is grown in the Carolinas and Tennessee.

Witch hazel is a perennial that drops its leaves each autumn. Its single root sends up several twisting stems that fork into many flexible, hairy branches. It blooms long after most other flowers have disappeared—from September to December, depending on location. This is how it got one of its common names, winterbloom. As a late bloomer, it makes a colorful addition to any garden.

The shrub's spidery yellow flowers appear at the same time that its previous year's fruits mature. Its woody seed pods burst open with an audible pop and propel their two hard black seeds up to 25 feet. The seeds are edible and have been compared with hazelnuts, hence the name snapping hazelnut.

Witch hazel grows from seeds or twig cuttings. Refrigerate seeds at around 40°F for several months before planting to encourage germination. Cuttings generally produce roots in about 10 weeks.

Witch hazel grows best in moist, rich, sandy or peaty soil under partial shade, but it tolerates poorer soil and full sun. Harvest the leaves and twigs at any time and dry them.

Yarrow

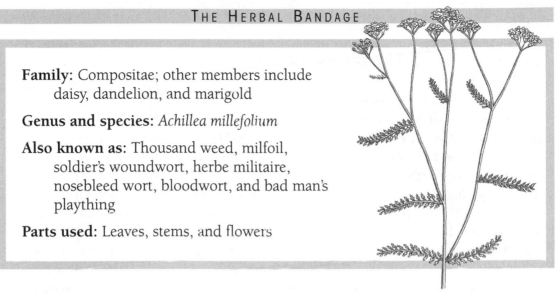

Family: Compositae; other members include daisy, dandelion, and marigold

Genus and species: *Achillea millefolium*

Also known as: Thousand weed, milfoil, soldier's woundwort, herbe militaire, nosebleed wort, bloodwort, and bad man's plaything

Parts used: Leaves, stems, and flowers

Legend has it that during the Trojan War, Achilles stopped the bleeding of his fellow soldiers' wounds by applying yarrow's fernlike leaves. Scientists have discovered that the mythological hero may have been onto something.

Yarrow contains substances that may stop bleeding and may have pain-relieving and anti-inflammatory properties helpful in wound treatment. Yarrow also appears to have potential as a digestive aid, menstrual remedy, and mild sedative.

Healing History

Achilles defined yarrow's use in herbal healing for more than 2,500 years. Dioscorides, a 1st-century physician attached to Roman legions, recommended rubbing the crushed plant on wounds.

The herb's many popular names— herbe militaire, nosebleed wort, soldier's woundwort, and bloodwort—attest to its use as a blood stopper during the Middle Ages. (The word *wort* is Old English for "plant.") Perhaps from an association with brawling, yarrow also became linked to ruffians, earning the name bad man's plaything.

Around Achilles' time, ancient Chinese physicians were prescribing Asian yarrow to treat inflammations, bleeding, heavy menstrual flow, dog bites, and snakebites. The Chinese also used yarrow in the ritual of the I Ching, the oracle consulted to predict the future. Coins are typically used today, but the traditional way to cast the I Ching involved dried yarrow stems. India's Ayurvedic physicians recommended yarrow to treat fevers.

Sixteenth-century British herbalist John Gerard suggested yarrow for "swellings . . . of the privie parts." In the 17th century, John Parkinson advised, "If it be put into the nose, assuredly it will stop the bleeding of it." And his contemporary Nicholas Culpeper wrote, "An ointment of the leaves cures wounds . . . restrains violent bleedings . . . is good for inflammations and ulcers . . . and is excellent for the piles [hemorrhoids]."

Colonists introduced yarrow into North America. Native Americans adopted it enthusiastically as an external treatment for wounds and burns and as an internal treatment for colds, sore throats, arthritis, toothaches, insomnia, and indigestion.

America's 19th-century Eclectic physicians, forerunners of today's naturopaths, considered yarrow a "tonic upon the venous system" but downplayed its age-old role in wound treatment. Their text King's American Dispensatory (1898) recommended the herb for bloody urine, incontinence, hemorrhoids, menstrual cramps, diarrhea, dysentery, and "hemorrhage where the bleeding is small in amount."

Contemporary herbalists recommend yarrow as an "herbal Band-Aid." They also prescribe it for fevers and urinary tract infections and as a digestive aid.

Therapeutic Uses

If Achilles had had some yarrow on hand when his vulnerable heel was wounded, he might have survived the Trojan War.

Wounds. Yarrow contains many chemicals that support its traditional use as a wound treatment. Two of them, achilletin and achilleine, spur blood coagulation. Several more—azulene, camphor, chamazulene, eugenol, menthol, quercetin, rutin, and salicylic acid—have anti-inflammatory and pain-relieving action. Several others—tannins, terpeniol, and cineol—are antiseptic.

Digestive problems. Chamazulene, one of the chemicals in yarrow (and chamomile), helps relax the smooth muscle tissue of the digestive tract. This makes the herb an antispasmodic.

Commission E, the expert panel that evaluates herbal medicines for the German counterpart of the FDA, endorses yarrow as a digestive aid.

Women's health concerns. Antispasmodics relax not only the digestive tract but also other smooth muscles, such as the uterus. This lends some credence to yarrow's use in treating menstrual cramps.

Stress, anxiety, and insomnia. Yarrow contains a small amount of a hypnotic chemical called thujone, the effects of which have been compared to marijuana. The thujone in yarrow may account for the herb's traditional use as a sedative.

In large amounts, thujone is poisonous, but the recommended amounts of yarrow do not supply enough of the compound to cause harm.

Intriguing Possibility

Two animal studies have shown that yarrow protects the liver from toxic chemical damage, and a scientifically conducted trial in India found that yarrow helps treat hepatitis. If you have liver disease, ask your physician about using yarrow in addition to standard therapies.

Rx Recommendations

To treat wounds, press fresh leaves and flowers into cuts and scrapes until you can wash and bandage them. To help promote healing, apply the herb externally to clean wounds and inflamed skin.

For an infusion to soothe digestive upset and possibly act as a tranquilizer, use 1 to 2 teaspoons of dried herb per cup of boiling water. Steep for 10 to 15 minutes, then strain. Drink up to 3 cups a day. Yarrow tastes tangy and bitter, with some astringency. To improve the flavor, add honey, sugar, or lemon or mix the herb with an herbal beverage blend.

As a homemade tincture, use ½ to 1 teaspoon up to three times a day.

When using commercial preparations, follow the package directions.

Do not give medicinal yarrow preparations to children under age 2. For older children and adults over age 65, start with low-strength preparations and increase the strength if necessary.

The Safety Factor

High doses of yarrow may turn urine dark brown. This is harmless and should not cause alarm.

The medical literature contains no reports of toxicity from yarrow, but people who are allergic to ragweed may develop a rash from contact with the plant.

Wise-Use Guidelines

Thujone-free yarrow extracts have been approved by the FDA for use in beverages. For adults who are not pregnant or nursing and are not taking pharmaceutical tranquilizers or sedatives, yarrow is considered safe in the amounts typically recommended.

You should use medicinal amounts of yarrow only in consultation with your doctor. If it causes minor discomforts, such as a rash or diarrhea, reduce the dosage or stop using it altogether. Let your doctor know if you experience unpleasant effects or if the symptoms for which you're using the herb do not improve significantly within 2 weeks.

Growing Information

Yarrow is an attractive 3-foot perennial covered with delicate hairs. Its feathery leaves are divided into what seem like thousands of tiny leaflets; hence its names thousand weed and milfoil (a corruption of *mille feuille*, the French term for 1,000 leaves). Yarrow's numerous tiny white flowers develop in dense clusters on flat-topped, umbrella-like stalks in summer.

Yarrow grows easily from seeds or root divisions planted in spring or fall. Sow seeds just under the surface of fine soil and keep them moist until they germinate, usually within 2 weeks. Thin seedlings to 12-inch spacing. Yarrow adapts to many soil types but needs good drainage and does best in moderately rich soil under full sun. Divide plants every few years to keep them growing vigorously.

Harvest yarrow when the plants are in bloom and hang them to dry.

CHAPTER 6

Using the Healing Herbs

A QUICK REFERENCE GUIDE

When you have a cold, which herbs should you reach for? How about when you have a headache? Anxiety? Indigestion?

This quick reference guide can help you make the right choice. It organizes the herbs discussed throughout the book into three categories: (1) conditions; (2) healing actions, such as antibiotic, decongestant, and so on; and (3) other uses, such as insect repellent and weight control.

Consumer Precautions

Before using any herb medicinally, read its profile in chapter 5, especially the information on safety and side effects. Also read chapter 2, which contains some general safe-use guidelines. Follow all of the recommendations in both chapters.

The charts below list only the most potentially hazardous herb side effects. Other side effects are possible. In addition, any herb may cause an allergic reaction.

Healing herbs are best used in consultation with a physician. This is especially true if you have a chronic condition such as asthma, arthritis, cancer, diabetes, heart disease, or high blood pressure.

Herbal oils are highly concentrated and should not be ingested unless you're under the care of a naturopath or professional herbalist. Even a small amount—a teaspoon—can be toxic. Never allow children to ingest herbal oils.

A Special Note to Women

With few exceptions, pregnant and nursing women should not ingest medicinal amounts of healing herbs because of the possibility of harming the fetus or infant.

Most herbal digestive aids have antispasmodic action—that is, they help to relax the smooth muscle lining the digestive tract. The uterus is also a smooth muscle, so it may be affected by antispasmodic herbs. But many of these herbal digestive aids have traditionally been used to stimulate the uterus and promote menstruation, so it's possible that taking large amounts of these herbs may, over time, increase the risk of miscarriage.

This contradiction appears to be dose-related. Made with a dose of 1 to 2 teaspoons of freshly grated root, ginger tea is a safe, effective treatment for the morning sickness of pregnancy. In extremely large doses, however—20 to 40 teaspoons of root—it may induce uterine contractions.

The antispasmodic herbs are popular ingredients in cooking. Pregnant and nursing women may feel free to use culinary amounts of these herbs.

It's by no means clear from the research to date that all herbal digestive aids stimulate the uterus when taken in large doses, but given the traditional uses of antispasmodic herbs, pregnant women—and women who are trying to conceive—are best advised not to take medicinal amounts.

Conditions and Their Herbal Remedies

Condition	Herb(s)	Special Precaution(s)
Acne	*For external use:* Tea tree	As little as a teaspoon of *tea tree* oil can be toxic. Do not ingest it, and keep it out of the reach of children.
AIDS	Garlic St. John's wort	If you are taking antidepressant medication or a protease inhibitor, consult a physician before using *St. John's wort*.
Alzheimer's disease	Ginkgo	None
Antidepressant-induced sexual problems	Ginkgo	None
Anxiety	Catnip Celery Chamomile Kava Lemon balm Motherwort Passionflower Scullcap Yarrow	Long-term use of *celery* may deplete potassium stores. *Lemon balm* interferes with thyroid-stimulating hormone. If you have an underactive thyroid (hypothyroidism), consult a physician before using it.
Arthritis	Angelica Black haw Boneset Chamomile	*Angelica* may cause a rash in sensitive people who are exposed to direct sunlight. *Fenugreek* has estrogenic action. People who have a history of blood clots (thromboembolisms),

Condition	Herb(s)	Special Precaution(s)
Arthritis (cont.)	Chaparral Echinacea Evening primrose Fenugreek Gentian Ginger Horsetail Juniper Licorice Meadowsweet Nettle Red pepper St. John's wort Turmeric Vervain White willow	inflammation of blood vessels (thrombophlebitis), heart disease, or stroke should consult their physicians before using it. Long-term use of *horsetail, juniper, nettle,* and *vervain* may deplete potassium stores. Long-term use of *licorice* may cause water retention, elevated blood pressure, and a hormone imbalance (pseudoaldosteronism). *Meadowsweet* and *white willow* contain aspirin-like compounds. If you are aspirin-sensitive, consult a physician before using these herbs. If you are taking antidepressant medication, consult a physician before using *St. John's wort.* *Vervain* may depress heart rate and constrict bronchial passages. If you have heart disease, high blood pressure, diabetes, or asthma, consult a physician before using it.
Asthma	Angelica Cocoa (chocolate) Coffee Kola Maté Tea	*Angelica* may cause a rash in sensitive people who are exposed to direct sunlight. *Cocoa (chocolate), coffee, kola, maté,* and *tea* all contain caffeine, which may cause jitters, irritability, insomnia, and addiction.
Athlete's foot	Tea tree	As little as a teaspoon of *tea tree* oil can be toxic. Do not ingest it, and keep it out of the reach of children.
Bad breath	Alfalfa Parsley	Long-term use of large amounts of *parsley* may deplete potassium stores.
Benign prostate enlargement	Nettle Saw palmetto	Long-term use of *nettle* may deplete potassium stores.
Bleeding	Blackberry Shepherd's purse Witch hazel Yarrow	*Shepherd's purse* may cause powerful uterine contractions.
Breast tenderness	Evening primrose	None

Condition	Herb(s)	Special Precaution(s)
Bronchitis (*see also* Cough)	Barberry Echinacea Garlic	None
Burns (*see also* Pain)	*For external use:* Aloe Chamomile Comfrey Echinacea Gotu kola Marshmallow Passionflower St. John's wort Yarrow	Flush burns with cold water before applying herbal medicines. Extensive burns that raise blisters or char the skin require professional attention.
Cancer prevention	Alfalfa Apple Bilberry Blackberry Cranberry Garlic Ginseng Raspberry Tea (green) Turmeric	*Tea* contains caffeine, which may cause jitters, irritability, insomnia, and addiction.
Cancer treatment	Mistletoe Tea (green)	*Mistletoe* may slow heart rate and affect blood pressure. If you have heart disease, diabetes, high blood pressure, or a history of stroke, consult your physician before using it. *Tea* contains caffeine, which may cause jitters, irritability, insomnia, and addiction.
Canker sores	Licorice	Long-term use of *licorice* may cause water retention, elevated blood pressure, and a hormone imbalance (pseudoaldosteronism).
Cataract prevention	Bilberry Blackberry Cranberry Raspberry Turmeric	None

Condition	Herb(s)	Special Precaution(s)
Cholera	Barberry Goldenseal	None
Cirrhosis	Ginseng Licorice Milk thistle	Long-term use of *licorice* may cause water retention, elevated blood pressure, and a hormone imbalance (pseudoaldosteronism).
Colds and flu (*see also* Cough)	Boneset Echinacea Garlic Ginger Hyssop Marshmallow Meadowsweet Slippery elm	*Meadowsweet* contains aspirin-like compounds. If you are aspirin-sensitive, consult a physician before using it.
Cold sores (*see* Herpes and cold sores)		
Colic	Dill Slippery elm	None
Congestive heart failure (*see also* Diuretic in "Healing Actions" table)	Hawthorn	None
Conjunctivitis	Barberry	None
Constipation	Apple Buckthorn Cascara sagrada Psyllium Rhubarb Senna Vervain	*Buckthorn, cascara sagrada, rhubarb,* and *senna* may cause abdominal distress. *Vervain* may depress heart rate and constrict bronchial passages. If you have heart disease, high blood pressure, diabetes, or asthma, consult a physician before using it.
Cough	Angelica Cocoa (chocolate) Coffee Ephedra Eucalyptus Fenugreek Horehound Hyssop	*Angelica* may cause a rash in sensitive people who are exposed to direct sunlight. *Cocoa (chocolate), coffee, kola, maté,* and *tea* all contain caffeine, which may cause jitters, irritability, insomnia, and addiction. *Ephedra* may raise blood pressure and cause jitters, irritability, and insomnia. People with high blood

Condition	Herb(s)	Special Precaution(s)
	Kola Licorice Marshmallow Maté Mullein Pennyroyal Peppermint Slippery elm Tea Thyme	pressure, heart or kidney disease, or a history of stroke should not use it. In very large doses, ephedra may cause potentially fatal heart problems. *Fenugreek* has estrogenic action. People who have a history of blood clots (thromboembolisms), inflammation of blood vessels (thrombophlebitis), heart disease, or stroke should consult their physicians before using it. Long-term use of *licorice* may cause water retention, elevated blood pressure, and a hormone imbalance (pseudoaldosteronism).
Depression	St. John's wort	If you are already taking antidepressant medication, consult a physician before using *St. John's wort*.
Diabetes	Apple Celery Evening primrose Fenugreek Garlic Ginseng Red pepper Sage	Long-term use of *celery* may deplete potassium stores. *Fenugreek* has estrogenic action. People who have a history of blood clots (thromboembolisms), inflammation of blood vessels (thrombophlebitis), heart disease, or stroke should consult their physicians before using it.
Diarrhea	Apple Barberry Bayberry Blackberry Dill Goldenseal Meadowsweet Mullein Psyllium Raspberry Rhubarb Slippery elm Tea Uva-ursi	*Bayberry* may change the body's sodium-potassium balance. If you have high blood pressure, heart disease, diabetes, kidney disease, or a history of stroke, consult a physician before using it. *Meadowsweet* contains aspirin-like compounds. If you are aspirin-sensitive, consult a physician before using it. Large doses of *rhubarb* have a laxative effect and may cause abdominal distress. *Tea* contains caffeine, which may cause jitters, irritability, insomnia, and addiction. Long-term use of *uva-ursi* may deplete potassium stores.
Dizziness	Ginger Ginkgo	None

Condition	Herb(s)	Special Precaution(s)
Ear infection	Echinacea Garlic	None
Eczema	Evening primrose	None
Emphysema	Eucalyptus Ginseng Peppermint	None
Fever	Bayberry Black haw Meadowsweet White willow	*Bayberry* may change the body's sodium-potassium balance. If you have high blood pressure, heart disease, diabetes, kidney disease, or a history of stroke, consult a physician before using it. *Meadowsweet* and *white willow* contain aspirin-like compounds. If you are aspirin-sensitive, consult a physician before using these herbs.
Fibromyalgia	Red pepper	None
Flu (*see* Colds and flu)		
Food poisoning prevention	Rosemary Sage Thyme	None
Food poisoning treatment	Angelica Apple Barberry Bayberry Burdock Catnip Chamomile Cinnamon Clove Dill Echinacea Garlic Ginseng Goldenseal Meadowsweet Mullein Peppermint	*Angelica* may cause a rash in sensitive people who are exposed to direct sunlight. *Bayberry* may change the body's sodium-potassium balance. If you have high blood pressure, heart disease, diabetes, kidney disease, or a history of stroke, consult a physician before using it. *Meadowsweet* contains aspirin-like compounds. If you are aspirin-sensitive, consult a physician before using it.

Condition	Herb(s)	Special Precaution(s)
Gallstone prevention	Coffee Dandelion	*Coffee* contains caffeine, which may cause jitters, irritability, insomnia, and addiction. Long-term use of *dandelion* may deplete potassium stores.
Gas	Dill	None
Giardiasis	Barberry Elecampane Goldenseal	None
Glaucoma prevention	Bilberry Blackberry Cranberry Raspberry	None
Gout (*see also* **Pain**)	Celery Nettle	Long-term use of *celery* and *nettle* may deplete potassium stores.
Gum disease prevention	Goldenseal Myrrh	None
Hay fever	Nettle Parsley	Long-term use of *nettle* and *parsley* may deplete potassium stores.
Headache	Eucalyptus Feverfew (for migraine) Meadowsweet Red pepper (for cluster headache) White willow	*Meadowsweet* and *white willow* contain aspirin-like compounds. If you are aspirin-sensitive, consult a physician before using these herbs.
Hearing loss	Gingko	None
Heart disease (*see also* **High blood pressure** *and* **High cholesterol**)	Alfalfa Bilberry Blackberry Cranberry Evening primrose Garlic Ginger Ginkgo Hawthorn	*Meadowsweet* and *white willow* contain aspirin-like compounds. If you are aspirin-sensitive, consult a physician before using these herbs. *Soybean* has estrogenic action. People who have a history of blood clots (thromboembolisms), inflammation of blood vessels (thrombophlebitis), heart disease, or stroke should consult their physicians before using it.

Condition	Herb(s)	Special Precaution(s)
Heart disease (cont.)	Meadowsweet Motherwort Raspberry Soybean Tea (green) Turmeric White willow	*Tea* contains caffeine, which may cause jitters, irritability, insomnia, and addiction.
Hemorrhoids	*For external use:* Blackberry Mullein Psyllium Shepherd's purse Slippery elm Tarragon Witch hazel *For internal use:* Horse chestnut	*Shepherd's purse* may cause powerful uterine contractions.
Hepatitis	Licorice Milk thistle	Long-term use of *licorice* may cause water retention, elevated blood pressure, and a hormone imbalance (pseudoaldosteronism).
Herpes and cold sores	*For external use:* Comfrey Hyssop Lemon balm Licorice Peppermint Uva-ursi *For internal use:* Echinacea Garlic Ginseng Lemon balm	Long-term use of *licorice* may cause water retention, elevated blood pressure, and a hormone imbalance (pseudoaldosteronism). Long-term use of *uva-ursi* may deplete potassium stores. *Lemon balm* interferes with thyroid-stimulating hormone. If you have an underactive thyroid (hypothyroidism), consult a physician before using it.
High blood pressure (*see also* Diuretic in "Healing Actions" table)	Barberry Black cohosh Cat's claw Celery Garlic Ginger Ginseng	*Black cohosh* may depress heart rate. If you have congestive heart failure, consult a physician before using it. It also has estrogenic action. People who have a history of blood clots (thromboembolisms), inflammation of blood vessels (thrombophlebitis), heart disease, or stroke should consult their physicians before using it.

Condition	Herb(s)	Special Precaution(s)
	Mistletoe Motherwort Turmeric Valerian	Long-term use of *celery* may deplete potassium stores. *Mistletoe* may slow heart rate and affect blood pressure. If you have heart disease, diabetes, high blood pressure, or a history of stroke, consult your physician before using it.
High cholesterol	Alfalfa Apple Cat's claw Celery Fenugreek Garlic Ginger Ginseng Psyllium Red pepper Scullcap Soybean Tea Turmeric	Long-term use of *celery* may deplete potassium stores. *Fenugreek* and *soybean* have estrogenic action. People who have a history of blood clots (thromboembolisms), inflammation of blood vessels (thrombophlebitis), heart disease, or stroke should consult their physicians before using them. *Tea* contains caffeine, which may cause jitters, irritability, insomnia, and addiction.
Hives	Nettle Parsley	Long-term use of *nettle* and *parsley* may deplete potassium stores.
Impotence (caused by poor bloodflow)	Ginkgo Ginseng	None
Infertility, male	Ginseng	None
Insomnia	Celery Hop Lavender Lemon balm Motherwort Passionflower Scullcap Valerian Yarrow	Long-term use of *celery* may deplete potassium stores. *Lemon balm* interferes with thyroid-stimulating hormone. If you have an underactive thyroid (hypothyroidism), consult a physician before using it.
Intermittent claudication	Ginkgo	None
Irritable bowel syndrome	Peppermint	None

Condition	Herb(s)	Special Precaution(s)
Jet lag	Cocoa (chocolate) Coffee Ephedra Ginseng Kola Maté Tea	*Cocoa (chocolate), coffee, kola, maté,* and *tea* all contain caffeine, which may cause jitters, irritability, insomnia, and addiction. *Ephedra* may raise blood pressure and cause jitters, irritability, and insomnia. People with high blood pressure, heart or kidney disease, or a history of stroke should not use it. In very large doses, ephedra may cause potentially fatal heart problems.
Kidney stone prevention	Coffee Horsetail	*Coffee* contains caffeine, which may cause jitters, irritability, insomnia, and addiction. Long-term use of *horsetail* may deplete potassium stores.
Lead poisoning	Apple Garlic	None
Leprosy (Hansen's disease)	Garlic Gotu kola	None
Macular degeneration	Bilberry Blackberry Cranberry Ginkgo Raspberry	None
Menopausal discomforts	Black cohosh Fennel Fenugreek Licorice Red clover Soybean	Long-term use of *licorice* may cause water retention, elevated blood pressure, and a hormone imbalance (pseudoaldosteronism). All of these herbs have estrogenic action. Women who have been advised not to take birth control pills or hormone replacement therapy should consult their physicians before using them.
Menstrual cramps (*see also* Pain)	Black cohosh Black haw Chaste tree Fennel Fenugreek Feverfew Red clover Yarrow	*Black cohosh, fennel, fenugreek,* and *red clover* have estrogenic action. Women who have been advised not to take birth control pills or hormone replacement therapy should consult their physicians before using these herbs.

Condition	Herb(s)	Special Precaution(s)
Menstruation, delayed	Celery Chaste tree Fenugreek Motherwort Parsley Pennyroyal Rhubarb Shepherd's purse	Long-term use of *celery* or *parsley* may deplete potassium stores. *Fenugreek* has estrogenic action. Women who have been advised not to take birth control pills or hormone replacement therapy should consult their physicians before using it. Large doses of *rhubarb* have a laxative effect and may cause abdominal distress. *Shepherd's purse* may cause powerful uterine contractions.
Menstruation, heavy	Chaste tree Shepherd's purse	*Shepherd's purse* may cause powerful uterine contractions.
Migraine	Feverfew	None
Morning sickness	Ginger Raspberry	None
Motion sickness	Ginger	None
Mouth sores	Blackberry	None
Mushroom poisoning	Milk thistle	None
Nausea	Ginger	None
Osteoporosis prevention	Soybean	*Soybean* has estrogenic action. Women who have been advised not to take birth control pills or hormone replacement therapy should consult their physicians before using it.
Pain (*see also* Anesthetic in "Healing Actions" table)	Black haw Coffee Meadowsweet Passionflower Red pepper Vervain White willow	*Coffee* contains caffeine, which may cause jitters, irritability, insomnia, and addiction. *Meadowsweet* and *white willow* contain aspirin-like compounds. If you are aspirin-sensitive, consult a physician before using these herbs. *Vervain* may depress heart rate and constrict bronchial passages. If you have heart disease, high blood pressure, diabetes, or asthma, consult a physician before using it.

Condition	Herb(s)	Special Precaution(s)
Pinkeye (*see* Conjunctivitis)		
Poison ivy, oak, and sumac	Aloe	None
Postpartum hemorrhage	Shepherd's purse	*Shepherd's purse* may cause powerful uterine contractions.
Premenstrual syndrome (PMS)	Black cohosh Buchu Celery Chaste tree Dandelion Evening primrose Horsetail Juniper Nettle Parsley Sarsaparilla Uva-ursi	*Black cohosh* has estrogenic action. Women who have been advised not to take birth control pills or hormone replacement therapy should consult their physicians before using it. *Buchu, celery, dandelion, horsetail, juniper, nettle, parsley, sarsaparilla,* and *uva-ursi* are diuretics and may deplete potassium stores.
Prostate cancer	Fennel Red clover Saw palmetto	*Fennel* and *red clover* have estrogenic action. People who have a history of blood clots (thromboembolisms), inflammation of blood vessels (thrombophlebitis), heart disease, or stroke should consult their physicians before using them.
Psoriasis	Echinacea Gotu kola	None
Scalds (*see* Burns)		
Sore throat	Fenugreek Licorice Marshmallow Mullein Sage Slippery elm	Long-term use of *licorice* may cause water retention, elevated blood pressure, and a hormone imbalance (pseudoaldosteronism). *Fenugreek* has estrogenic action. People who have a history of blood clots (thromboembolisms), inflammation of blood vessels (thrombophlebitis), heart disease, or stroke should consult their physicians before using it.
Stress	Catnip Celery	Long-term use of *celery* can deplete potassium stores.

Condition	Herb(s)	Special Precaution(s)
	Chamomile Ginseng Kava Lemon balm Motherwort Passionflower Scullcap Yarrow	*Lemon balm* interferes with thyroid-stimulating hormone. If you have an underactive thyroid (hypothyroidism), consult a physician before using it.
Stroke prevention and treatment	Bilberry Blackberry Cranberry Garlic Ginger Ginkgo Meadowsweet Raspberry Turmeric White willow	*Meadowsweet* and *white willow* contain aspirin-like compounds. If you are aspirin-sensitive, consult a physician before using these herbs.
Sunburn (*see* Burns)		
Tinnitus (ringing in the ears)	Ginkgo	None
Toothache	*For external use, on gums only:* Clove oil	Herbal oils are highly concentrated. As little as a teaspoon may be toxic if ingested. Keep herbal oils away from children.
Tooth decay prevention	Peppermint Tea	*Tea* contains caffeine, which may cause jitters, irritability, insomnia, and addiction.
Ulcers	Chamomile Garlic Licorice Papaya	Long-term use of *licorice* may cause water retention, elevated blood pressure, and a hormone imbalance (pseudoaldosteronism).
Urinary incontinence	Cranberry	None
Urinary tract infection prevention	Cranberry Horsetail	Long-term use of *horsetail* may deplete potassium stores.

Condition	Herb(s)	Special Precaution(s)
Urinary tract infection treatment	Barberry Garlic Meadowsweet Uva-ursi	*Meadowsweet* contains aspirin-like compounds. If you are aspirin-sensitive, consult a physician before using it. Long-term use of *uva-ursi* may deplete potassium stores.
Varicose veins	Bilberry Blackberry Cranberry Gotu kola Horse chestnut Raspberry Tarragon	None
Wounds	*For external use:* Aloe Blackberry Comfrey Eucalyptus Fenugreek Gotu kola Horsetail Lavender Marshmallow St. John's wort Shepherd's purse Slippery elm Tea tree Uva-ursi Witch hazel Yarrow *For internal use:* Echinacea Garlic	Long-term use of *horsetail* and *uva-ursi* may deplete potassium stores. If you are taking antidepressant medication, consult a physician before using *St. John's wort*. *Shepherd's purse* may cause powerful uterine contractions. As little as a teaspoon of *tea tree* oil can be toxic. Do not ingest it, and keep it out of the reach of children.
Yeast infection (candidiasis)	Barberry Chamomile Cinnamon Dandelion Echinacea Garlic Tea tree	Long-term use of *dandelion* may deplete potassium stores. As little as a teaspoon of *tea tree* oil can be toxic. Do not ingest it, and keep it out of the reach of children.

Healing Actions of Herbs

Use	Herb(s)	Special Precaution(s)
Anesthetic	*For external use:* Clove Cinnamon Peppermint	Never ingest herbal oils. As little as a teaspoon can be toxic.
Antibiotic (antibacterial)	Apple Barberry Bayberry Boneset Burdock Catnip Chamomile Cinnamon Clove Dill Echinacea Garlic Ginseng Goldenseal Licorice Meadowsweet Myrrh Peppermint St. John's wort Tea tree	*Bayberry* may change the body's sodium-potassium balance. If you have high blood pressure, heart disease, diabetes, kidney disease, or a history of stroke, consult a physician before using it. Long-term use of *licorice* may cause water retention, elevated blood pressure, and a hormone imbalance (pseudoaldosteronism). *Meadowsweet* contains aspirin-like compounds. If you are aspirin-sensitive, consult a physician before using it. If you are taking antidepressant medication, consult a physician before using *St. John's wort*. As little as a teaspoon of *tea tree* oil can be toxic. Do not ingest it, and keep it out of the reach of children.
Antibiotic (antifungal)	Aloe Barberry Burdock Chamomile Cinnamon Clove Dandelion Echinacea Garlic Goldenseal Licorice St. John's wort Tea tree	Long-term use of *dandelion* may deplete potassium stores. Long-term use of *licorice* may cause water retention, elevated blood pressure, and a hormone imbalance (pseudoaldosteronism). If you are taking antidepressant medication, consult a physician before using *St. John's wort*. As little as a teaspoon of *tea tree* oil can be toxic. Do not ingest it, and keep it out of the reach of children.

Use	Herb(s)	Special Precaution(s)
Antibiotic (antiparasitic, antiprotozoan)	Barberry Bayberry Clove Echinacea Elecampane Garlic Goldenseal Turmeric	*Bayberry* may change the body's sodium-potassium balance. If you have high blood pressure, heart disease, diabetes, kidney disease, or a history of stroke, consult a physician before using it.
Antidepressant	Coffee St. John's wort	*Coffee* contains caffeine, which may cause jitters, irritability, insomnia, and addiction. If you are already taking antidepressant medication, consult a physician before using *St. John's wort.*
Antihistamine	Clove Nettle	Long-term use of *nettle* may deplete potassium stores.
Anti-inflammatory	Angelica Black haw Boneset Cat's claw Chamomile Chaparral Echinacea Fenugreek Gentian Ginger Horsetail Juniper Licorice Meadowsweet St. John's wort Turmeric Vervain White willow	*Angelica* may cause a rash in sensitive people who are exposed to direct sunlight. Long-term use of *horsetail, juniper,* and *vervain* may deplete potassium stores. Long-term use of *licorice* may cause water retention, elevated blood pressure, and a hormone imbalance (pseudoaldosteronism). *Meadowsweet* and *white willow* contain aspirin-like compounds. If you are aspirin-sensitive, consult a physician before using these herbs. If you are taking antidepressant medication, consult a physician before using *St. John's wort.* *Vervain* may depress heart rate and constrict bronchial passages. If you have heart disease, high blood pressure, diabetes, or asthma, consult a physician before using it.
Antiperspirant	Sage	None
Antiseptic	*For external use in treating minor burns and wounds:* Aloe Apple	Long-term use of *licorice* may cause water retention, elevated blood pressure, and a hormone imbalance (pseudoaldosteronism).

Use	Herb(s)	Special Precaution(s)
	Blackberry Catnip Chamomile Chaparral Cinnamon Clove Eucalyptus Garlic Hop Lemon balm Licorice Myrrh Passionflower Peppermint Rosemary Sage St. John's wort Tarragon Thyme Turmeric Yarrow *For internal use:* Echinacea Ginseng	If you are taking antidepressant medication, consult a physician before using *St. John's wort.*
Antiviral	Boneset Cat's claw Chamomile Cinnamon Echinacea Ginger Ginseng Lemon balm St. John's wort	*Lemon balm* interferes with thyroid-stimulating hormone. If you have an underactive thyroid (hypothyroidism), consult a physician before using it. If you are taking antidepressant medication, consult a physician before using *St. John's wort.*
Decongestant	Angelica Cocoa (chocolate) Coffee Ephedra Eucalyptus Kola Maté Pennyroyal	*Angelica* may cause a rash in sensitive people who are exposed to direct sunlight. *Cocoa (chocolate), coffee, kola, maté,* and *tea* all contain caffeine, which may cause jitters, irritability, insomnia, and addiction. *Ephedra* may raise blood pressure and cause jitters, irritability, and insomnia. People with high blood

Use	Herb(s)	Special Precaution(s)
Decongestant (cont.)	Peppermint Rosemary Tea	pressure, heart or kidney disease, or a history of stroke should not use it. In very large doses, ephedra may cause potentially fatal heart problems.
Diuretic	Buchu Celery Dandelion Horsetail Juniper Nettle Parsley Sarsaparilla Uva-ursi	Long-term use of diuretic herbs may deplete potassium stores. Do not use diuretics for weight loss.
Laxative	Apple Buckthorn Cascara sagrada Coffee Psyllium Rhubarb Senna Vervain	*Buckthorn, cascara sagrada, rhubarb,* and *senna* may cause abdominal distress. If you find yourself using these herbs more than twice a month, consult a physician. *Coffee* contains caffeine, which may cause jitters, irritability, insomnia, and addiction. *Vervain* may depress heart rate and constrict bronchial passages. If you have heart disease, high blood pressure, diabetes, or asthma, consult a physician before using it.
Sedative	Celery Hop Lavender Lemon balm Motherwort Passionflower Scullcap Valerian Yarrow	Long-term use of *celery* may deplete potassium stores. *Lemon balm* interferes with thyroid-stimulating hormone. If you have an underactive thyroid (hypothyroidism), consult a physician before using it.
Stimulant	Cocoa (chocolate) Coffee Ephedra Ginseng Kola Maté Tea	*Cocoa (chocolate), coffee, kola, maté,* and *tea* all contain caffeine, which may cause jitters, irritability, insomnia, and addiction. *Ephedra* may raise blood pressure and cause jitters, irritability, and insomnia. People with high blood pressure, heart or kidney disease, or a history of stroke should not use it. In very large doses, ephedra may cause potentially fatal heart problems.

Use	Herb(s)	Special Precaution(s)
Tranquilizer	Catnip Celery Chamomile Lavender Lemon balm Motherwort Passionflower Scullcap Yarrow	Long-term use of *celery* may deplete potassium stores. *Lemon balm* interferes with thyroid-stimulating hormone. If you have an underactive thyroid (hypothyroidism), consult a physician before using it.

Other Uses of Herbs

Use	Herb(s)	Special Precaution(s)
Athletic performance enhancement	Coffee Ginseng	*Coffee* contains caffeine, which may cause jitters, irritability, insomnia, and addiction.
Digestive support	Angelica Caraway Catnip Chamomile Cinnamon Clove Cocoa (chocolate) Dandelion Dill Fennel Feverfew Gentian Ginger Hop Horehound Lavender Lemon balm Marshmallow Papaya Passionflower Pennyroyal Peppermint Red pepper Rosemary	*Angelica* may cause a rash in sensitive people who are exposed to direct sunlight. *Cocoa (chocolate)* contains caffeine, which may cause jitters, irritability, insomnia, and addiction. Long-term use of *dandelion* may deplete potassium stores. *Fennel* has estrogenic action. People who have a history of blood clots (thromboembolisms), inflammation of blood vessels (thrombophlebitis), heart disease, or stroke should consult their physicians before using it. *Lemon balm* interferes with thyroid-stimulating hormone. If you have an underactive thyroid (hypothyroidism), consult a physician before using it.

Use	Herb(s)	Special Precaution(s)
Digestive support (cont.)	Sage Slippery elm Thyme Turmeric Yarrow	
Immune system stimulation	*For external use:* Aloe *For internal use:* Astragalus Barberry Boneset Cat's claw Chamomile Echinacea Garlic Ginger Ginseng Goldenseal Gotu kola Licorice Marshmallow Mistletoe St. John's wort	Long-term use of *licorice* may cause water retention, elevated blood pressure, and a hormone imbalance (pseudoaldosteronism). *Mistletoe* may slow heart rate and affect blood pressure. If you have heart disease, diabetes, high blood pressure, or a history of stroke, consult your physician before using it. If you are taking antidepressant medication, consult a physician before using *St. John's wort*.
Insect repellent	Eucalyptus Lavender Pennyroyal	As little as a teaspoon of *pennyroyal* oil can be toxic. Do not ingest it, and keep it out of the reach of children.
Labor stimulation	Blue cohosh Shepherd's purse	Using herbs to induce labor requires medical supervision.
Lactation support	Chaste tree	None
Liver protection	Astragalus Barberry Ginseng Licorice Milk thistle Turmeric	Long-term use of *licorice* may cause water retention, elevated blood pressure, and a hormone imbalance (pseudoaldosteronism).
Memory improvement	Ginkgo Ginseng	None

Use	Herb(s)	Special Precaution(s)
Weight control	Coffee Ephedra	*Coffee* contains caffeine, which may cause jitters, irritability, insomnia, and addiction. *Ephedra* may raise blood pressure and cause jitters, irritability, and insomnia. People with high blood pressure, heart or kidney disease, or a history of stroke should not use it. In very large doses, ephedra may cause potentially fatal heart problems. Both of these herbs should be used for weight control only under medical supervision.

References

Because of space limitations, only the books used as sources for *The New Healing Herbs* are listed here. For a complete bibliography, including medical journal articles, send your request plus a check or money order for $5 (for reproduction, postage, and handling) to Self-Care Associates, P.O. Box 460066, San Francisco, CA 94146-0066. Please allow 3 weeks for delivery.

American Pharmaceutical Association. *Handbook of Nonprescription Drugs.* Washington, D.C.: American Pharmaceutical Association, 1996.

Bassman, L. *The Whole Mind: The Definitive Guide to Complementary Treatments for Mind, Mood, and Emotion.* Novato, Calif.: New World Library, 1998.

Beinfield, H., and E. Korngold. *Between Heaven and Earth: A Guide to Chinese Medicine.* New York: Ballantine, 1991.

Blumenthal, M., et al. *The Complete German Commission E Monographs: Therapeutic Guide to Herbal Medicines.* Austin, Tex.: American Botanical Council and Integrative Medicine Communications, 1998.

Boyle, W. *Herb Doctors: Pioneers in 19th-Century American Botanical Medicine.* East Palestine, Ohio: Buckeye Naturopathic Press, 1988.

Brinker, F. J. *The Toxicology of Botanical Medicines.* 2nd ed. Portland, Ore.: Eclectic Medical Institute, 1987.

Brown, D. *Herbal Prescriptions for Better Health.* Rocklin, Calif.: Prima Publishing, 1996.

Burton Goldberg Group. *Alternative Medicine: The Definitive Guide.* Fife, Wash.: Future Medicine, 1994.

Castleman, M. *Nature's Cures.* Emmaus, Pa.: Rodale Press, 1996.

Chin, W. Y., and H. Keng. *An Illustrated Dictionary of Chinese Medicinal Herbs.* Sebastopol, Calif.: CRCS Publications, 1992.

Collinge, W. *The American Holistic Health Association Complete Guide to Alternative Medicine.* New York: Warner Books, 1996.

Conrow, R., and A. Hecksel. *Herbal Pathfinders: Voices of the Herb Renaissance.* Santa Barbara, Calif.: Woodbridge Press, 1983.

Coulter, H. L. *Divided Legacy.* Berkeley, Calif.: Homeopathic Educational Services, 1982.

Crenshaw, T. *The Alchemy of Love and Lust.* New York: Putnam, 1996.

Culpeper, N. *Culpeper's Complete Herbal and English Physician.* 1826 ed. Avon, England: Pitman Press, 1981.

Cummings, S., and D. Ullman. *Everybody's Guide to Homeopathic Medicines.* New York: Tarcher-Putnam, 1997.

Cumston, C. G. *An Introduction to the History of Medicine.* New York: Dorset Press, 1987.

Der Marderosian, A., and L. Liberti. *Natural Product Medicine.* Philadelphia: George F. Stickley, 1988.

DeSmet, P. A., ed. *Adverse Effects of Herbal Drugs.* Berlin: Springer-Verlag, 1993.

De Waal, M. *Medicinal Herbs in the Bible.* York Beach, Maine: Samuel Weiser, 1984.

Dobelis, I. N., ed. *Magic and Medicine of Plants.* Pleasantville, N.Y.: Reader's Digest, 1986.

Duke, J. A. *Ginseng: A Concise Handbook.* Algonac, Mich.: Reference Publications, 1989.

———. *The Green Pharmacy.* Emmaus, Pa.: Rodale Press, 1997.

———. *Handbook of Medicinal Herbs.* Boca Raton, Fla.: CRC Press, 1985.

Ehrenreich, B. and D. English. *Witches, Midwives, and Nurses: A History of Women Healers.* Detroit: Black and Red, 1973.

Eskinazi, D., et al., eds. *Botanical Medicine: Efficacy, Quality Assurance, and Regulation.* Larchmont, N.Y.: Mary Ann Liebert, 1999.

Facts and Comparisons. *Drug Facts and Comparisons, 1999 and 2000.* St. Louis, Mo.: Facts and Comparisons Publishing Group, 1999 and 2000.

Felter, H. W., and J. U. Lloyd. *King's American Dispensatory.* 18th ed., 1898. Portland, Ore.: Eclectic Medical Publications, 1983.

Foster, S. *Echinacea Exalted!* Brixley, Mo.: Ozark Beneficial Plant Project, 1985.

———. *Herbal Bounty.* Salt Lake City: Peregrine Smith Books, 1984.

Foster, S., and J. A. Duke. *A Field Guide to Medicinal Plants: Eastern and Central North America* (Peterson Field Guide #40). Boston: Houghton Mifflin, 1990.

Foster, S., and V. E Tyler. *Tyler's Honest Herbal.* 4th ed. New York and London: Haworth Herbal Press, 1999.

Fratkin, J. *Chinese Herbal Patent Formulas.* Boulder, Colo.: Shya Publications, 1986.

Fugh-Berman, A. *Alternative Medicine: What Works.* Tucson.: Odonian Press, 1996.

Fulder, S. *Ginseng: Magical Herb of the East.* Northamptonshire, England: Thorsons Publishing, 1988.

Funfgeld, E. W., ed. *Rokan (Ginkgo Biloba): Recent Results in Pharmacology and Clinic.* Berlin: Springer-Verlag, 1988.

Gilman, A. G., et al, eds. *Goodman and Gilman's The Pharmacological Basis of Therapeutics.* 7th ed. New York: Macmillan, 1985.

Graedon, J., and T. Graedon. *Graedon's Best Medicine: From Herbal Remedies to High-Tech Rx Breakthroughs.* New York: Bantam Books, 1991.

Grieve, M. *A Modern Herbal.* New York: Dover, 1971.

Griffith, H. W. *The Complete Guide to Vitamins, Minerals, Supplements, and Herbs.* Tucson: Fisher Books, 1988.

Hallowell, M. *Herbal Healing: A Practical Introduction.* Bath, England: Ashgrove Press, 1985.

Harris, B. C. *Comfrey: What You Need to Know.* New Canaan, Conn: Keats Publishing, 1982.

Harris, L. J. *The Book of Garlic.* Berkeley, Calif.: Aris Books, 1979.

Herbrandson, D. *Shaker Herbs and Their Medicinal Uses.* New Gloucester, Maine: Shaker Heritage Society, Sabbathday Lake, 1985.

Heyn, B. *Ayurvedic Medicine.* Northamptonshire, England: Thorsons Publishing, 1987.

Hobbs, C. *The Ginsengs: A Users Guide.* Santa Cruz, Calif.: Botanica Press, 1996.

———. *Herbal Remedies for Dummies.* Foster City, Calif.: IDG Books, 1998.

Hoffman, D. *The Holistic Herbal.* Dorset, England: Element Books, 1983.

Hou, J. P. *Ginseng: The Myth and the Truth.* North Hollywood, Calif.: Wilshire Book Co., 1978.

Keville, K., and M. Green. *Aromatherapy: A Complete Guide to the Healing Art.* Freedom, Calif.: Crossing Press, 1995.

Kiangsu Institute of Modern Medicine. *Encyclopedia of Chinese Drugs,* vol. 2. Shanghai: Shanghai Scientific and Technical Publications, 1977.

Kloss, J. *Back to Eden.* Loma Linda, Calif.: Back to Eden Books, 1988.

Koch, H. P., and L. D. Lawson, eds. *Garlic: The Science and Therapeutic Application of Allium Sativum and Related Species.* Baltimore: Williams and Wilkins, 1996.

Kowalchik, C., and W. H. Hylton, eds. *Rodale's Illustrated Encyclopedia of Herbs.* Emmaus, Pa.: Rodale Press, 1987.

Kreig, M. B. *Green Medicine: The Search for Plants That Heal.* Chicago: Rand McNally, 1964.

Lad, V., and D. Frawley. *The Yoga of Herbs.* Santa Fe: Lotus Press, 1986.

Law, D. *The Concise Herbal Encyclopedia.* New York: St. Martin's Press, 1973.

Leung, A. Y. *Encyclopedia of Common Natural Ingredients Used in Food, Drugs, and Cosmetics.* New York: John Wiley & Sons, 1980.

Lewis, W., and M. P. F. Elvin-Lewis. *Medical Botany.* New York: John Wiley & Sons, 1974.

Lust, J. *The Herb Book.* New York: Bantam, 1974.

Marti-Ibaez, F. *The Epic of Medicine.* New York: Bramhall House, 1962.

McCaleb, R., et al. *The Herb Research Foundation's Encyclopedia of Popular Herbs.* Roseville, Calif.: Prima Publishing, 2000.

McGuffin, M., et al., eds. *American Herbal Products Association Botanical Safety Handbook.* Boca Raton, Fla.: CRC Press, 1997.

McIntyre, M. *Herbal Medicine for Everyone.* London: Penguin, 1988.

Medical Economics. *PDR for Herbal Medicines.* Montvale, N.J.: Medical Economics, 1998.

Micozzi, M. S. *Fundamentals of Complementary and Alternative Medicine.* New York: Churchill Livingstone, 1996.

Millspaugh, C. F. *American Medicinal Plants.* 1892 ed. New York: Dover, 1974.

Morse, F. *The Story of the Shakers.* Woodstock, Vt.: Countryman Press, 1986.

Mowrey, D. B. *Next Generation Herbal Medicine.* Lehi, Utah: Cormorant Books, 1988.

———. *The Scientific Validation of Herbal Medicine.* Lehi, Utah: Cormorant Books, 1986.

Murray, M. *Natural Alternatives to Over-the-Counter and Prescription Drugs.* New York: William Morrow, 1994.

———. *The 21st Century Herbal.* Bellevue, Wash.: Vita-Line, 1987.

Murray, M., and J. Pizzorno. *Encyclopedia of Natural Medicine.* Rocklin, Calif.: Prima Publishing, 1991.

Olsen, C. *Australian Teatree Oil Guide.* Pagosa Springs, Colo.: Kali Press, 1997.

Pendergrast, M. *Uncommon Grounds: The History of Coffee and How It Transformed Our World.* New York: Basic Books, 1999.

Pizzorno, J., and M. Murray. *A Textbook of Natural Medicine.* Kenmore, Wash.: Bastyr University Publications, 1996.

Reid, D. P. *Chinese Herbal Medicine.* Boston: Shambhala, 1987.

Riddle, J. M. *Eve's Herbs: A History of Contraception and Abortion in the West.* Cambridge, Mass.: Harvard University Press, 1997.

Schechter, S. *Fighting Radiation with Foods, Herbs, and Vitamins.* Brookline, Mass.: East West Health Books, 1988.

Simon, J. E., and L. Grant, eds. *Proceedings of the First National Herb Growing and Marketing Conference.* West Lafayette, Ind.: Purdue University Cooperative Extension Service, 1987.

————. *Proceedings of the Second National Herb Growing and Marketing Conference.* West Lafayette, Ind.: Purdue University Cooperative Extension Service, 1987.

Simon, J. E., et al. *Proceedings of the Fourth National Herb Growing and Marketing Conference.* Silver Spring, Pa.: International Herb Growers and Marketers Association, 1989.

Spencer, J. W., and J. J. Jacobs. *Complementary/Alternative Medicine: An Evidence-Based Approach.* St. Louis: Mosby, 1999.

Spoerke, D. *Herbal Medications.* Santa Barbara, Calif.: Woodbridge Press, 1980.

Starr, P. *The Social Transformation of American Medicine.* New York: Basic Books, 1982.

Stuart, M., ed. *The Encyclopedia of Herbs and Herbalism.* New York: Grosset & Dunlap, 1979.

Strehlow, W., and G. Hertzka. *Hildegard of Bingen's Medicine.* Santa Fe: Bear, 1988.

Tannahill, R. *Food in History.* New York: Stein & Day, 1973.

Tierra, M. *The Way of Herbs.* New York: Pocket Books, 1983.

Tyler, V. *Herbs of Choice: The Therapeutic Use of Phytomedicinals.* New York: Hawthorn Press, 1994.

Tyler, V. E., et al. *Pharmacognosy.* 9th ed. Philadelphia: Lea and Febiger, 1988.

Ullman, D. *The Consumer's Guide to Homeopathy.* New York: G. P. Putnam's Sons, 1995.

Weed, S. S. *Wise Woman Herbal for the Childbearing Years.* Woodstock, N.Y.: Ash Tree Publishing, 1985.

Weil, A. *Natural Health, Natural Medicine.* Boston: Houghton Mifflin, 1990.

Weiner, M., and J. A. Weiner. *Herbs That Heal.* Mill Valley, Calif: Quantum Books, 1994.

Weiner, M. A. *Earth Medicine, Earth Food.* New York: Macmillan, 1980.

————. *The People's Herbal.* New York: Perigee/Putnam, 1984

————. *Weiner's Herbal.* New York: Stein & Day, 1980.

Weiss, G., and S. Weiss. *Growing and Using the Healing Herbs.* Emmaus, Pa.: Rodale Press, 1985.

Weiss, R. F. *Herbal Medicine.* Beaconsfield, England: Beaconsfield Publishers, 1988.

Werbach, M., and M. Murray. *Botanical Influences on Illness.* Tarzana, Calif.: Third Line Press, 1994.

Wheelwright, E. G. *Medicinal Plants and Their History.* New York: Dover, 1974.

White, L., and S. Mavor. *Kids, Herbs, and Health.* Loveland, Colo.: Interweave Press, 1998.

Willard, T. *Textbook of Modern Herbology.* Calgary, Alberta: Progressive Publishing, 1988.

Wren, R. C. *Potter's New Cyclopaedia of Botanical Drugs and Preparations.* Essex, England: C. W. Daniel, 1988.

Zhu, C-H. *Clinical Handbook of Chinese Prepared Medicines.* Brookline, Mass.: Paradigm Publications, 1989.

Index

American colonists (*cont.*)
 herbs used by (*cont.*)
  horehound, 240–41
  hyssop, 250
  lemon balm, 267
  marshmallow, 277
  meadowsweet, 282–83
  motherwort, 294
  mullein, 297
  passionflower, 313
  pennyroyal, 317
  rosemary, 348
  sage, 351
  St. John's wort, 355
  uva-ursi, 398
  valerian, 403
  vervain, 407
  witch hazel, 414–15
 history of herbal healing and,
  25–26
Anaphylaxis, 125–26
Androgens, 131–32
Anemia
 from alfalfa, 58
 angelica for, 65
Angelica, 6, 63–66, **63**
Anise, 274
Anthocyanosides
 in bilberry, 79–80
 in blackberry, 83–84
 in cranberry, 156–57
 in raspberry, 330
Anthraquinones
 in aloe, 44, 61–62
 in buckthorn, 44, 102–3
 in cascara sagrada, 44,
  111
 in rhubarb, 342–43
 in senna, 44, 369
Antibiotics
 barberry, 74
 bayberry, 77
 blue cohosh, 95
 catnip, 114–15
 garlic, 199
 goldenseal, 227
 hop, 238
 St. John's wort, 357

Anticoagulants
 angelica, 65
 feverfew and, 195
 garlic, 39, 43, 202
 ginkgo and, 215
 ginseng and, 223
 motherwort, 295
 shepherd's purse and, 373
 turmeric, 397
Anticonvulsant, valerian as, 404
Antidepressant-related sexual
  problems, ginkgo for, 214
Antidotes, 14, 105
Anti-inflammatories
 aloe, 60
 angelica, 65
 barberry, 75
 black cohosh, 89
 blue cohosh, 95
 boneset, 98
 burdock, 105
 comfrey, 153
 dandelion, 160
 fenugreek, 190
 meadowsweet, 283–84
 myrrh, 300
 scullcap, 366
 uva-ursi, 400
 vervain, 407
 white willow, 411–12
Antiseptics
 chaparral, 128
 cinnamon, 134
 clove, 137
 eucalyptus, 178
 goldenseal, 226
 thyme, 391
 uva-ursi, 399
Antispasmodics
 caraway, 108
 chamomile, 124–25
 feverfew, 194
 passionflower, 314
 peppermint, 323
 yarrow, 418
Anxiety
 catnip for, 114
 celery seed for, 121

chamomile for, 124
from coca, 142
from coffee, 148–49
hop for, 238
kava for, 257
lavender for, 263–64
motherwort for, 294
passionflower for, 314
scullcap for, 366
yarrow for, 418
Aphrodisiacs
 chaste tree, 131–32
 ginseng, 221
 lavender, 262
 saw palmetto and, 361–62
Apigenin, 124
Apiol, 310–11
Appetite
 gentian for, 203
 ginseng for, 221
Apple, 67–70, **67**
Aquavit, 108
Arab herbalists
 herbs used by
  alfalfa, 56
  aloe, 60
  blackberry, 82
  coffee, 145
  garlic, 197
  gentian, 203
  lemon balm, 266
  marshmallow, 276
  myrrh, 299
  sage, 350
 history of herbal healing and, 15
Aromatherapy
 Egyptian herbalists and, 10–11
 history of herbal healing and,
  4–5
 lavender and, 262–63
Arrhythmia
 diagnosing, 294
 hawthorn for, 234
 horehound and, 241
 peppermint and, 323–24
Arthritis. *See also* Osteoarthritis;
  Rheumatoid arthritis
 angelica for, 65

red clover, 333
St. John's wort, 354–55
shepherd's purse, 371
history of herbal healing and, 11–12
Green tea, 384–87
Growing herbs, 50. *See also specific herbs*
Gum disease, chaparral for, 128

H

HA, 167
Halcion, 267, 404
Hansen's disease
garlic for, 200–201
gotu kola for, 231
Harmala compounds, 315
Harvesting herbs, 49–50
Hawthorn, 233–35, **233**
Hay fever
clove for, 137
juniper and, 254
nettle for, 304
HDL, 366
Headache
aspirin for, 41
eucalyptus for, 178
from ginkgo, 215
migraine, feverfew for, 193–95
peppermint for, 323
red pepper for, 339
from saw palmetto, 364
spearmint for, 323
Healing action of herbs, 435–39. *See also specific herbs*
Health problems and their herbal remedies, 421–34. *See also specific problems*
Heart attack
aspirin for, 412
cat's claw for, 117
garlic for, 199–200, 202
passionflower for, 314
red wine for, 140
white willow for, 412
Heartburn, from cocoa, 142

Heart disease
alfalfa for, 57
apple for, 68
coca and, 141
evening primrose for, 181
ginger for, 208
ginkgo for, 213
hawthorn for, 234–35
motherwort for, 294
passionflower for, 314
red pepper for, 339
tea for, 386
turmeric for, 396
vervain and, 408
Helmbold's Compound Extract of Buchu, 100
Hemlock, poison, 38
Hemorrhage, postpartum, goldenseal for, 227
Hemorrhoids
blackberry for, 84
horse chestnut for, 243–44
hyssop for, 250
mullein for, 297–98
psyllium for, 325–26
witch hazel for, 415
Hepatitis
licorice for, 273
milk thistle for, 287
tea for, 386
uva-ursi for, 400
yarrow for, 418
Herbs. *See also* Adulteration of herbs; *specific herbs*
in baths, 48
buying, 50–51
classification system for, 22
compresses, 48
conditions and, 421–34
consumer precautions, 420
double standard and, 40–41
drying, 45–46
external preparations, 48
forms of
capsules, 48
decoctions, 47
infusions, 46–47
oils, 43

ointments, 48
powder, 46
fragrant, 4–5, 10–11
growing, 50
harvesting, 49–50
healing actions of, 435–39
interactions with pharmaceuticals, 43
as laxatives, 44
medicinal, sources of, 44
other uses of, 439–41
potency, 41
preparing, 46–48
problematic, 44
publications about, 51
reactions to, general, 42–43
reference books, 442–44
reference guide, 420–21, 421–34
as sedatives, 44
as stimulants, 44
storing, 45–46
tincture, 47–48
as tranquilizers, 44
Herbal Ecstasy, 175
Herpalieve, 153
Herpes
hyssop for, 250
lemon balm for, 267
licorice for, 273
mullein for, 297
High blood pressure
barberry for, 74
black cohosh for, 89
blue cohosh and, 95
buchu for, 101
celery for, 120–21
cinnamon for, 134
coffee and, 149
dandelion for, 159–60
elecampane for, 171
gentian and, 205
ginseng for, 220
goldenseal and, 228
gotu kola for, 231
horehound for, 241
juniper for, 252–53
mistletoe for, 290–91

Mouthwash
chaparral in, 128
myrrh in, 300
Moxie, 203–4
Moxie Nerve Food, 204
Mucilage, 190, 297, 326
Mullein, 296–98, **296**
Multi-infarct dementia (MID),
ginkgo for, 211–13
Multiple sclerosis, evening
primrose for, 182
Mushroom poisoning, milk thistle
for, 287
Myricitrin, 77
Myristicin, 310
Myrrh, 299–301, **299**

N

Nardil, 292
National Formulary, 98, 114, 166,
297, 314, 334, 366, 403,
415
Native American herbalists
herbs used by
barberry, 73–74
bayberry, 76
black cohosh, 5, 87
blue cohosh, 94
boneset, 97
catnip, 113–14
chaparral, 127
echinacea, 165
ephedra, 173
evening primrose, 180
gentian, 203–4
ginseng, 218
goldenseal, 225
hop, 237
horse chestnut, 243
juniper, 252
licorice, 271
mints, 321
mistletoe, 290
nettle, 303
sarsaparilla, 359
saw palmetto, 362

senna, 368
slippery elm, 375
witch hazel, 414
yarrow, 418
history of herbal healing and,
24–25
Nature's Remedy, 111
Naturopathy, 31, 395
Nausea. *See also* Morning
sickness; Motion sickness
from barberry, 75
from bayberry, 77–78
from black cohosh, 89–90
from boneset, 99
from gentian, 205
from ginkgo, 215
from goldenseal, 228
from senna, 369
from uva-ursi, 400
NDGA, 127
Nepetalactone isomers, 114
Nettle, 302–5, **302**
Neuropathy, diabetic
evening primrose for, 182
red pepper for, 339
Nicorette, 247
Nicotine, 247
Nicotine gum, 247
Nitroglycerin, 39
Nonsteroidal anti-inflammatory
drugs (NSAIDs), 304, 396
Nordihydroguaiaretic acid
(NDGA), 127
Numzit, 137
Nursing. *See* Breastfeeding

O

Obesity. *See* Overweight; Weight
loss
Oils, herbal, 43
Ointments, herbal, 48
Onion, 20
Oolong tea, 384, 386–87
Ophthiole, 74
Orabase, 137
Orajel, 137

Oral hygiene, clove for, 137
Organ transplantation, ginkgo for,
214–15
Ornamental blue passionflower,
315
Osteoarthritis, red pepper for, 338
Osteoporosis
coffee and, 144, 150–51
black cohosh for, 89
soybean for, 379
OTC pharmaceuticals, 35–36
Overactive thyroid
ephedra and, 176
lemon balm for, 268
Over-the-counter (OTC)
pharmaceuticals, 35–36
Overweight. *See also* Weight loss
cocoa and, 141
coffee for, 148
dandelion for, 160
ephedra for, 174–75
fennel for, 186
Oxalic acid, 343
Oxindole alkaloids, 116
Oxytocin, 95

P

PAs, 41, 99, 153–54
PAF, 215
Pain relievers
black haw, 92
cinnamon, 134
coffee, 147
meadowsweet, 283–84
myrrh, 300
peppermint, 322
red pepper, 338
spearmint, 322
vervain, 407
white willow, 411–12
Pain King, 27
Palpitations, 294. *See also*
Arrhythmia
Papain, 307
Papaya, 306–8, **306**
Paraguay tea, 279–81

Protease inhibitors, 38
Prozac, 356
Pseudoaldosteronism, licorice
  and, 274
Pseudoephedrine, 5, 174
Psoralens, 65–66, 121, 311–12
Psoriasis
  aloe for, 60
  barberry for, 74
  gotu kola for, 231
  red pepper for, 338
Psyllium, 62, 112, 325–28, **325**,
  367
Pulegone, 318
Pygeum, 304
Pyrrolizidine alkaloids (PAs), 41,
  99, 153–54

Q

Qi, 71
Queen of Hungary's Water,
  347–48
Quinine, 193

R

Radiation therapy
  echinacea and, 168–69
  ginseng for, 221
  mistletoe and, 291
Ragweed allergy, 129
Raspberry, 6, 329–32, **329**
Rauwolfia serpentina, 9
Reactions, to herbs, 42–43. *See*
  also specific herbs
Red clover, 333–35, **333**
Red Cross Toothache Medication,
  137
Red pepper, 76, 336–40, **336**
Reference books, herbal, 442–44
Reference guide, herbal, 420–21,
  421–34
Reglan, 208
Remifemin, 88–89
Rennin, 307

Resources for herbal healing, 34,
  442–44
Resperine, 9
Respiratory problems. *See also*
  specific types
  angelica for, 64–65
  ephedra for, 174
  marshmallow for, 277
  tea for, 386
  tea tree for, 389
Reye's syndrome, 93, 285
Rezulin, 39–40
Rheumatoid arthritis
  evening primrose for, 182
  horsetail for, 247
Rhizomists, 12–13
Rhubarb, 341–43, **341**
Rhynchophylline, 116
Ringing in the ears
  ginkgo for, 214
  from uva-ursi, 400
Roman chamomile, 123, 126
Roman herbalists. *See also* Galen;
  Pliny the Elder
  herbs used by
    apple, 67
    blackberry, 82
    fenugreek, 188
    garlic, 197
    gentian, 203
    ginger, 207
    hawthorn, 233
    horehound, 240
    horsetail, 246
    licorice, 270
    mints, 320–21
    nettle, 302
    parsley, 309–10
    red clover, 333
    St. John's wort, 354–55
    shepherd's purse, 371
    vervain, 406
  history of herbal healing and,
    12–15
Rose, 344–46, **344**
Rose hips, 344–46
Rosemary, 347–49, **347**
Rutin, 382

S

SAD, 356
Safety issues. *See also specific herbs*
  aging and, 43
  breastfeeding and, 43, 120–21
  children and, 43
  complexity of, 38
  dosages, 41–42
  double standard and, 40–41
  with ephedra, 39, 175–76
  FDA and, 39–40
  with garlic, 39
  guidelines, 42–44
  interactions with
    pharmaceuticals, 43
  media and, 38–40
  nursing women, 43, 420–21
  with pharmaceuticals, 39–41
  pregnancy and, 43, 420–21
  with problematic herbs, 44
  with St. John's wort, 38–39
  with senna, 39
Saffron, 113
Sage, 350–53, **353**
St. John's wort, 38–39, 41, 43,
  354–58, **354**
Salicin, 92–93, 283, 409, 411–12
Salicylate, 284
Salicylic acid, 283, 411
Saliva, 337
Salysat, 352
Saponins, 58, 360–61
Sarsaparilla, 19, 55, 359–61, **359**
Sarsapogenin, 361
Saw palmetto, 362–64, **362**
Saw palmetto extract, 363
Scabies, turmeric for, 395
Scarlet fever, catnip for, 113
Scrofula, 297
Scullcap, 365–67, **365**
Scurvy
  in Age of Exploration, 24–25
  nettle for, 304
  vitamin C for, 25, 304
Seasonal affective disorder (SAD),
  356

catnip, 113
Chinese herbalists and, 385
ginger, 209–10
green, 384–87
history of herbal healing and, 19
oolong, 384, 386–87
tannins in, 385–86
Tea bush, 384
Tea tree, 388–89, **388**
Technology, backlash against, 34
Testosterone, 132, 361
Thalidomide scandal, 35
Theobromine, 141
Theodosius, 406
Theophrastus, 12
Theophylline, 141
Thomson, Samuel A., 27–28, 76, 225, 317, 337, 375, 403
3-n-butyl phthalide, 120
Thromboembolism, red clover and, 335
Thrombophlebitis, red clover and, 335
Thujone, 353, 418
Thyme, 390–93, **390**
Thymol, 391–92
Thyroid, thyme and, 392
Tincture, 47–48
Tinnitis
ginkgo for, 214
from uva-ursi, 400
Toenail infections, tea tree for, 389
Tofu, 377–78, <u>378</u>
Tooth problems
catnip for, 113
chaparral for, 128
clove for, 137
cocoa and, 143
tarragon for, 382
tea for, 386
Toothpaste, myrrh in, 300
Toxin exposure, apple for, 69. *See also* Poisoning
Toxin-induced liver damage, milk thistle for, 288

Tranquilizers
alcohol and, 44
feverfew, 194
herbs as, 44
kava, 257
lemon balm, 267
scullcap, 366
Tranylcypromine, 292
Treacle, 14–15
Triazolam, 267, 404
Trifolium Compounds, 334
Troglitazone, 39–40
Tuberculosis
garlic for, 199
hop for, 238
mullein for, 296–97
red clover for, 335
Turmeric, 394–97, **394**
Tyler, Varro E., 105, 114, 226, 241, 297, 350, 398
Tyramines, 142, 292

U

Ulcers
alfalfa and, 56–57
bilberry for, 81
chamomile for, 123–24
coffee and, 149
garlic for, 199
ginger for, 208–9
licorice for, 271–72
papaya for, 307
red pepper for, 337
thyme for, 392
turmeric for, 396
Ultimate X-phoria, 175
Underactive thyroid, lemon balm and, 268
Uric acid, 120
Urinary problems, horsetail for, 247
Urinary tract infections (UTIs)
buchu for, 100
cranberry for, 155–57
dill for, 163

meadowsweet for, 284
nettle for, 303
uva-ursi for, 399
Ursolic acid, 399
USDA, 129, 380
U.S. Pharmacopoeia, 30, 35, 98, 110, 114, 127, 159, 204, 226, 237, 277, 310, 317, 360, 366, 398, 403, 415
Utication, 302
UTIs. *See* Urinary tract infections
Uva-ursi, 6, 398–401, **398**

V

Valepotriates, 114, 403
Valerian, 114, 402–5, **402**
Valium, 257, 404
Varicose veins
bilberry for, 80–81
blackberry for, 84
gotu kola for, 231–32
horse chestnut for, 243–44
hyssop for, 250
tarragon for, 382
Venereal disease, 55. *See also specific types*
Vertigo, ginkgo for, 214
Vervain, 406–8, **406**
Viagra, 39
Vicks VapoRub, 322
Viruses. *See also* Colds and flu
cat's claw for, 117
lemon balm for, 267
Vision improvement, bilberry for, 79. *See also* Cataracts
Vitamin B$_6$, 131
Vitamin C
in cranberry, 155
in dandelion, 160
kidney problems and, 346
in maté, 280
in nettle, 304
in rose hips, 344–46
for scurvy, 25, 304
in yellow cedar bark tea, 25

Vitamin E, 83, 156
Voltaren, 304
Vomiting. *See* Nausea

W

Walnuts, 19
Water hemlock, 66
Water retention, glycyrrhetinic
    acid and, 272
Weight loss. *See also* Overweight
    buchu for, 101
    coffee for, 148
    diuretics and, 101, 186, 305,
        311–12, 361, 400
    fennel for, 186
    uva-ursi for, 400
Well-being, improved, ginseng
    for, 219
Weiss, Rudolph Fritz, 235, 254,
    290–91, 297, 303, 357,
    372, 392
West African herbalists, 259
White willow, 6, 282, 407–13, **407**
Whooping cough
    elecampane for, 171
    eucalyptus for, 178
Witch hazel, 414–16, **414**
Witch-hunts, 17–18
Withdrawal, from valerian, 404–5
Women herbalists, 6–7, 17–18
Women's health problems. *See also*
        specific problems
    alfalfa for, 57
    caraway and, 108

catnip for, 114–15
celery for, 121
chamomile for, 125
elecampane for, 171
ephedra for, 175
fennel for, 186
fenugreek for, 189–90
feverfew for, 193–94
gentian for, 204
ginger for, 209
goldenseal for, 227
hop for, 238
juniper for, 253
lavender for, 264
lemon balm for, 268
motherwort for, 294
parsley for, 311
passionflower for, 314
peppermint for, 323
rhubarb for, 342
rosemary for, 348
sage for, 352
sarsaparilla for, 360
slippery elm for, 375
spearmint for, 323
thyme for, 392
uva-ursi for, 399
white willow for, 412
yarrow for, 418
Wounds
    aloe for, 59–60
    apple for, 69
    blackberry for, 84
    chaparral for, 128
    comfrey for, 153–54
    echinacea for, 168

eucalyptus for, 178
fenugreek for, 189–90
gentian for, 203
gotu kola for, 230–32
horsetail for, 246–47
hyssop for, 250
lavender for, 264–65
lemon balm for, 267–68
licorice for, 274
marshmallow for, 277
passionflower for, 314
peppermint for, 323
sage for, 351–52
St. John's wort for, 357
shepherd's purse for, 372
slippery elm for, 375
tea tree for, 388–89
turmeric for, 395, 397
uva-ursi for, 399–400
yarrow for, 418–19

Y

Yarrow, 417–19, **417**
Yeast infections. *See also*
        Infections
    aloe for, 61
    dandelion for, 160
    echinacea for, 168
    goldenseal for, 227
    licorice for, 273
    tea tree for, 389
Yerba maté, 279–81

About the Author

The *Library Journal* has called Michael Castleman "one of the nation's top health writers." He has been herbal medicine columnist for *Herb Quarterly* magazine since 1988. His articles on herbal medicine have appeared in many publications and online services, including *Herbs for Health*, *Herb Companion*, *Prevention*, *Reader's Digest*, *Natural Health*, *New Woman*, *American Health*, *Healthy Living*, PlanetRx.com, and Salon.com.

Castleman is also the author of 10 consumer medical books with a combined total of more than 2 million copies in print. Among them are *Blended Medicine*, a home medical guide that combines the best of mainstream and alternative medicine for 100 common conditions; *Nature's Cures*, an exploration of the science behind 30 alternative therapies; and *There's Still a Person in There* (with Matthew Naythons, M.D., and Dolores Gallagher-Thompson, Ph.D.), a family guide to Alzheimer's disease.

A former adjunct professor at the University of California, Berkeley, Graduate School of Journalism, where he taught medical writing, Castleman has won numerous awards for excellence in journalism. In 1996, he received a National Magazine Award nomination for his coverage of breast cancer.

Castleman lives in San Francisco with his wife and two children.

615.321   Castleman, Michael.
CASTLEM
          The new healing
          herbs.

$17.95

DATE			

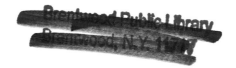

BAKER & TAYLOR